Blue Book of Clinical Research Evidence in Acupuncture and Moxibustion

(2015-2024)

World Federation of Acupuncture-Moxibustion Societies

National Clinical Research Center for Chinese Medicine Acupuncture and Moxibustion

Editor in Chief　LIU Baoyan

中华医学电子音像出版社
CHINESE MEDICAL MULTIMEDIA PRESS

北　京

Editorial Committee

Consultant Gordon H. Guyatt

Editor in Chief LIU Baoyan

Associate Editors ZHANG Yanjun, WANG Jingui, YANG Jinsheng, YANG Longhui, XU Nenggui, YANG Yuyang, SHI Jiangwei, LU Liming, SHEN Yan

Editorial Board Member (Sort by Chinese surname strokes)

WANG Wei (Wuhan, China), WANG Hua, WANG Shu, WANG Jingui, WANG Shengfeng, WANG Fuchun, FANG Jianqiao, SHI Guangxia, SHI Jiangwei, LIU Cunzhi, LIU Zhishun, LIU Weihong, LIU Jianping, LIU Baoyan, YAN Shiyan, XU Nenggui, SUN Feng, SUN Xin, SUN Yuanjie, SUN Jianhua, LU Wenli, SU Tongsheng, DU Yuanhao, DU Zhicheng, LI Ying, YANG Jun, YANG Shuo, YANG Longhui, YANG Yuyang, YANG Jinsheng, WU Jiani, WU Huangan, GANG Weijuan, HE Liyun, YU Yongfu, YU Shuguang, SHEN Yan, ZHANG Wangjian, ZHANG Yonggang, ZHANG Ruyang, ZHANG Yanjun, LU Liming, CHEN Zheng, CHEN Bo, CHEN Wen, ZHOU Xu, FANG Yigong, MENG Zhihong, ZHAO Hong, ZHAO Xing, ZHAO Ling, ZHAO Jiping, HAO Yang, RONG Peijing, HU Siyuan, FEI Yutong, YAO Chen, QIN Guoyou, NI Guangxia, YIN Haibo, GUO Yi, GUO Shengnan, TAO Liyuan, CUI Zhuang, ZHANG Wei, YAN Xiaoyan, LIANG Fanrong, GE Long, ZENG Fang, LEI Li, ZHAI Jingbo

Academic Support *Chinese Journal of Acupuncture and Moxibustion (Electronic Edition)*, *World Journal of Acupuncture-Moxibustion*

People involved in writing (Sort by Chinese surname strokes)

MA Qingtao, WANG Wei (Tianjin, China), WANG Song, DENG Shizhe, XING Jingjing, LIU Jian, LIU Wei, LIU Chaoda, SUN Chun, DU Shihao, LI Boxuan, YANG Hongling, ZHANG Yanan, CHEN Yaqiong, FAN Baochao, NIE Dehui, XU Fan, XU Zhijie, HUANG Hongwen, DONG Yu

World Federation of Acupuncture-Moxibustion Societies

The World Federation of Acupuncture-Moxibustion Societies (WFAS) is an international federation that unites organizations specializing in acupuncture, moxibustion and traditional Chinese medicine. WFAS began its preparation in 1984 when a proposal of its establishment was submitted to the State Council of the People's Republic of China by four major ministries and commissions: The former Ministry of Health of China, the China Association for Science and Technology, the Ministry of Foreign Affairs of the People's Republic of China, and the former State Science and Technology Commission of the People's Republic of China. After approval by the State Council, it was established in November 1987, led by China and under the guidance of the World Health Organization (WHO), with its headquarters located in Beijing, China.

WFAS is an international non-governmental organization representing acupuncture societies. In 1998, it established official working relations with WHO and became an A Liaison to the Technical Committee on Traditional Chinese Medicine of the International Organization for Standardization (ISO/TC249), and enjoys a special consultative status with the Economic and Social Council of the United Nations. Currently, WFAS has 272 member organizations from over 70 countries and regions.

The purpose of WFAS: To promote the understanding and cooperation between the acupuncture and moxibustion communities in the world, to strengthen international academic exchanges, to further develop the acupuncture and moxibustion medicine, to continuously improve the status and role of acupuncture and moxibustion medicine in the world's medical and health care, and to make contributions to human health.

The mission of WFAS: To organize the world academic conferences, seminars and symposiums on acupuncture; to encourage all kinds of academic communications by facilitating friendly exchange among international acupuncture communities; to fulfill the obligations accompanied by the official relations with WHO including the implementation of WHO global strategy on traditional medicine; to give publicity to acupuncture and fight for acupuncture legalization in all countries; to enhance acupuncture education so as to cultivate more competent professionals; to facilitate acupuncture service; to publish journals to spread acupuncture information; to formulate and promote international standards on acupuncture; and to undertake other tasks necessary to achieve the objectives of this association.

The Science and Technology Working Committee of the World Federation of Acupuncture-Moxibustion Societies (Science and Technology Working Committee) is one of the subcommittees. The committee is chaired by Professor XU Nenggui (China) and Professor Gordon H. Guyatt (Canada). The deputy director member include Professor WEI Guoqing (Australia), Professor

ZHANG Yuqing (U.S.A.), Professor WANG Shaobai (U.S.A.), Professor TANG Chunzhi (China), Professor LU Liming (China), and Professor SHI Jiangwei (China).

In the past few years, the Science and Technology Working Committee, closely following the national science and technology development strategy, has actively carried out various tasks. Many studies have been published in international prestigious medical journals, such as *The BMJ*, *Annals of Internal Medicine, Autophagy*, and *Nature Communications*, etc., showcasing the team's outstanding achievements in the field of acupuncture. The Science and Technology Working Committee has conducted more than 30 academic training and free clinic activities domestically, enhancing academic exchanges while promoting the inheritance and dissemination of Lingnan traditional Chinese medicine acupuncture. It has also jointly conducted scientific research and the promotion of new technologies with several hospitals, including Yunnan Zhaotong Central Hospital, Guangzhou Central Hospital, Zhongshan Third Hospital, and Shenzhen Bao'an Pure Traditional Chinese Medicine Treatment Hospital. It has launched the "Three-Name Project" to promote new technologies and joint research with Shenzhen Bao'an Pure Traditional Chinese Medicine Treatment Hospital. It has also carried out multidisciplinary research jointly with Guangzhou Research Institute of Xi'an University of Electronic Science and Technology and Harbin Institute of Technology (Shenzhen) and other institutions, forming a leading domestic research team in acupuncture treatment, clinical research methodology, computer science, artificial intelligence, biomedicine, and clinical medicine. This team is interdisciplinary, multi-level, and a leader in the country, promoting the development of interdisciplinary studies in acupuncture imaging. Collaborating with several domestic and international universities, key laboratories have been established, including the Guangdong Provincial Department of Education Key Laboratory and the Greater Bay Area Key Laboratory for the Combination of Acupuncture and Stem Cell Therapy for Central Nervous Degenerative Diseases, achieving fruitful results.

In the future, under the guidance of WFAS, the Science and Technology Working Committee will continue to promote innovation and exchange and collaboration in the research work of acupuncture, and build a communication and cooperation bridge for acupuncture researchers at home and abroad. Through innovative research work, it will promote the clinical application and promotion of acupuncture and moxibustion, facilitate the internationalization of acupuncture and moxibustion, and enhance the domestic and international influence of acupuncture and moxibustion research. Attaching importance to the training of young scientific and technological workers, providing necessary support and incentive measures, to build a platform for young acupuncture and moxibustion science and technology workers to display their talents.

National Clinical Research Center for Chinese Medicine Acupuncture and Moxibustion

In May 2019, an *Announcement of Identifying the Fourth Group of National Clinical Research Centers* was jointly released by the Ministry of Science and Technology of the People's Republic of China, the National Health Commission of the People's Republic of China, the Logistics Department of Central Military Commission and the National Medical Products Administration. According to the announcement, 18 hospitals covering 10 disease fields are recognized as National Clinical Research Centers. Finally, the First Teaching Hospital of Tianjin University of Traditional Chinese Medicine is successfully approved as a National Clinical Research Center for Chinese Medicine Acupuncture and Moxibustion.

The First Teaching Hospital of Tianjin University of Traditional Chinese Medicine was established in 1954. It is the earliest and largest Traditional Chinese Medicine (TCM) medical organization set up in Tianjin. Besides, it is the Founding Unit of the National Medical Center, the National Clinical Research Center for Chinese Medicine Acupuncture and Moxibustion, the Hospital of National Regional Medical Center Construction, the Key TCM Hospital of National TCM Inheritance and Innovation Project, the National TCM Clinical Teaching and Training Demonstration Center and the National TCM Service Export Base. Furthermore, the hospital is the National Clinical Research Base of TCM, the National Regional TCM (Specialty) Medical Center, the National TCM Dominant Specialty Construction Unit, one of the first group of National Standardized Training Bases for TCM Residents, the National Comprehensive Training Base for TCM Talents, the Base of National TCM Epidemic Prevention and Control and Emergency Medical Rescue, and the National TCM Culture Publicity and Education Base. Moreover, the hospital is one of the first group of the National First-Class Hospitals, the Top 100 Hospital in China, and the National Reliable Demonstration Hospital.

The hospital is composed of three campuses, namely Nankai campus, Xiqing campus and Jinghai campus. The hospital covers an area of about 358 247 square meters. Besides, it has 45 clinical and technical departments and 2 600 beds. The annual outpatient and emergency department visits exceed 3.03 million, and more than 70 000 patients are discharged each year.

The hospital has more than 3 200 employees, including two academicians of the Chinese Academy of Engineering, three masters of TCM, five national famous TCM doctors, five Qi-Huang scholars, four young Qi-Huang scholars, 20 experts with special allowances from the State Council, eight young/middle-aged experts with outstanding contributions at national level, 37 instructors for academic experience inheritance of national senior TCM experts, 23 national clinical talents of TCM, five experts awarded by the Tianjin Municipal People's Government and 33 famous TCM doctors of Tianjin. Besides, there are two innovation teams of the Ministry of

Education, one national inheritance and innovation team of TCM, 48 doctoral supervisors, and 234 master supervisors.

The hospital stays committed to putting people's health first and pays attention to the health management of the whole life cycle. Besides, the hospital adheres to the integration of prevention, medical treatment and rehabilitation, and attaches equal importance to TCM and western medicine. The hospital is committed to "Five Specialties" (specialties, special diseases, experts, special medicine and professional skills), highlighting the characteristics of TCM. Additionally, the hospital has carried out extensive diagnosis and treatment with TCM characteristics, and has improved the diagnosis and treatment ability of integrated TCM and western medicine. The hospital has formed a number of unique diagnosis and treatment programs by combining TCM with western medicine for difficult diseases, such as strokes and their complications and coronary heart diseases, giving full play to the unique role of TCM in the prevention and treatment of common diseases, frequent diseases and chronic diseases.

The hospital strives for the peak of disciplines and specialties, and forms a discipline group led by acupuncture and moxibustion. The hospital has two national key disciplines, four national key clinical specialties, three high-level key disciplines of TCM of the National Administration of Traditional Chinese Medicine, six regional treatment centers of traditional Chinese medicine (specialties) of the National Administration of Traditional Chinese Medicine, 10 key disciplines of the National Administration of Traditional Chinese Medicine, 13 dominant specialties of traditional Chinese medicine of the National Administration of Traditional Chinese Medicine, and 13 key specialties of the National Administration of Traditional Chinese Medicine.

The hospital has a scientific research workstation for TCM postdoctors. And the hospital is authorized by the State Council for the doctoral degree of the first-level discipline of TCM. Besides, the hospital has one national teaching team. In addition, the hospital is a comprehensive base for high-level TCM talents training of the National Administration of Traditional Chinese Medicine, one of the first group of the standardized training bases for TCM resident physicians and general practitioners, the national base for standardized training of residents in TCM and key specialties in TCM general practice, and the national TCM clinical teaching and training demonstration center.

The hospital has always adhered to the path of "revitalizing the hospital with science and technology". The hospital has a number of national science and technology platforms such as the National Clinical Research Center for Chinese Medicine Acupuncture and Moxibustion, the National Clinical Research Base of TCM, the National Drug Clinical Trial Institution, and 16 provincial and ministerial science and technology platforms such as the Key Laboratory of Acupuncture Therapy for Encephalopathy of the National Administration of Traditional Chinese Medicine. Besides, the Clinical Research Center of TCM is established. In the past five years, the hospital has undertaken 31 major scientific research tasks such as the national major scientific and technological project "major new drug creation", the national key research and development program "modernization of TCM", and the key projects of the National Natural Science

Foundation of China. The hospital has taken the lead in undertaking 63 clinical trial projects for new Chinese medicine, and won five national science and technology progress awards and 16 first prizes of provincial and ministerial science and technology pogress prizes. Based on the academic influence evaluation of disciplines (specialties) of TCM hospitals in 2023, the hospital ranked the 8th in comprehensive ranking, acupuncture ranked the 1st, TCM Tuina and TCM pediatrics ranked the 2nd, and TCM cardiology ranked the 3rd. Furthermore, the hospital ranked the 75th in the Science and Technology Evaluation Metrics (STEM) of Chinese hospitals in 2022.

The hospital has successively established cooperative relations with more than 40 countries such as the United States, Russia, Germany, Japan, and South Korea. In addition, the hospital has held 16 international symposiums on acupuncture and moxibustion and the first China-ASEAN International Forum on Traditional Medicine. Moreover, the hospital has built three overseas centers.

The hospital stays committed to the guidance of XI Jinping Thought on Socialism with Chinese Characteristics for a New Era, the hospital's motto of "being kind in heart and being good in action", and the purpose of "developing careers, serving the society, maintaining health and benefiting mankind". With discipline construction as the guide, reform and innovation as the driving force, and talent team and modern management as the support, we will build a higher level of teaching and research-oriented TCM hospital, creating a new future of high-quality development.

The department of acupuncture and moxibustion is the leading department of the hospital. The department is comprised of 15 inpatient wards, outpatient clinics of north and south campuses of the hospital, the acupuncture research institute, and the editorial department of *Chinese Journal of Acupuncture and Moxibustion (Electronic Edition)*. The department has undergone 70 years of development and innovation under the leadership of Professor SHI Xuemin, an academician of the Chinese Academy of Engineering and a master of TCM. The department has become the largest clinical research and teaching base for acupuncture and an international exchange center in China. There are 1 000 beds, more than 600 000 outpatients annually, and more than 20 000 discharged patients each year. The department has treated 33 million stroke patients in total, so the clinical service ability of acupuncture and moxibustion ranks first nationwide.

The department of acupuncture and moxibustion has been established as National Key Discipline (2002), Key Discipline of National Administration of Traditional Chinese Medicine (2001), High-Level Key Discipline of Traditional Chinese Medicine (2023), Top Priority" Discipline of Tianjin (2005), the National Acupuncture Clinical Research Center (1988), the National Traditional Chinese Medicine Clinical Research Base (2008), a National Clinical Key Specialty Construction Unit (2011), Regional Acupuncture Diagnosis and Treatment Center of the National Administration of Traditional Chinese Medicine (2018) and Advantageous Specialty of National Administration of Traditional Chinese Medicine (2021, 2024).

Currently, the department has four stable research directions, including the scientific connotation and innovative research of Xing Nao Kai Qiao therapy (activating the brain and opening the orifices), clinical evaluation and mechanism research on advantageous diseases, standardization of acupuncture, and interdisciplinary innovation in acupuncture. In recent years, it has undertaken 432 scientific research projects at various levels. There are 69 national projects focused on acupuncture treatment for advantageous diseases, such as stroke, hypertension and cognitive impairment, and 105 provincial and ministerial level projects. Besides, the department has won one national science and technology progress award, three first prizes of provincial and ministerial level, 24 second prizes of provincial and ministerial level, and 27 third prizes of provincial and ministerial level.

The talent team is an innovative team of "Yangtze scholars and innovation team development plan" of the Ministry of Education of the People's Republic of China. The team includes one academician of the Chinese Academy of Engineering, one master of TCM, one national famous TCM doctor, and five experts with special allowances from the State Council. There are four postdoctoral cooperative supervisors, 10 doctoral supervisors, 47 master's supervisors, five presidents/chairmen of secondary societies, and 10 vice presidents/vice chairmen of secondary societies. Furthermore, the department has built the largest collaborative innovation network in China, with 218 network collaboration units, covering 31 provinces, municipalities and autonomous regions across the country. There is a famous Chinese saying that China leads the world in acupuncture and Tianjin leads China in acupuncture. The department has always been in a leading position in acupuncture at home and abroad. In the 2021-2023 academic influence selection of disciplines (specialties) in TCM hospitals organized by the China Association of Chinese Medicine and the China Academy of Chinese Medical Sciences, the department has successively ranked first in acupuncture in China, leading the development of the acupuncture.

Under the background of increasing emphasis on evidence-based medicine in the global medical system, the publication of *Blue Book of Clinical Research Evidence in Acupuncture and Moxibustion (2015-2024)* marks a higher level research of acupuncture and moxibustion. We will take the curative effect as the guidance, discuss the mechanism and principle of acupuncture and moxibustion in depth, and strive to provide patients with more scientific treatment prescription.

Academician HAN Jisheng

The publication of *Blue Book of Clinical Research Evidence in Acupuncture and Moxibustion (2015-2024)* is another important impetus to the scientization and standardization of acupuncture and moxibustion. We will continue to explore the potential of acupuncture and moxibustion, transform sufficient clinical experience into evidence of clinical efficacy, empower traditional medicine with science, and make greater contributions to human health!

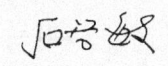

Academician SHI Xuemin

Blue Book of Clinical Research Evidence in Acupuncture and Moxibustion (2015-2024) is not only a summary of the clinical research results of acupuncture and moxibustion in the past ten years, but also a scientific basis for the future development of acupuncture and moxibustion. We hope that these high-quality evidence-based evidences will be transformed and applied to promote the integration and innovation of acupuncture and moxibustion with modern medicine, enrich the research content of health medicine in the new era, and benefit the health and well-being of mankind!

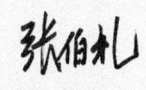

Academician ZHANG Boli

Preface

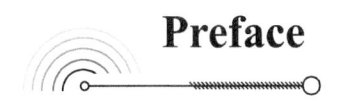

Since ancient times, acupuncture has served as a continuous thread, weaving together the wisdom and practices of Eastern and Western medicine. In the 21st century, this ancient art and science is revealing a renewed vitality and depth. I, Gordon Guyatt, a long-time advocate and researcher of evidence-based medicine, am privileged to witness the profound changes in this field. I am honored to write the foreword for this *Blue Book of Clinical Research Evidence in Acupuncture and Moxibustion (2015-2024)*.

Over the past decade, high-impact acupuncture clinical research published by Chinese and international scholars has not only provided the global medical community with rich data and insights but also transformed acupuncture from a traditional expertise-based practice to an evidence-based medical science. These studies, like bright beacons, illuminate the scientific path of acupuncture, presenting it with the evidence-based medicine framework and broadening acupuncture's application.

This book carefully selects the most representative and influential clinical studies on acupuncture in the last decade by both Chinese and international scholars. Insightful expert commentaries highlight the application and effectiveness of acupuncture in pain management, Neurological, Gastroenterological disorders, etc. These clinical studies explore the efficacy and safety of acupuncture, providing solid scientific evidence for future research.

It is with immense pleasure that I share these research highlights with you through this book. Whether you are a patient, healthcare practitioner, researcher, or curious explorer of traditional medicine, you will find new insights and reflections from these studies. Let us embark on this journey together, experiencing the sparks that emerge from the fusion of acupuncture and modern science and witnessing the perfect harmony of ancient wisdom with contemporary medicine.

I hope that the *Blue Book of Clinical Research Evidence in Acupuncture and Moxibustion (2015-2024)* will bridge Eastern and Western medicine, contributing to the advancement of global healthcare.

Yours sincerely,

Gordon H. Guyatt
Founder of Evidence Based Medicine
Fellow of the Royal Canadian Academy of Sciences
Professor of McMaster University

Foreword

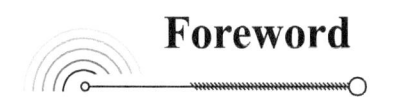

Acupuncture and moxibustion, which originated in China and with a long history and profound cultural heritage, has been spread and applied in 196 countries and regions, gradually becoming integrated into the mainstream medical system. However, the global legislation pertaining to acupuncture and moxibustion treatment remains insufficient, and the practitioners of acupuncture and moxibustion in many countries and regions have yet to obtain legal status. Therefore, providing and promoting high-quality clinical and basic research results of acupuncture and moxibustion and formulating and publicizing relevant standards and norms of acupuncture and moxibustion have become top priorities for the promotion of the internationalization of acupuncture and moxibustion.

The World Federation of Acupuncture-Moxibustion Societies (WFAS) and National Clinical Research Center for Chinese Medicine Acupuncture and Moxibustion in China, supported by the Science and Technology Working Committee of WFAS and *Chinese Journal of Acupuncture and Moxibustion (Electronic Edition)*, have systematically summarized the clinical research of acupuncture and moxibustion in the past ten years. Fifty-two high-impact clinical studies of acupuncture and moxibustion from January 2015 to July 2024 were selected from the Science Citation Index (SCI) database, and 60 experts and scholars from the fields of acupuncture and moxibustion and clinical methodology and statistics were invited to study these articles in depth, focusing on the clinical value, design methods and characteristics, and impact on the development of acupuncture and moxibustion, also including existing problems and suggestions. Based on this, the *Blue Book of Clinical Research Evidence in Acupuncture and Moxibustion* (hereinafter referred to as *Blue Book*) was issued at the 7th International Symposium on Acupuncture and Moxibustion held in London, UK. The *Blue Book* also contained the *Tianjin Consensus on Clinical Research of Traditional Chinese Medicine Initiated by Researchers* and its key interpretations, aiming at improving the level of clinical research of acupuncture and moxibustion, generating evidence of high quality, and promoting the dissemination and application of acupuncture and moxibustion with real and reliable scientific data.

The WFAS plans to issue the *Blue Book* every year to incorporate the latest developments and progress of acupuncture clinical research for most acupuncture practitioners and to provide comprehensive, accurate, and scientific data supporting high-quality research evidence for public health intervention, acupuncture related legislation, and its entry into medical insurance and the mainstream medical system. Professor Gordon H. Guyatt, the founder of evidence-based medicine and chairman of the Science and Technology Working Committee of WFAS, wrote a preface for the *Blue Book*, expecting that acupuncture and moxibustion can pave its own unique path of clinical research guided by the notions and methods of evidence-based medicine. We would like to extent our appreciation to all colleagues and collaborators for their diligent efforts in creating the *Blue Book*.

LIU Baoyan

President of World Federation of Acupuncture-Moxibustion Societies

Academician of International Eurasian Academy of Sciences (IEAS)

Faculty Member of China Academy of Chinese Medical Sciences

Contents

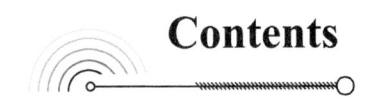

Chapter 1 Progress of Clinical Research on Acupuncture in the Last Decade ⋯⋯⋯⋯⋯⋯ 1

Chapter 2 **Comments of Clinical Trials of Acupuncture and Moxibustion in SCI Journals** ⋯⋯⋯⋯⋯⋯ 13

Section 1 Introduction and Comments of *Acupuncture for Combat-Related Posttraumatic Stress Disorder: A Randomized Clinical Trial* ⋯⋯⋯⋯⋯⋯ 13

Section 2 Introduction and Comments of *Acupuncture and Sleep Quality Among Patients With Parkinson Disease: A Randomized Clinical Trial* ⋯⋯⋯⋯⋯⋯ 15

Section 3 Introduction and Comments of *Acupuncture for Chronic Radiation-Induced Xerostomia in Head and Neck Cancer: A Multicenter Randomized Clinical Trial* ⋯⋯⋯⋯⋯⋯ 16

Section 4 Introduction and Comments of *Effect of Acupuncture vs Sham Acupuncture on Patients With Poststroke Motor Aphasia: A Randomized Clinical Trial* ⋯⋯⋯⋯⋯⋯ 18

Section 5 Introduction and Comments of *Effect of Acupuncture for Methadone Reduction: A Randomized Clinical Trial* ⋯⋯⋯⋯⋯⋯ 20

Section 6 Introduction and Comments of *Effect of Acupuncture on Neurogenic Claudication Among Patients With Degenerative Lumbar Spinal Stenosis: A Randomized Clinical Trial* ⋯⋯⋯⋯⋯⋯ 22

Section 7 Introduction and Comments of *Effect of Acupuncture for Temporomandibular Disorders: A Randomized Clinical Trial* ⋯⋯⋯⋯⋯⋯ 24

Section 8 Introduction and Comments of *Self-Administered Acupressure for Probable Knee Osteoarthritis in Middle-Aged and Older Adults: A Randomized Clinical Trial* ⋯⋯⋯⋯⋯⋯ 25

Section 9 Introduction and Comments of *Efficacy of Acupuncture for Chronic Spontaneous Urticaria: A Randomized Controlled Trial* ⋯⋯⋯⋯⋯⋯ 27

Section 10 Introduction and Comments of *Acupuncture and Doxylamine-Pyridoxine for Nausea and Vomiting in Pregnancy: A Randomized, Controlled, 2 × 2 Factorial Trial* ⋯⋯⋯⋯⋯⋯ 28

Section 11 Introduction and Comments of *Electroacupuncture vs Sham Electroacupuncture in the Treatment of Postoperative Ileus After Laparoscopic Surgery for Colorectal Cancer: A Multicenter, Randomized Clinical Trial* ⋯⋯⋯⋯⋯⋯ 30

Section 12 Introduction and Comments of *Electroacupuncture for Motor Dysfunction and Constipation in Patients With Parkinson's Disease: A Randomised Controlled Multi-centre trial* ⋯⋯⋯⋯⋯⋯ 31

Section 13 Introduction and Comments of *Effects of Electroacupuncture for Opioid-Induced Constipation in Patients With Cancer in China: A Randomized Clinical Trial* ⋯⋯⋯⋯⋯⋯ 33

Section 14 Introduction and Comments of *Acupuncture vs Massage for Pain in Patients Living With Advanced Cancer: The IMPACT Randomized Clinical Trial* ⋯⋯⋯⋯⋯⋯ 34

Section 15 Introduction and Comments of *Efficacy and Safety of Auricular Acupuncture for Depression: A Randomized Clinical Trial* ⋯⋯⋯⋯⋯⋯ 36

Section 16 Introduction and Comments of *Effect of Acupuncture on Postoperative Ileus After Laparoscopic Elective Colorectal Surgery: A Prospective, Randomised, Controlled Trial* ⋯⋯⋯⋯⋯⋯ 38

Section 17	Introduction and Comments of *Acupuncture Improves the Symptoms, Intestinal Microbiota, and Inflammation of Patients With Mild to Moderate Crohn's Disease: A Randomized Controlled Trial*	39
Section 18	Introduction and Comments of *Effect of Electroacupuncture on Insomnia in Patients With Depression: A Randomized Clinical Trial*	41
Section 19	Introduction and Comments of *Effectiveness of Acupuncture for Anxiety Among Patients With Parkinson Disease: A Randomized Clinical Trial*	43
Section 20	Introduction and Comments of *Effectiveness of Acupuncture for Pain Control After Cesarean Delivery: A Randomized Clinical Trial*	44
Section 21	Introduction and Comments of *Acupuncture for the Treatment of Diarrhea-Predominant Irritable Bowel Syndrome: A Pilot Randomized Clinical Trial*	46
Section 22	Introduction and Comments of *Comparison of Acupuncture vs Sham Acupuncture or Waiting List Control in the Treatment of Aromatase Inhibitor-Related Joint Pain: A Randomized Clinical Trial*	48
Section 23	Introduction and Comments of *Effect of Adjunctive Acupuncture on Pain Relief Among Emergency Department Patients With Acute Renal Colic Due to Urolithiasis: A Randomized Clinical Trial*	49
Section 24	Introduction and Comments of *Effect of Acupoint Hot Compress on Postpartum Urinary Retention After Vaginal Delivery: A Randomized Clinical Trial*	51
Section 25	Introduction and Comments of *Effectiveness of Electroacupuncture or Auricular Acupuncture vs Usual Care for Chronic Musculoskeletal Pain Among Cancer Survivors: The PEACE Randomized Clinical Trial*	52
Section 26	Introduction and Comments of *Efficacy of Acupuncture for Chronic Prostatitis/Chronic Pelvic Pain Syndrome: A Randomized Trial*	54
Section 27	Introduction and Comments of *Effect of Briefing on Acupuncture Treatment Outcome Expectations, Pain, and Adverse Side Effects Among Patients With Chronic Low Back Pain: A Randomized Clinical Trial*	56
Section 28	Introduction and Comments of *Effect of Acupuncture on Atrial Fibrillation Stratified by CHA_2DS_2-VASc Score—A Nationwide Cohort Investigation*	57
Section 29	Introduction and Comments of *Greater Somatosensory Afference With Acupuncture Increases Primary Somatosensory Connectivity and Alleviates Fibromyalgia Pain via Insular γ-Aminobutyric: A Randomized Neuroimaging Trial*	58
Section 30	Introduction and Comments of *Efficacy of Intensive Acupuncture Versus Sham Acupuncture in Knee Osteoarthritis: A Randomized Controlled Trial*	60
Section 31	Introduction and Comments of *Electroacupuncture vs Prucalopride for Severe Chronic Constipation: A Multicenter, Randomized, Controlled, Noninferiority Trial*	62
Section 32	Introduction and Comments of *Manual Acupuncture Versus Sham Acupuncture and Usual Care for Prophylaxis of Episodic Migraine Without Aura: Multicentre, Randomised Clinical Trial*	63
Section 33	Introduction and Comments of *Effect of Acupuncture for Postprandial Distress Syndrome: A Randomized Clinical Trial*	65
Section 34	Introduction and Comments of *Electroacupuncture Trigeminal Nerve Stimulation Plus Body Acupuncture for Chemotherapy-Induced Cognitive Impairment in Breast Cancer Patients: An Assessor-Participant Blinded, Randomized Controlled Trial*	67

Contents

Section 35　Introduction and Comments of *Effect of Acupuncture vs Sham Procedure on Chemotherapy-Induced Peripheral Neuropathy Symptoms: A Randomized Clinical Trial* ········ 68

Section 36　Introduction and Comments of *Effect of Electroacupuncture vs Sham Treatment on Change in Pain Severity Among Adults With Chronic Low Back Pain: A Randomized Clinical Trial* ········ 70

Section 37　Introduction and Comments of *Acupuncture as Adjunctive Therapy for Chronic Stable Angina: A Randomized Clinical Trial* ········ 72

Section 38　Introduction and Comments of *Effect of True and Sham Acupuncture on Radiation-Induced Xerostomia Among Patients With Head and Neck Cancer: A Randomized Clinical Trial* ········ 75

Section 39　Introduction and Comments of *Acupuncture Versus Cognitive Behavioral Therapy for Insomnia in Cancer Survivors: A Randomized Clinical Trial* ········ 76

Section 40　Introduction and Comments of *Effect of Acupuncture vs Sham Acupuncture or Waitlist Control on Joint Pain Related to Aromatase Inhibitors Among Women With Early-Stage Breast Cancer: A Randomized Clinical Trial* ········ 78

Section 41　Introduction and Comments of *Effect of Acupuncture vs Sham Acupuncture on Live Births Among Women Undergoing in Vitro Fertilization: A Randomized Clinical Trial* ········ 80

Section 42　Introduction and Comments of *Effect of Electroacupuncture on Urinary Leakage Among Women With Stress Urinary Incontinence: A Randomized Clinical Trial* ········ 82

Section 43　Introduction and Comments of *Effect of Acupuncture and Clomiphene in Chinese Women With Polycystic Ovary Syndrome: A Randomized Clinical Trial* ········ 84

Section 44　Introduction and Comments of *The Long-Term Effect of Acupuncture for Migraine Prophylaxis: A Randomized Clinical Trial* ········ 85

Section 45　Introduction and Comments of *Rewiring the Primary Somatosensory Cortex in Carpal Tunnel Syndrome With Acupuncture* ········ 87

Section 46　Introduction and Comments of *A Randomised Controlled Trial Examining the Effect of Acupuncture at the EX-HN3 (Yintang) Point on Pre-operative Anxiety Levels in Neurosurgical Patients* ········ 89

Section 47　Introduction and Comments of *Acupuncture As an Integrative Approach for the Treatment of Hot Flashes in Women With Breast Cancer: A Prospective Multicenter Randomized Controlled Trial (AcCliMaT)* ········ 90

Section 48　Introduction and Comments of *Acupuncture for Chronic Severe Functional Constipation: A Randomized Trial* ········ 92

Section 49　Introduction and Comments of *Acupuncture for Menopausal Hot Flashes: A Randomized Trial* ········ 94

Section 50　Introduction and Comments of *Transcutaneous Acupoint Electrical Stimulation Pain Management After Surgical Abortion: A Cohort Study* ········ 95

Section 51　Introduction and Comments of *Electroacupuncture Versus Gabapentin for Hot Flashes Among Breast Cancer Survivors: A Randomized Placebo-Controlled Trial* ········ 97

Section 52　Introduction and Comments of *Alexander Technique Lessons or Acupuncture Sessions for Persons With Chronic Neck Pain* ········ 98

Chapter 3　Content and Interpretation of the *Tianjin Consensus on Clinical Research of Traditional Chinese Medicine Initiated by Researchers* ········ 100

Section 1　Tianjin Consensus on Clinical Research of Traditional Chinese Medicine Initiated by Researchers ········ 100

Section 2　Interpretation of the *Tianjin Consensus on Clinical Research of Traditional Chinese Medicine Initiated by Researchers* ········ 101

Appendix: Disease Index (ICD-11) ········ 104

Chapter 1

Progress of Clinical Research on Acupuncture in the Last Decade

Acupuncture plays an important role in the field of Chinese medicine. In recent years, it has gained substantial traction, with its applications now extending to 196 countries and regions worldwide. Its therapeutic scope is broad, encompassing the treatment of approximately 461 types of diseases and 972 conditions[1]. Recent advancements in the clinical research of acupuncture have been promising, with findings published in several prestigious international journals, including the *Journal of the American Medical Association*, *Annals of Internal Medicine*, and *The BMJ*. This indicates a growing interest within the international academic community in clinical research in the field of acupuncture. Here, we present the progress of acupuncture clinical trials over the past decade aiming to further enhance the level of international clinical research in this area. We hope this summary will illuminate the trends and characteristics of international acupuncture clinical research.

1. A Decadal Review: Visualization and Analysis of Acupuncture Clinical Trials in Science Citation Index (SCI) Journals

In this study, Web of Science was utilized as the data source to retrieve literature on acupuncture clinical trials indexed in the SCI from January 2015 to July 2024. CiteSpace 6.2. R6 and VOSviewer 1.6.20 were employed to visualize and analyze publication time, geographic distribution, keywords of worldwide acupuncture clinical trials.

1.1 Annual Publications Trends

The publication volume of acupuncture clinical trial literature has fluctuated over the past decade, yet it followed an overall upward trend. The highest number of publications was recorded in 2022, with significant growth also noted in 2020 and 2021. In China, the number of publications on acupuncture clinical trials experienced slight fluctuations between 2021 and 2023; however, a notable overall increase was evident, particularly with a strong recent growth trend (Figure 1).

1.2 Publication Volume and Collaborative Network Map in Different Countries

Most global acupuncture clinical trials are conducted in China and the United States. Over the past decade, China has led the field with a total of 1 823 publications, representing 59.15% of the total number of publications (1 823/3 082). The United States has contributed 423

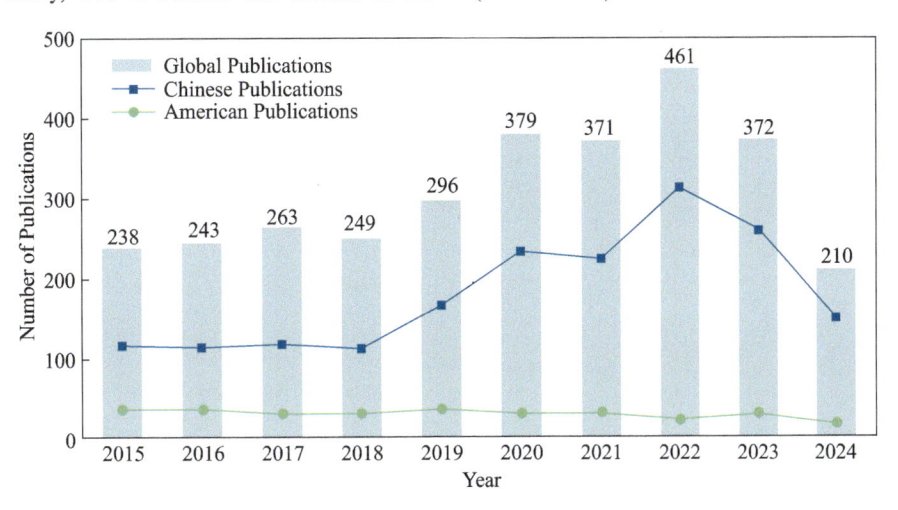

Figure 1 Annual Publication Trends of Acupuncture Clinical Trials in SCI Journals
Note: Data for 2024 are as of July 31.

publications, accounting for 14.02% of the total (423/3 082). South Korea has also made a marked impact, ranking third with 311 publications. Additionally, Australia (ranked fourth with 98 publications), Germany (ranked fifth with 94 publications), and Brazil (ranked sixth with 92 publications) have played important roles in acupuncture research. China has conducted extensive and fruitful research across a multitude of areas related to the clinical application of acupuncture and its integration with modern medical technology. Noteworthy contributions have been made in pain management, adjuvant chemotherapy, and rehabilitation. As shown in Figure 2, China, the birthplace of acupuncture, has engaged in collaborative research with numerous countries and regions worldwide, significantly enhancing global interest in acupuncture research. The United States has also excelled in acupuncture clinical research, particularly in the areas of pain management, psychosocial health, and integrative medicine. This has facilitated the integration of acupuncture with other treatment modalities and has created favorable conditions for acupuncture's international promotion. Furthermore, South Korean studies have focused on substantiating the efficacy of acupuncture for gynecological conditions, including menstrual irregularities and menopausal symptoms, while Australian research has focused on the effectiveness of acupuncture in managing chronic pain and sports injuries. Additionally, Turkey, the United Kingdom, and Japan have been actively engaged in related research, contributing to a diverse and globally oriented research ecosystem.

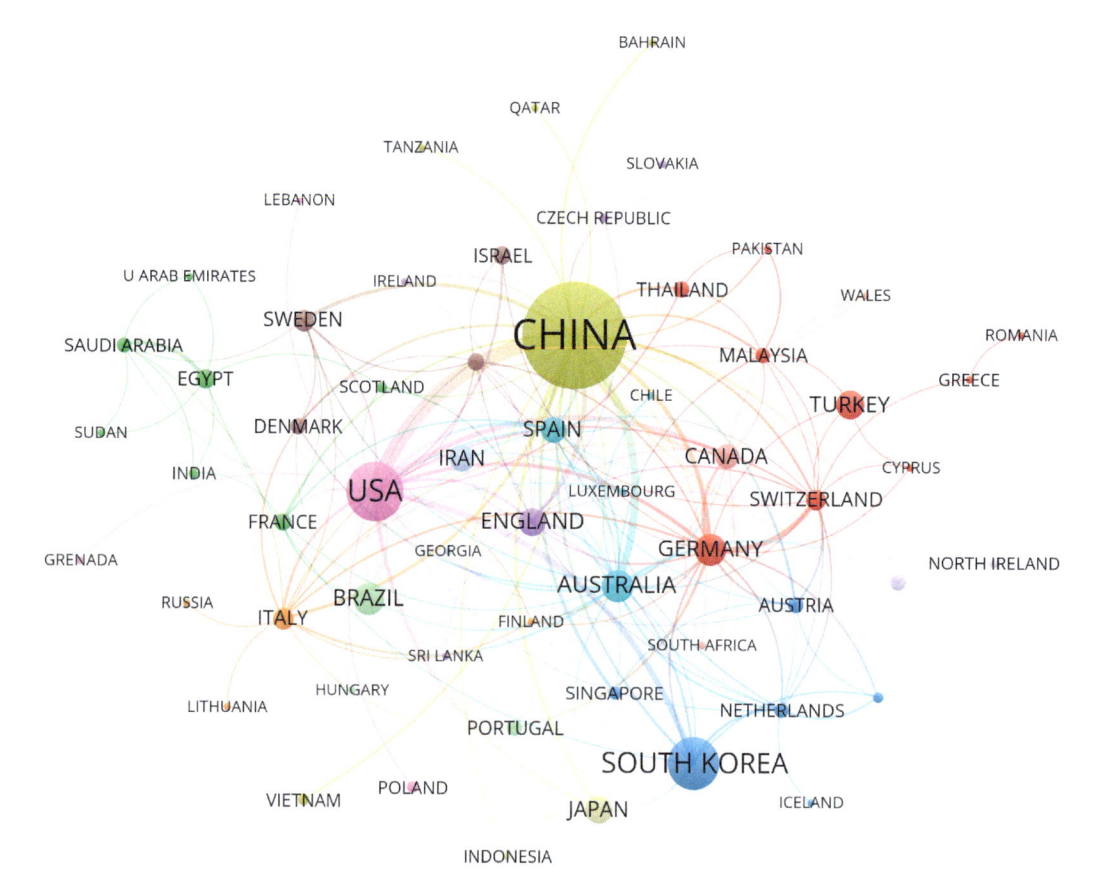

Figure 2 Publication Volume and Collaborative Network Map of Acupuncture Clinical Trials in SCI Journals in Different Countries

1.3 Co-occurrence Analysis of Keywords in Acupuncture Clinical Research

Figure 3 showed that among the research methods, randomized controlled trial (RCT) design is the primary approach for investigating and substantiating the efficacy of acupuncture, with a frequency of 417. This is followed by cohort studies (freq., 10) and case reports (freq., 8).

There are numerous forms of acupuncture beyond traditional acupuncture (freq., 1 167) and electroacupuncture (freq., 245). Recently, new techniques have emerged, including transcutaneous electrical acupoint stimulation (freq., 77), laser acupuncture (freq., 38), auricular acupuncture (freq., 35), and dry needling (freq., 30). These

Chapter 1　Progress of Clinical Research on Acupuncture in the Last Decade

novel approaches have garnered significant interest within the community. The differences in frequency indicate varying levels of importance attributed to these different acupuncture methods in research.

Within the broad frameworks of integrative medicine (freq., 47) and traditional Chinese medicine (freq., 96), the research scope of acupuncture has expanded beyond pain management to delve into the realm of psychosocial health, including conditions such as depression (freq., 61) and anxiety (freq., 59), as well as various chronic diseases. For anxiety and depression, acupuncture has been shown to significantly improve patients' psychological well-being by modulating the function of the autonomic nervous system (freq., 14).

Furthermore, in the field of cancer (freq., 37), acupuncture has demonstrated its distinctive efficacy in alleviating chemotherapy-related adverse effects, including chemotherapy-induced peripheral neuropathy (freq., 11) and cancer-related fatigue (freq., 11).

The findings of this research have expanded the applicability of acupuncture within the contemporary medical framework, providing a wider array of effective treatment options for diverse patient populations.

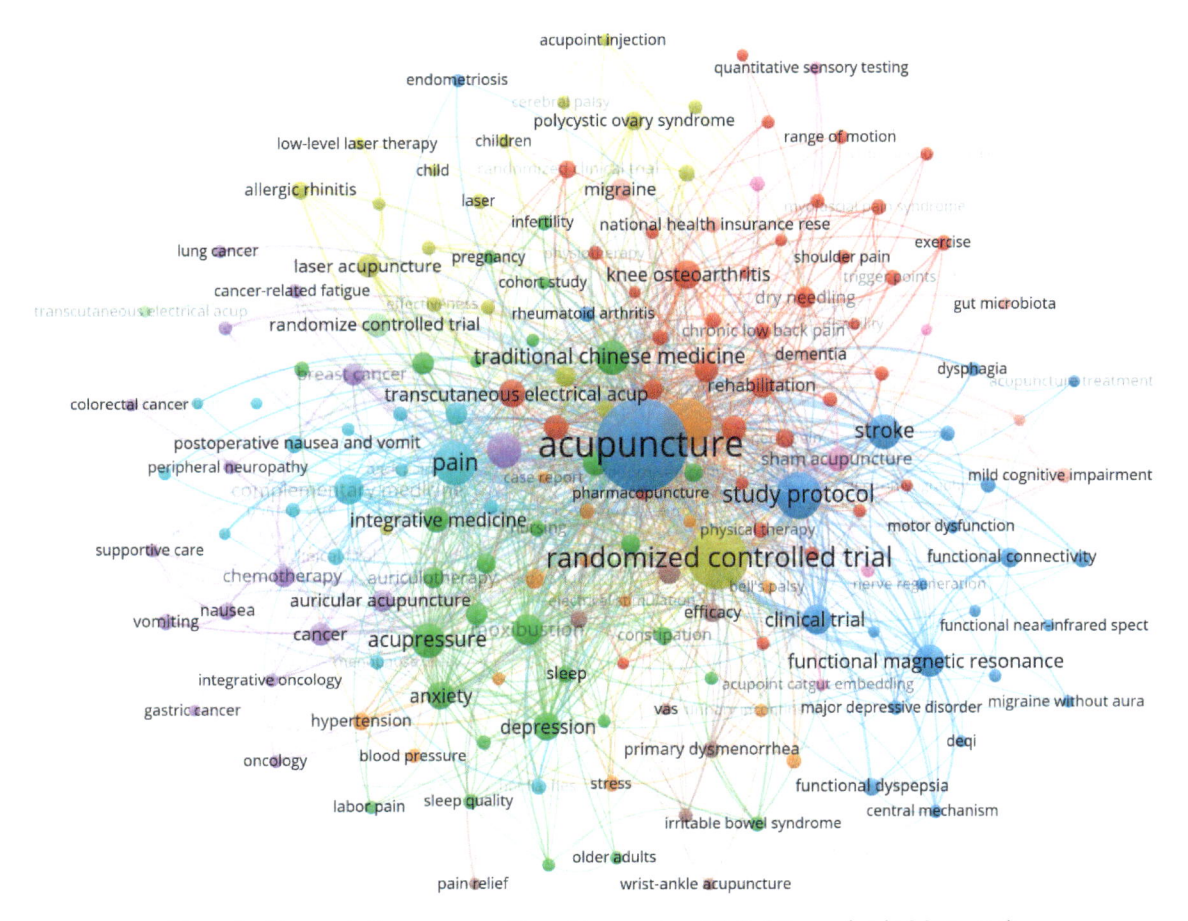

Figure 3　Keywords Co-occurrence Map of Acupuncture Clinical Researches in SCI Journals

1.4　Cluster Analysis of Keywords in Acupuncture Clinical Researches

(1) Cluster Analysis of Keywords in Acupuncture Clinical Researches in countries other than China

The 11 clusters can be broadly classified into four categories (Figure 4 and Table 1). Ⅰ. Indications for Acupuncture (Clusters #5, #6, #9): Pain disorders, such as myofascial pain syndrome, low back pain, knee osteoarthritis, and postoperative pain, are widely recognized as areas of strength for acupuncture and have garnered significant international attention. Ⅱ. Acupuncture Techniques (Clusters #2, #3, #4): This category primarily involves diverse acupuncture methods, including bee-sting acupuncture, auricular acupressure, and dry needling. Additionally, laser acupuncture, manual acupuncture, auricular acupuncture, acupuncture point embedding, and semi-permanent needles also provide a plethora of options for clinical application. Ⅲ. Role of Acupuncture in Disease Treatment (Clusters #0, #1, #8, #10): Acupuncture is often regarded as a complementary alternative therapy for conditions such as cancer and its complications (including

Blue Book of Clinical Research Evidence in Acupuncture and Moxibustion (2015-2024)

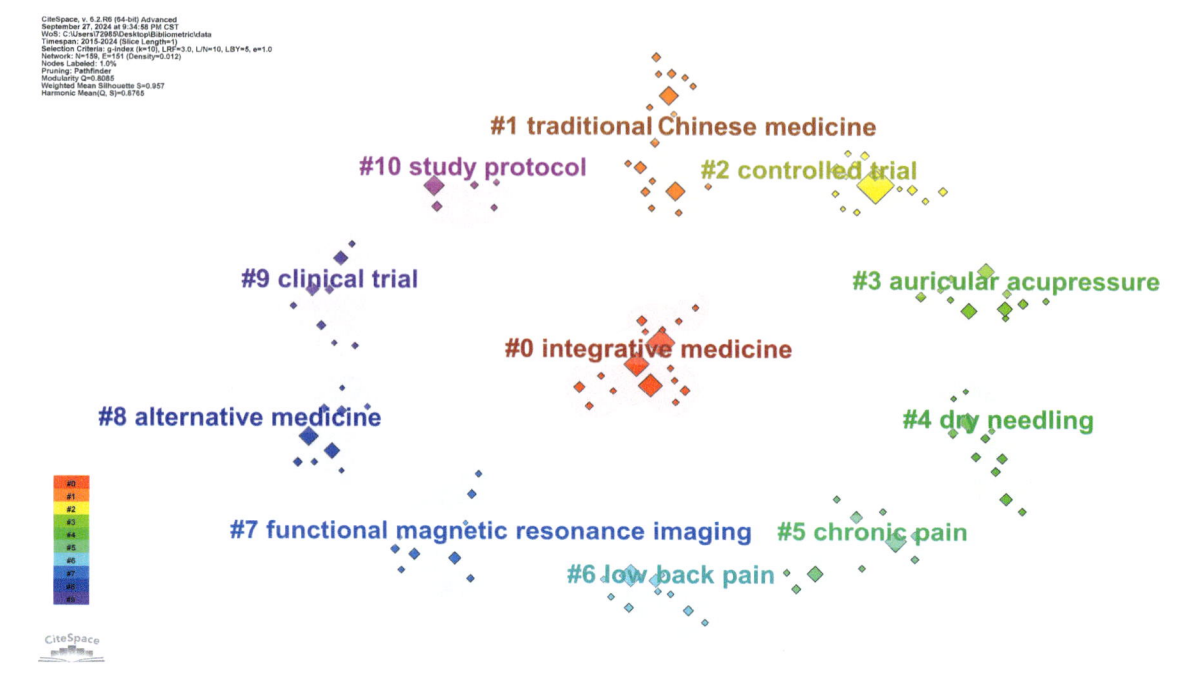

Figure 4 Keywords Co-occurrence Map of Acupuncture Clinical Researches in SCI Journals in Countries Other than China

gynecological and pediatric tumors), as well as for mild cognitive impairment. Ⅳ. Research on the Mechanisms of Acupuncture: Functional magnetic resonance imaging provides a new perspective for exploring acupoints specificity and comparing the efficacy of true over sham acupuncture.

Table 1 Clustering Labels for Keywords of Acupuncture Clinical Researches in SCI Journals in Countries Other than China

Group	Cluster Number	Label Name	Number of Keywords	Silhouette Value	Year	Main Keywords
Ⅰ	#5	chronic pain	10	0.955	2017	chronic pain; myofascial pain syndromes; thread embedding acupuncture; auricular acupuncture; anesthetic complications
	#6	low back pain	10	0.956	2019	low back pain; laser acupuncture; clinical trial protocol; controlled trial; postoperative pain
	#9	knee osteoarthritis	8	0.889	2017	knee osteoarthritis; manual therapy; laser acupuncture; auricular acupuncture; physical therapy
Ⅱ	#2	bee-sting acupuncture	14	1.000	2017	bee-sting acupuncture; controlled trial; chronic neck pain; heart rate variability; autonomic nervous system
	#3	auricular acupressure	11	0.871	2018	auricular acupressure; complementary therapy; dry needling; laser acupuncture; traditional acupuncture
	#4	dry needling	11	0.982	2016	dry needling; trigger points; chronic pain; chronic neck pain; lateral epicondylitis
Ⅲ	#0	integrative medicine	17	0.920	2019	integrative medicine; gynecological oncology; chemotherapy induced sleep disturbance; chemotherapy induced nausea; complementary medicine
	#1	traditional Chinese medicine	17	1.000	2018	traditional Chinese medicine; auriculotherapy; semi-permanent needles; tongue analysis; qualitative research

Chapter 1 Progress of Clinical Research on Acupuncture in the Last Decade

(Continued)

Group	Cluster Number	Label Name	Number of Keywords	Silhouette Value	Year	Main Keywords
Ⅲ	#8	alternative medicine	9	0.928	2017	alternative medicine; pediatric oncology; integrative medicine; supportive care; medication-resistant depression
	#10	complementary therapies	6	0.963	2019	complementary therapies; mild cognitive impairment; protocol; controlled trial; traditional medicine
Ⅳ	#7	functional magnetic resonance imaging	9	1.000	2018	functional magnetic resonance imaging; multivoxel pattern analysis; acupoint spatial discrimination; sham acupuncture; acupuncture expectancy

(2) Cluster Analysis of Keywords in Acupuncture Clinical Researches in China

The 11 clusters can be broadly classified into four categories (Figure 5 and Table 2). Ⅰ. Methodology of Acupuncture Researches (Clusters #0, #10): Currently, most acupuncture clinical research in China continues to focus on RCTs, the second are cohort studies. Ⅱ. Common Acupuncture Interventions (Clusters #2, #3): Scholars in China have conducted in-depth studies on various acupuncture interventions, including transcutaneous electrical acupoint stimulation, auricular acupressure, and subcutaneous needling. In contrast to their international counterparts, they have shown a keen interest in traditional methods such as the Qinglong tail-wagging acupuncture method, opposing needling, and thunder-fire moxibustion. Ⅲ. Indications for Acupuncture (Clusters #1, #4, #6, #8, #10): In recent years, acupuncture researches have encompassed clinical applications for varied conditions, including urinary incontinence, knee osteoarthritis, heart rate variability, functional anorectal pain, and degenerative spinal diseases. Ⅳ. Mechanisms of Acupuncture Effects (Clusters #7, #9): With the advancement of neuroimaging, particularly the extensive application of functional magnetic resonance imaging, there is a growing possibility of directly revealing the mechanisms behind effects of acupuncture. This trend is consistent in China and other countries.

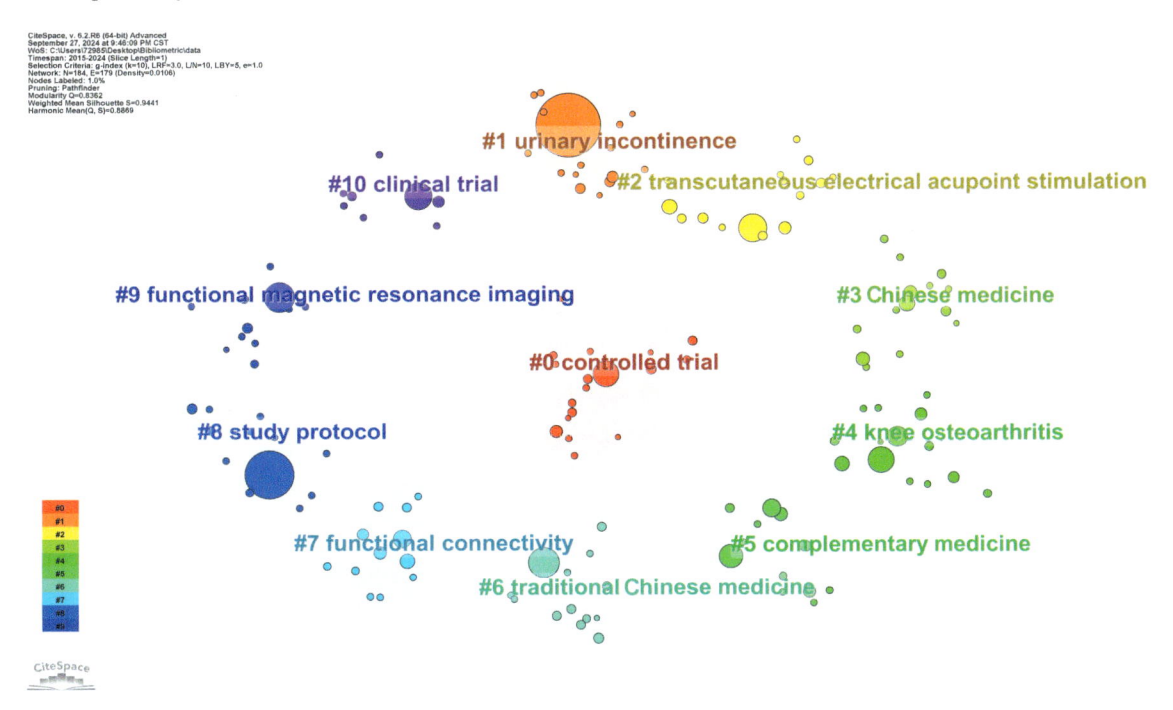

Figure 5 Keywords Co-occurrence Map of Acupuncture Clinical Researches in SCI Journals in China

Table 2 Clustering Labels for Keywords of Acupuncture Clinical Researches in SCI Journals in China

Group	Cluster Number	Label Name	Number of Keywords	Silhouette Value	Year	Main Keywords
I	#0	controlled trial	18	0.939	2019	controlled trial; adjuvant chemotherapy; cancer pain; opioid-induced constipation; nonpharmaceutical therapy
I	#5	cohort study	13	0.963	2019	cohort study; complementary medicine; musculoskeletal disorders; cervical spondylotic radiculopathy; thunder-fire moxibustion
II	#2	transcutaneous electrical acupoint stimulation	15	0.978	2018	transcutaneous electrical acupoint stimulation; breast cancer; postoperative analgesia; cancer-related fatigue; radical mastectomy
II	#3	auricular acupressure	14	0.988	2020	auricular acupressure; Chinese medicine; ischemic strokes; chronic tension-type headache; postoperative ileus
III	#1	urinary incontinence	17	1.000	2019	urinary incontinence; opposing needling; acupuncture; sham acupuncture; chronic insomnia disorder
III	#4	knee osteoarthritis	14	0.991	2019	knee osteoarthritis; clinical efficacy; Qinglong tail-wagging acupuncture method; total knee arthroplasty; sham acupuncture
III	#6	heart rate variability	13	0.937	2018	heart rate variability; traditional Chinese medicine; vagal activity; autonomic nervous system; needle sensation
III	#8	functional anorectal pain	12	1.000	2020	functional anorectal pain; BL31-BL34 (Baliao acupoints); elderly patients; study protocol; acupoint injection
III	#10	degenerative spinal disorders	9	0.839	2020	degenerative spinal disorders; postoperative pain; subcutaneous needling; controlled trial insomnia
IV	#7	functional connectivity	12	0.849	2019	functional connectivity; machine learning; multivariate pattern analyses; postprandial distress syndrome; major depressive disorder
IV	#9	functional magnetic resonance imaging	12	0.986	2019	functional magnetic resonance imaging; specific effect; nonspecific effect; low back pain; chronic pain

1.5 Trend Analysis of Keywords Over Time in Acupuncture Clinical Researches

(1) Trend Analysis of Keywords Over Time of Acupuncture Clinical Researches in the Countries Other Than China

The keywords timeline trend graph shown in Figure 6 illustrates the research hotspots and topics in acupuncture clinical researches in the countries other than China across the years. ①Between 2015 and 2016, the keywords "randomized controlled trial" (RCT, freq. 103) and "quality of life" (QoL, freq. 59) emerged as prominent themes. RCT is a crucial research method for exploring the specificity and efficacy of acupuncture, while QoL highlights unique advantages of acupuncture integrative regulating the human body's state and demonstrating acupuncture's effecacy. ②From 2017 to 2018, "auricular acupuncture" (freq. 16) and "auricular acupressure" (freq. 14) gradually became new research hotspots. ③From 2019 to 2024, "mild cognitive impairment" (freq. 7) and "functional magnetic resonance imaging" (freq. 8) have increasingly gained traction and are expected to take center stage. Given the lack of a "gold standard" drug for mild cognitive impairment and the challenges posed by the high costs and side effects of long-term western medical treatments, these factors significantly impact patient QoL[2]. Acupuncture may stimulate neural activity and adjust neural networks in the brain, potentially alleviating cognitive impairment.

(2) Trend Analysis of Keywords Over Time in Acupuncture Clinical Researches in China

The timeline trend graph of acupuncture clinical researches in China shown in Figure 7 illustrates the alternating trend in the keywords related to both Chinese and western acupuncture clinical studies. This trend reflects the ongoing exchange and integration of research directions across approaches. ①From 2015 to 2016, the keywords

Chapter 1 Progress of Clinical Research on Acupuncture in the Last Decade

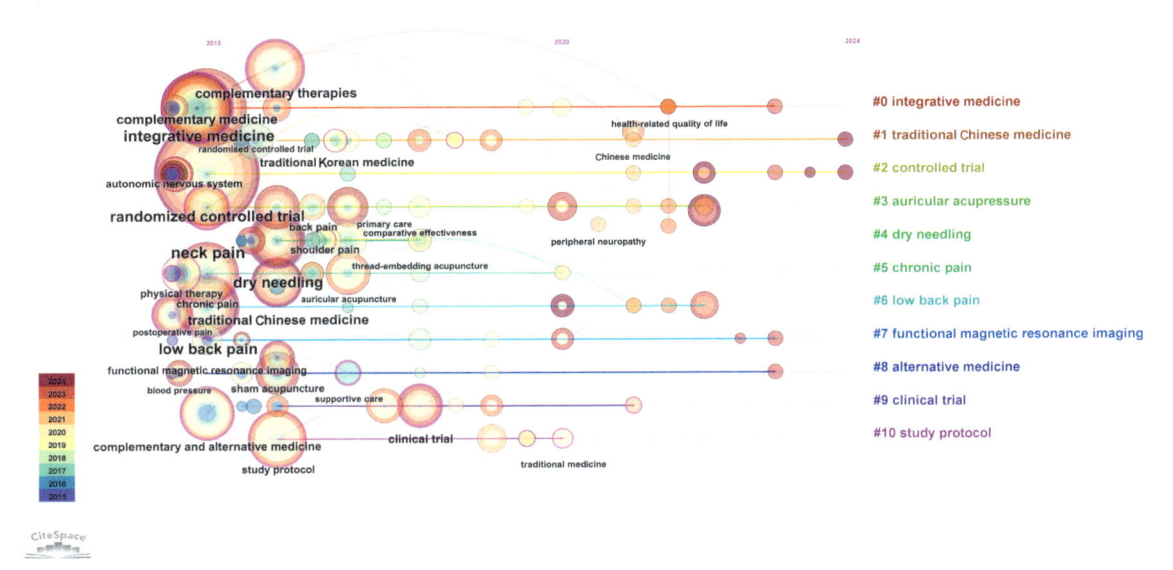

Figure 6 Keywords Timeline Trend Graph of Acupuncture Clinical Researches in SCI Journals in Countries Other than China

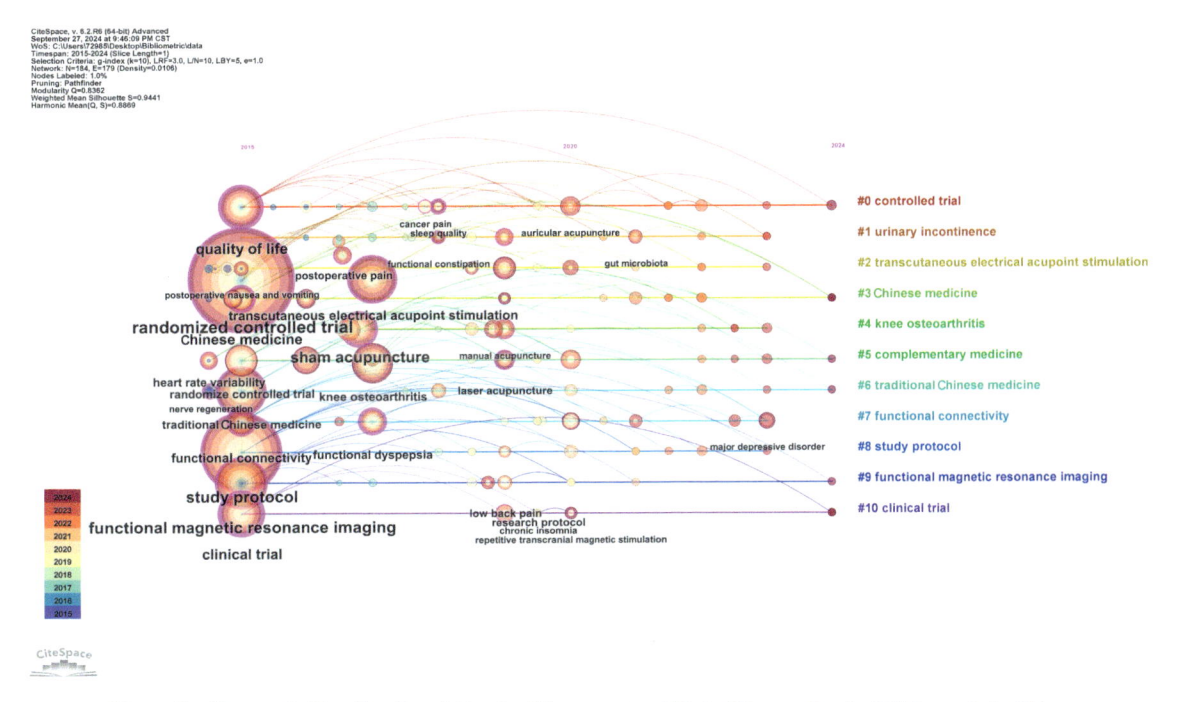

Figure 7 Keywords Timeline Trend Graph of Acupuncture Clinical Researches in SCI Journals in China

"study protocol" (freq. 180) and "functional magnetic resonance imaging" (freq. 70) occupied prominent positions in Chinese acupuncture clinical researches. This emphasizes the importance Chinese researchers place on the rigor of the study design and methodology, as well as their commitment to advancing the standardization of clinical research. Notably, China adopted functional magnetic resonance imaging technology earlier than the west to elucidate the mechanisms of acupuncture, underscoring China's leadership in this field. ②Between 2017 and 2019, "transcutaneous electrical acupoint stimulation" (freq. 59), a novel acupuncture technique, gained significant attention for its non-invasive stimulation of acupoints. Concurrently, keywords such as "knee osteoarthritis" (freq. 48) and "postoperative pain" (freq. 10) highlight the broad application of acupuncture in pain management. ③ From 2020 to 2024, "auricular acupuncture" (freq. 11) emerged as a key research hotspot in China. The auricular region is unique, as it is the only area on the body surface with vagus nerve distribution, containing nerve fibers that directly project to the nucleus of the solitary tract. This anatomical feature allows for the rapid evocation of auriculo-cerebral reflexes for modulation, leading to the development of auricular vagus nerve stimulators[3]. Auricular acupoints serve as a model for the communication and integration of classical TCM theories with modern science, acting as a bridge between TCM acupuncture and brain science. Furthermore, the diverse clinical applications of acupuncture have been fully recognized, with conditions such as primary dysmenorrhea (freq. 10), functional constipation (freq. 6), and colorectal cancer (freq. 7) showcasing the unique efficacy of acupuncture in treatment.

2. Analysis of Acupuncture Clinical Trials in SCI-indexed Journals with High Impact Factor Over the Past Decade

We conducted a systematic literature search on acupuncture clinical trials published in SCI-indexed journals with high impact factor over the past decade, ultimately including 52 papers. By analyzing publication trends, disease type distributions, sample sizes, interventions, and sham acupuncture settings, we summarized the characteristics of global scholars in designing acupuncture clinical trials, aiming to provide a reference for future high-quality acupuncture clinical trials.

2.1 Steady Increase in the Number of High-Quality Trials in China

The 52 papers involved contributions from nine countries. Among these, 31 articles (59.62% of the total) were published by Chinese teams, while 12 articles (23.08%) originated in America (Figure 8). Compared to previous studies[4,5], China has established a leading position in the number of high-quality acupuncture clinical trials, with this number continuing to grow. This achievement is attributed to the proactive research efforts of Chinese scholars who consistently utilize high-quality RCT evidence to construct a scientific clinical decision-making framework for acupuncture[6-8].

2.2 Expanding Types of Diseases Treated with Acupuncture

Pain disorders remain a major focus of high-quality acupuncture clinical trials. A study analyzing acupuncture RCTs published in journals with impact factors greater than 5 and indexed on PubMed between 2010 and 2018 identified tumors and pain as research hotspots[9]. In recent years, the range of diseases treated with acupuncture has gradually expanded from cancer and its complications to include digestive system disorders. Additionally, acupuncture has demonstrated its effecacy in treating

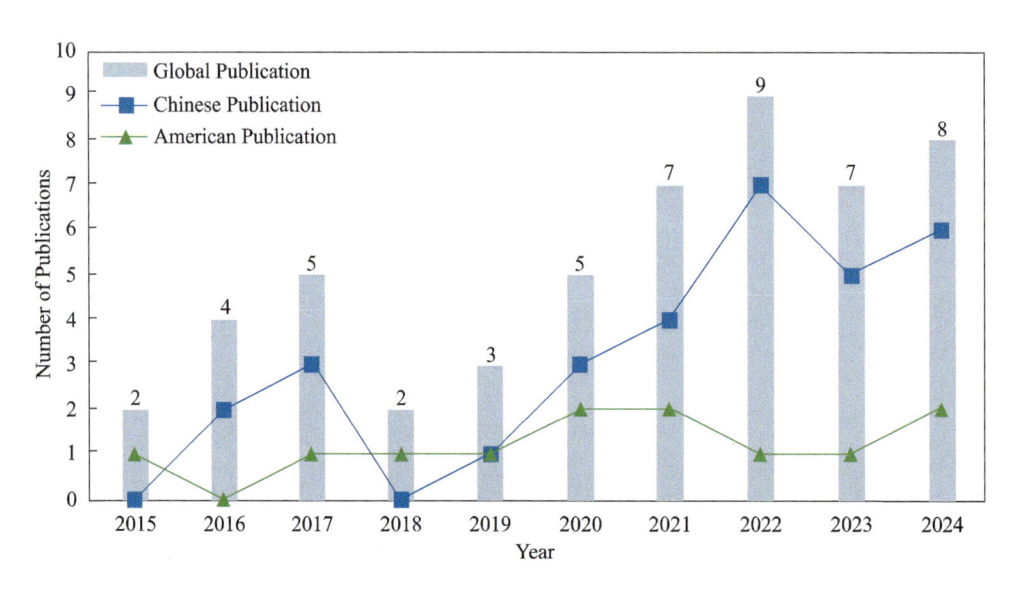

Figure 8 Trend Graph of Countries Publishing High-Quality Acupuncture Clinical Research Literature in the Past Decade
Note: Data for 2024 are as of July 31.

Chapter 1   Progress of Clinical Research on Acupuncture in the Last Decade

mental health disorders, cardiovascular diseases, pelvic floor disorders, and various dermatological conditions, indicating its potential for addressing a wide array of health issues. However, there remains need for more high-quality data derived from evidence-based medicine to support these findings (Figure 9).

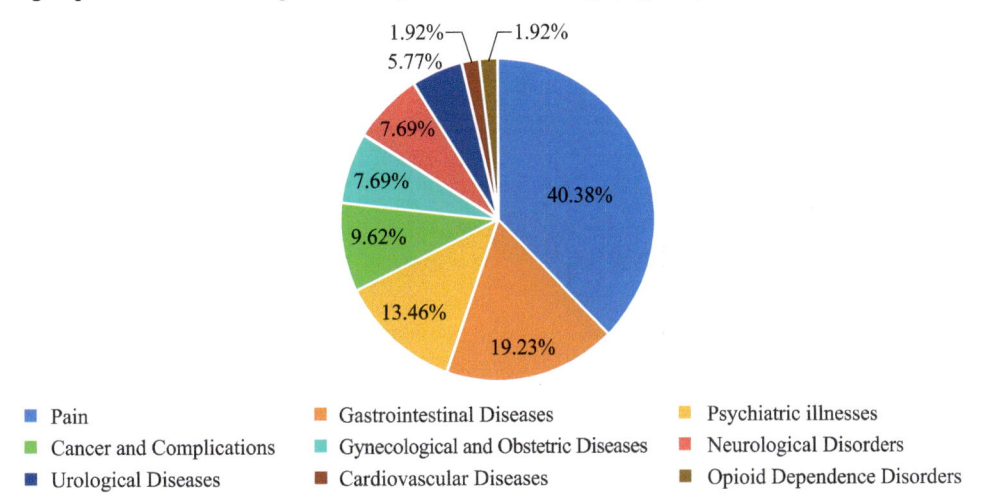

- Pain 40.38%
- Gastrointestinal Diseases 19.23%
- Psychiatric illnesses 13.46%
- Cancer and Complications 9.62%
- Gynecological and Obstetric Diseases 7.69%
- Neurological Disorders 7.69%
- Urological Diseases 5.77%
- Cardiovascular Diseases 1.92%
- Opioid Dependence Disorders 1.92%

Figure 9   Distribution of Diseases in High-Quality Acupuncture Clinical Research Literature Over the Past Decade
Note: Some papers address comorbidities, and this study includes such papers in multiple disease categories.

2.3   From Explanatory RCTs to Real-World Study: Development Trends and Paradigms in Acupuncture Clinical Trials

A total of 17 (32.69% of 52 papers) of the included references featured validation studies and superiority/on-inferiority studies. In these studies, groups were classified into acupuncture, sham acupuncture, and control groups (western medicine group/routine care group). Comparing acupuncture groups with sham acupuncture groups can help identify the specific effects and efficacy of acupuncture, while comparisons with western medicine or routine care groups can assess the superiority and safety of acupuncture. One study showed significant differences between China and the western countries concerning the needs, objectives, designs, pretests, investigators, acupuncture treatment protocols, sources of these protocols, methodological quality, results, conclusions, publication bias, and scope of RCT studies on acupuncture. This has resulted in a positive outcome rate of 71.43% for Chinese scholars compared to 59.18% for their foreign counterparts[10]. The differing reports of acupuncture results between Chinese and western researchers have underscored the importance of validating the acupuncture-specific effects, emerging as a key focus of clinical acupuncture research (37/52, 71.15%; Figure 10). Real-world studies emphasize evaluating

- superiority/non-inferiority studies: 61.53%
- validation studies: 71.15%

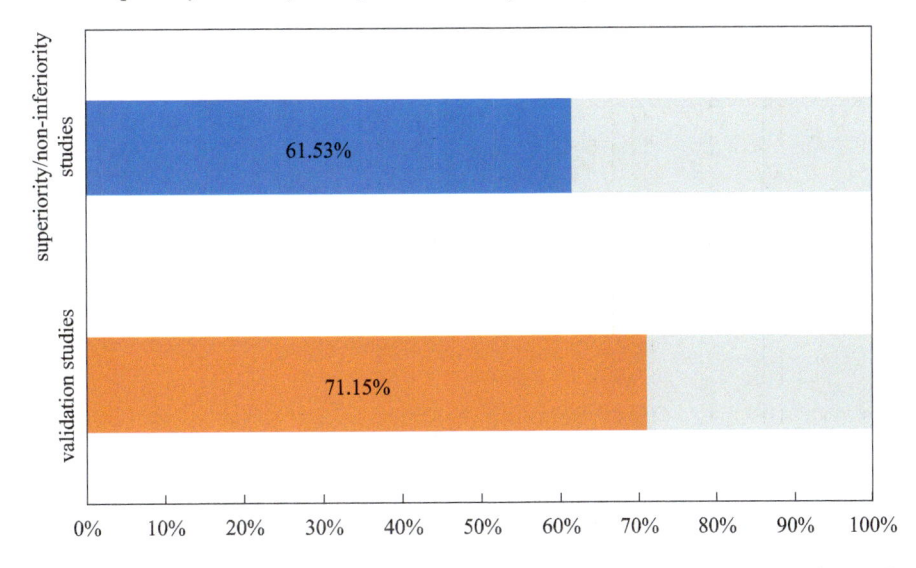

Figure 10   Distribution of Document Types in High-Quality Acupuncture Clinical Papers Over the Past Decade

· 9 ·

clinical outcomes of interventions in actual clinical settings, thereby contributing to high-quality, broadly applicable clinical evidence[11]. Given the unique characteristics of acupuncture, establishing a new research paradigm that adheres to its principles: From explanatory RCTs and pragmatic RCTs to clinical efficacy-oriented real-world studies, has become an urgent priority in the field of acupuncture.

2.4 Validation of Acupuncture Specific Effects: Controversies and Advances in the Placebo Acupuncture Design

Placebo acupuncture is an internationally recognized control method essential for validating the specific effects of acupuncture, playing a crucial role in ensuring the quality of RCTs[12]. However, the placebo acupuncture design remains a topic of considerable debate[13]. The primary design options for placebo acupuncture include sham needling at verum acupoints (without penetrating the skin), shallow needling at sham points, and shallow needling at non-treatment-related points. Sham needling may be less effective at achieving blinding and carries a higher risk of unblinding, yet it has the advantage of not breaking the skin, thus minimally activating the body's receptors and avoiding specific therapeutic effects[14]. The main distinction between shallow needling at sham points and shallow needling at non-therapeutically relevant points lies in the former having an accurately named point with a clear primary therapeutic effect. While both methods aim to exploit differences in site effects, shallow needling at sham points is more likely to yield negative results compared to no needling at all[12]. When designing sham needling, it is imperative to "maximize blinding while minimizing any potential effects", all while ensuring effective blinding. Therefore, it is recommended to adhere to the sham acupuncture reporting guidelines and a checklist in clinical trials (SHARE) guidelines for sham needling reporting to enhance transparency and rigor in the design[15].

In acupuncture RCTs, the designs of Streitberger and Park (Figure 11) dominated the choice of comfort needles. None of the devices punctures the skin but can produce a pain sensation like that of a needle prick. Studies have shown that both devices are effective in allowing blinded patient recruitment[11]. Of the 52 papers, 12 (23.08%) mentioned the use of the comfort needle device. In addition, researchers in China are actively developing novel placebo needle devices, and the results have been published in high quality international journals[16-18] (Figure 12).

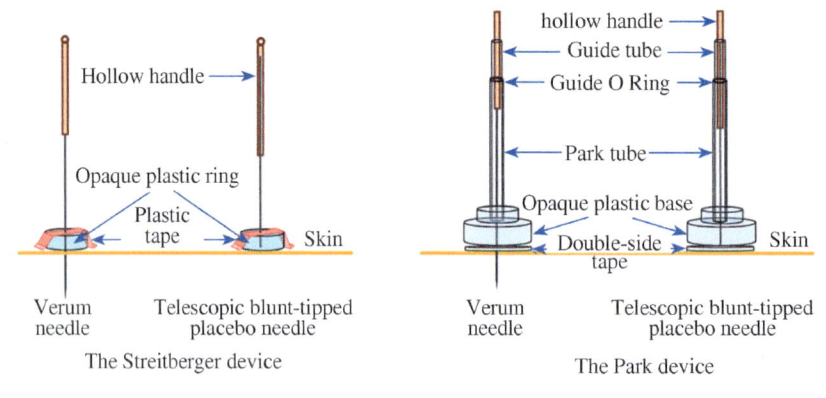

Figure 11 Schematic Diagram of the Streitberger and Park Sham Acupuncture Devices

3. Conclusion and Perspectives

China's excellence in the field of acupuncture studies has propelled the development of acupuncture clinical research worldwide, yielding remarkable achievements. High-quality acupuncture clinical trials have extensively explored various areas, including pain disorders, digestive disorders, and neurological conditions, highlighting the diverse potential applications of acupuncture. These trials employed a range of acupuncture methods, such as electroacupuncture, manual acupuncture, and laser acupuncture, to address the therapeutic needs of individuals with different conditions. Notably, sham acupuncture is a crucial component of these clinical trials, enhancing the quality of evidence for evaluating the effects of acupuncture treatments through scientifically rigorous control designs, thereby ensuring the accuracy and reliability of the study results. However, challenges are remained, including issues of duplication and subpar quality in some clinical trials, which contribute to a degree of waste in research resources.

At the 16th International Symposium on Acupuncture and Moxibustion held in Tianjin, China, in 2023, 30 experts in TCM and clinical research gathered for a retreat on the

Chapter 1 Progress of Clinical Research on Acupuncture in the Last Decade

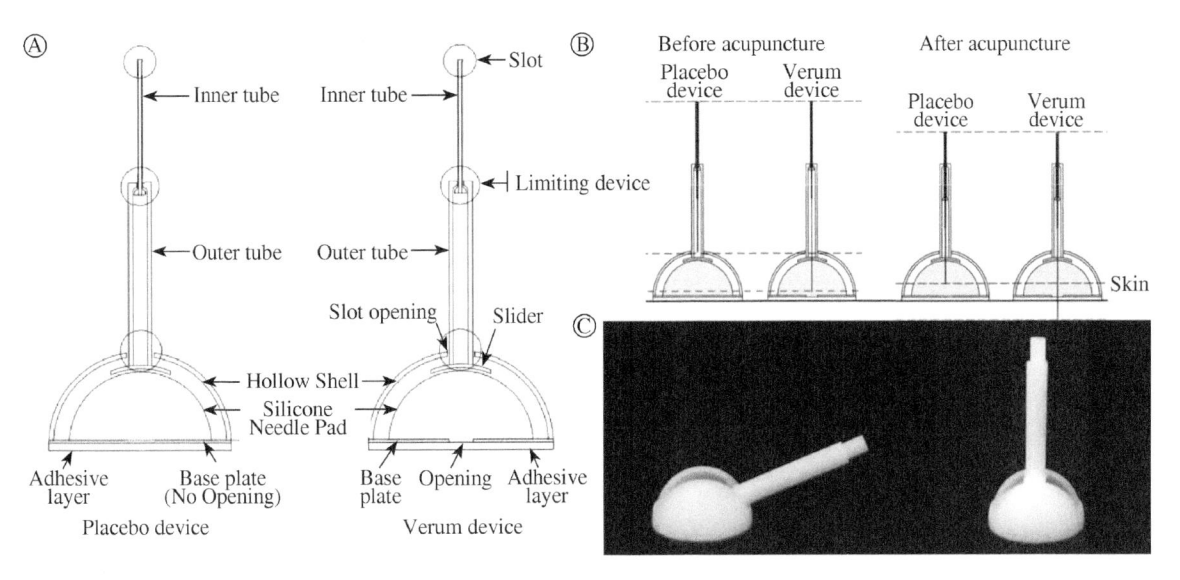

Figure 12 An Auxiliary Device for Double-Blind Sham Acupuncture Studies
Note: A. The schematic structure of the sham acupuncture and true acupuncture devices; B. The operation of sham acupuncture and true acupuncture; C. A physical image of the new auxiliary acupuncture device.

topic of researcher-initiated clinical research system of TCM. This event was led by President LIU Baoyan of the World Federation of Acupuncture-Moxibustion Societies and culminated in the formation of *Tianjin Consensus on Clinical Research of Traditional Chinese Medicine Initiated by Researchers*. The consensus aims to unite and organize members of the Chinese medicine community to explore and promote clinical research that aligns with the unique characteristics of TCM. It seeks to facilitate the widespread application of Chinese medicine globally and to fully realize its value in various healthcare settings.

In the future, we should enhance communication and collaboration among different countries and regions, establish interdisciplinary acupuncture clinical research teams, and integrate new technologies and methods from various fields into acupuncture research. This approach will promote acupuncture's diversified development and is crucial for improving its quality clinical studies. Based on traditional medical theories and modern scientific advancements, we can develop experimental paradigms and evaluation protocols that align with the unique characteristics of acupuncture research. This will help establish high-quality clinical evidence, broaden the spectrum of diseases treatable with acupuncture, optimize treatment protocols, and contribute to improving the health of humanity through the benefits of acupuncture.

Authors: SHI Jiangwei, SHEN Yan, FAN Guanwei, WANG Jingui, ZHANG Yanjun (First Teaching Hospital of Tianjin University of Traditional Chinese Medicine, National Clinical Research Center for Chinese Medicine Acupuncture and Moxibustion); LIU Baoyan, LIU Zhishun, HE Liyun (China Academy of Chinese Medical Sciences)

References

[1] YAN S Y, XIONG Z Y, LIU X Y, et al. Review of clinical research in acupuncture and moxibustion from 2010 to 2020 and prospects [J]. Zhongguo Zhen Jiu, 2022, 42 (1): 116-118, 120.

[2] KASPER S, BANCHER C, ECKERT A, et al. Management of mild cognitive impairment (MCI): The need for national and international guidelines [J]. World J Biol Psychiatry, 2020, 21 (8): 579-594.

[3] LI S Y, RONG P J, ZHANG Y, ET AL. Ideas of "Treating Encephalopathy With Ear Therapy" Based on the Auricular Point Vagus Nerve Electrical Stimulation Technique and Its Clinical Application [J]. Journal of Traditional Chinese Medicine, 2020, 61 (24): 2154-2158.

[4] HONG S H, WU F, DING S S, et al. Analysis on literature regarding acupuncture-moxibustion with high impact factor journal of SCI during the recent 5 years [J]. Zhongguo Zhen Jiu, 2015, 35 (3): 291-294.

[5] HONG S H, ZHANG Y Y, XU F. Analysis and Discussion of Acupuncture-related RCT Studies in High Impact Factor SCI Journals in Recent Seven Years [J]. Journal of Zhejiang Chinese Medical University, 2021, 45 (7): 718-725.

[6] DING N. Methodological study on the consensus process of clinical practice guidelines of

acupuncture-moxibustion [D]. Beijing: China Academy of Chinese Medical Sciences, 2023.

[7] QIU R J, WEI X X, GUAN Z Y, et al. Research status and progress of core outcome sets in the field of traditional Chinese medicine [J]. Chinese Journal of Evidence-Based Medicine, 2023, 23 (2): 211-220.

[8] LIN J Y, SHEN T W, JI Z C, et al. Quality analysis of the literature on randomised controlled clinical trials of acupuncture in China in the last 5 years [J/OL]. Shanghai Journal of Acupuncture and Moxibustion, 2024: 1-9 [2024-09-26]. https://doi.org/10.13460/j.issn.1005-0957.2024.11.0004.

[9] SHI Y Z, ZHOU S Y, ZHENG Q H, et al. Characteristics Analysis of Randomized Controlled Trials Regarding Acupuncture with International High Quality [J]. World Chinese Medicine, 2018, 13 (7): 1580-1583.

[10] GANG W J, GONG C Z, JING X H. Acupuncture randomized controlled trials: comparing China-based vs. Western-based studies [J]. Zhongguo Zhen Jiu,, 2022, 42 (1): 3-7, 22.

[11] FAN W M, SUN C Y, ZHANG J L, et al. An investigation into improved methods for clinical randomised controlled trials of acupuncture [J]. Shanghai Journal of Acupuncture and Moxibustion, 2024, 43 (1): 104-110.

[12] ZHANG Z X. Evaluation of Factors and Rationality of Sham Acupuncture Settings Based on Foreign High-Quality Acupuncture Clinical Trials [D]. Tianjin: Tianjin University of Traditional Chinese Medicine, 2023.

[13] GUO Q L, LIU Q G, ZHAN H, et al. Application and Consideration of Placebo-Acupuncture Control in Clinical Research [J]. Journal of Clinical Acupuncture and Moxibustion, 2017, 33 (11): 1-3.

[14] LIU J H, MA N, DONG X, et al. Analysis of the current state of research and application of the consolation needling control design [J]. Shanghai Journal of Acupuncture and Moxibustion, 2022, 41 (3): 318-322.

[15] LIU X Y, MA P H, LIU B Y, et al. Interpretation of Sham Acupuncture REporting (SHARE) guidelines and a checklist in clinical trials [J]. Chinese Journal of Evidence-Based Medicine, 2024, 24 (7): 838-844.

[16] FAN J Q, LU W J, TAN W Q, et al. Effectiveness of Acupuncture for Anxiety Among Patients With Parkinson Disease: A Randomized Clinical Trial [J]. JAMA Network Open, 2022, 5 (9): e2232133.

[17] YAN M, FAN J, LIU X, et al. Acupuncture and Sleep Quality Among Patients With Parkinson Disease: A Randomized Clinical Trial [J]. JAMA Network Open, 2024, 7 (6): e2417862.

[18] WANG Y T, LIU X, XU Z Q, et al. An auxiliary device for double-blind placebo acupuncture research [J]. Zhongguo Zhen Jiu, 2022, 42 (3): 351-354.

Chapter 2

Comments of Clinical Trials of Acupuncture and Moxibustion in SCI Journals

Section 1　Introduction and Comments of *Acupuncture for Combat-Related Posttraumatic Stress Disorder: A Randomized Clinical Trial*

1. Introduction

IMPORTANCE　Current interventions for posttraumatic stress disorder (PTSD) are efficacious, yet effectiveness may be limited by adverse effects and high withdrawal rates. Acupuncture is an emerging intervention with positive preliminary data for PTSD.

OBJECTIVE　To compare verum acupuncture with sham acupuncture (minimal needling) on clinical and physiological outcomes.

DESIGN, SETTING, AND PARTICIPANTS　This was a 2-arm, parallel-group, prospective blinded randomized clinical trial hypothesizing superiority of verum to sham acupuncture. The study was conducted at a single outpatient-based site, the Tibor Rubin VA Medical Center in Long Beach, California, with recruitment from April 2018 to May 2022, followed by a 15-week treatment period. Following exclusion for characteristics that are known PTSD treatment confounds, might affect biological assessment, indicate past nonadherence or treatment resistance, or indicate risk of harm, 93 treatment-seeking combat veterans with PTSD aged 18 to 55 years were allocated to group by adaptive randomization and 71 participants completed the intervention protocols.

INTERVENTIONS　Verum and sham were provided as 1-hour sessions, twice weekly, and participants were given 15 weeks to complete up to 24 sessions.

MAIN OUTCOMES AND MEASURES　The primary outcome was pretreatment to posttreatment change in PTSD symptom severity on the Clinician-Administered PTSD Scale-5 (CAPS-5). The secondary outcome was pretreatment to posttreatment change in fear-conditioned extinction, assessed by fear-potentiated startle response. Outcomes were assessed at pretreatment, midtreatment, and posttreatment. General linear models comparing within and between-group were analyzed in both intention-to-treat and treatment-completed models.

RESULTS　A total of 85 male and 8 female veterans (mean [SD] age, 39.2 [8.5] years) were randomized. There was a large treatment effect of verum (Cohen d, 1.17), a moderate effect of sham (d, 0.67), and a moderate between-group effect favoring verum (mean [SD] Δ7.1 [11.8]; t_{90}=2.87, d, 0.63; P=0.005) in the intention-to-treat analysis. The effect pattern was similar in the treatment-completed analysis: Verum d, 1.53; sham d, 0.86; between-group mean (SD) Δ, 7.4 (11.7); t_{69}=2.64; d, 0.63; P=0.01. There was a significant pretreatment to posttreatment reduction of fear-potentiated startle during extinction (ie, better fear extinction) in the verum but not the sham group and a significant correlation (r=0.31) between symptom reduction and fear extinction. Withdrawal rates were low.

CONCLUSIONS AND RELEVANCE　The acupuncture intervention used in this study was clinically efficacious and favorably affected the psychobiology of PTSD in combat veterans. These data build on extant literature and suggest that clinical implementation of acupuncture for PTSD, along with further research about comparative efficacy, durability, and mechanisms of effects, is warranted.

2. Expert Comments

Comment 1

Pharmacotherapy and psychotherapy are effective for PTSD, but patient compliance is poor. This trial enrolled soldiers with PTSD as participants in a novel investigation that further expands the clinical scope of acupuncture.

In the acupuncture group, treatment was administered twice a week for approximately 15 weeks (24 times), and the needle was retained for 30 minutes each time, meeting the intensity requirements for clinical efficacy. The acupuncture program included semi-standardized acupoint selection, combined with teaching materials, expert consensus, and patient evaluation, four syndromes were summed to determine the main treatment points, and before each treatment, acupuncture doctors formed four diagnoses and selected a group of corresponding points. The supine and prone positions were alternated to avoid point fatigue. The acupoints, distributed bilaterally, were connected with electroacupuncture at 2/100 Hz. The formulation and implementation of the acupuncture treatment plan could reflect the characteristics of traditional Chinese medicine. However, the depth and current frequency were not reported in the clinical study protocol and results report.

To facilitate blinding, micro-acupuncture was used as sham acupuncture, and the acupoints, depth, and stimulation intensity were set to minimize the biological therapeutic effect. Non-meridian and non-acupoints should be used as the operation sites (approximately 2 cm beside the meridian acupoint in the acupuncture group), different body shapes across patients should be considered, and key anatomical landmarks should be avoided. The acupuncture points were shallowly punctured to a depth of no more than 0.25 inches. Sham acupuncture only simulated the feeling of skin being punctured, without manipulation and deqi, with the indicator light of the electroacupuncture instrument being on but without current output. To further facilitate blinding, the number of acupoints selected and frequency of treatment were the same as those in the acupuncture group, and the layout of the diagnosis and treatment environment, preparation of articles, operation process, and communication with patients were carried out in accordance with the standard process. The selection of the control group was appropriate and the process was duly implemented.

Comment 2

(1) Study design and process implementation

The study used a randomized controlled trial design to evaluate the clinical and biological effects of acupuncture on combat-related PTSD. A two-group parallel comparison approach was utilized, hypothesizing that true acupuncture would be superior to sham acupuncture in reducing PTSD symptoms and enhancing fear extinction responses. The internal validity of the results was enhanced by conducting the study in strict compliance with ethical standards and minimizing bias through adaptive randomization and double blinding. Overall, the study design demonstrated a high level of rigor in terms of controlling variables and reducing interfering factors, especially regarding the multi-level evaluation system, including the evaluation of clinical signs and symptoms (eg, CAPS-5 score) and physiological response (eg, fear-enhanced startle response), which increased the results' power and comprehensiveness. However, there are areas for improvement. First, the fact that this was a single-center study may have limited the external validity of the results. Second, while adaptive randomization was employed to ensure group balance, the generalizability of the results may be limited owing to the specific nature of the study sample (ie, limited to combat veterans). In addition, the study lacked long-term follow up, preventing a full assessment of the long-term efficacy of acupuncture.

(2) Selection and application of clinical research methodology and statistical methods

In terms of clinical research methodology, the study selected a confirmatory randomized controlled trial design, combined with blind and sham acupuncture for control, which provided a scientific basis for evaluating the specific effect of acupuncture. The primary analysis employed an intention-to-treat and completion treatment model, ensuring robust and reliable results. Generalized linear models and repeated measures analysis of variance were used for statistical analysis, effectively controlling the correlations and providing adequate power for detecting between-group differences. The study further validated the clinical significance of the results by assessing the magnitude of the treatment effect using Cohen's *d* effect sizes.

Nevertheless, there remain some issues that need to be addressed regarding the statistical methodology. First, while the study assessed the effects of reducing PTSD symptoms, it was not possible to adequately adjust for multiple hypothesis testing, which may have increased the risk of type I errors. Second, the study's handling of dropout participant data, despite the intention-to-treat analysis, may have led to bias given the complexity of the reasons for dropout. Finally, the effectiveness of sham acupuncture received limited discussion, as sham acupuncture itself may produce certain physiological effects, which warrant caution regarding the interpretation of the results.

In summary, this study had obvious advantages in terms of design and methodological application, especially in terms of randomization, blinding, and multi-dimensional outcome assessment. However, there are areas for improvement in terms of external validity, detailed handling of statistical methods, and discussion of sham acupuncture. Overall, the study provided valuable evidence for the use of acupuncture in the treatment of PTSD, but caution should be exercised in the generalizability and evaluation of the rigor of the conclusions. Future studies should further explore the long-term nature of the efficacy of acupuncture and its comparative effectiveness against other treatments.

Chapter 2   Comments of Clinical Trials of Acupuncture and Moxibustion in SCI Journals

Section 2   Introduction and Comments of *Acupuncture and Sleep Quality Among Patients With Parkinson Disease: A Randomized Clinical Trial*

1. Introduction

IMPORTANCE   Poor sleep quality greatly impairs quality of life and accelerates deterioration in patients with Parkinson disease (PD), but current remedies remain limited. Acupuncture, used as an adjunctive therapy with anti-Parkinson medications, has shown positive effects in patients with PD. However, high-quality clinical evidence to support the effectiveness of acupuncture for patients with PD and poor sleep quality is lacking.

OBJECTIVE   To assess the safety and efficacy of real acupuncture (RA) vs sham acupuncture (SA) as an adjunctive therapy for patients with PD who have poor sleep quality.

DESIGN, SETTING, AND PARTICIPANTS   This single-center randomized clinical trial was performed at The First Affiliated Hospital of Guangzhou University of Chinese Medicine in China from February 18, 2022, to February 18, 2023. Patients with PD and sleep complaints were recruited and randomized (1 : 1) to receive RA or SA treatment for 4 weeks. Data analysis was performed from April 12 to August 17, 2023.

INTERVENTION   Treatment with RA or SA for 4 weeks.

MAIN OUTCOMES AND MEASURES   The main outcome was the change in Parkinson Disease Sleep Scale (PDSS) scores measured at baseline, after 4 weeks of treatment, and at 8 weeks of follow-up.

RESULTS   Of the 83 participants enrolled, 78 (94.0%) completed the intervention and were included in the analysis. Their mean (SD) age was 64.1 (7.9) years; 41 (52.6%) were men and 37 (47.4%) were women. A significant increase in PDSS scores from baseline was observed for both the RA group (29.65 [95% CI, 24.65-34.65]; $P<0.001$) and the SA group (10.47 [95% CI, 5.35-15.60]; $P<0.001$). Compared with the SA group, the RA group had a significant increase in PDSS scores after 4 weeks of treatment (19.75 [95% CI, 11.02-28.49]; $P<0.001$) and at 8 weeks of follow-up (20.24 [95% CI, 11.51-28.98]; $P<0.001$).

CONCLUSIONS AND RELEVANCE   In this randomized clinical trial, acupuncture proved beneficial in improving sleep quality and quality of life among patients with PD. These findings suggest that the therapeutic effects of acupuncture could continue for up to 4 weeks.

2. Expert Comments

Comment 1

Sleep disturbance is a common non-motor symptom in PD and a common side effect of PD medications. Sleep disorders severely impact the quality of life of patients with PD and accelerate the deterioration of motor and non-motor symptoms, critically influencing patient outcomes. However, at present, although the drugs for sleep disorders in patients with PD can improve sleep to some extent, they are often accompanied by side effects; hence, it is urgent to develop novel safe and effective therapies. Previous studies have indicated that acupuncture can be used to treat insomnia and improve sleep disorders in patients with PD, but the quality of research and evidence is low. Therefore, this study addressed the key factors and treatment challenges that affect the outcomes of patients with PD using a high-quality clinical trial design to provide high-quality research evidence based on analyzing the status of clinical research on acupuncture treatment of PD sleep disorders.

Referring to previous studies, this study selected commonly used acupoints from the tranquilizing mind and spleen and stomach meridians for the acupuncture treatment plan, and the acupoint location was based on the Chinese national standard. The needle selection, treatment frequency, and course of treatment were reported; especially, the operation method of a true/false acupuncture auxiliary device was employed to ensure patient blinding. However, there remain areas of improvement. The selection of acupoints in the treatment plan differed from that in the cited study without explanation. The acupuncture method of the selected acupoints may have followed the principles of conventional acupuncture, but there was no reporting of the details of the operation of each acupoint and the qualification requirements for the acupuncturist. Although it is noted that the data analysis was performed on patients who received at least 1 week of treatment, the compliance of patients with the acupuncture treatment was not reported in the results, which may have underestimated the acupuncture's efficacy.

To conclude, the study addressed a well-defined topic, and the report of the acupuncture intervention was more detailed regarding the difficulties and key points of clinical treatment of patients with PD. However, further improvements are needed in reporting the rationality of the acupuncture treatment plan, acupuncture operation, qualifications of the acupuncturist, and patient compliance.

Comment 2

This was a single-center randomized controlled trial. The intervention included acupuncture treatment. The report strictly adhered to consolidated standards of reporting trials (CONSORT). The inclusion criteria, acupuncture operations in the experimental and control groups, and design of acupoints and non-acupoints were clearly described. The study used a simple randomized, single-blind design, in which the patients were unaware of the grouping. In addition, the blinding of the statistical analyst was emphasized. The sample size of the study was estimated based on the results of a pilot trial; the study power was set at 90%, and the dropout rate was estimated at 20%. The results were reported in the order of availability analysis, efficacy comparison, and safety evaluation of randomized controlled trial. The baseline data of the two groups were first described, followed by a comparability analysis, with statistical inference results (P values) reported accordingly. The analysis of efficacy indicators in this study indicated that a full dataset analysis was conducted, with 40 complete cases in the experimental group and 38 complete cases in the control group, meeting the protocol set. However, the article also described the use of random filling to obtain a full dataset for analysis, but the number of reported data cases was 40 and 38, which may cause some confusion for readers. The statistical method section states the principle basis of method selection and describes that combined with the effect data obtained at three time points in the study, according to the repeated measurement design, a linear mixed-effect model to analyze the group effect, time effects, and interaction was chosen, with the results presented using line charts.

Overall, this study was a single-center randomized controlled trial with a reasonable design, standardized report, reasonable statistical description and inference methods, clear report logic, and reasonable inferences.

Section 3　Introduction and Comments of *Acupuncture for Chronic Radiation-Induced Xerostomia in Head and Neck Cancer: A Multicenter Randomized Clinical Trial*

1. Introduction

IMPORTANCE　Patients with head and neck cancer who undergo radiotherapy can develop chronic radiation-induced xerostomia. Prior acupuncture studies were single center and rated as having high risk of bias, making it difficult to know the benefits of acupuncture for treating radiation-induced xerostomia.

OBJECTIVE　To compare true acupuncture (TA), sham acupuncture (SA), and standard oral hygiene (SOH) for treating radiation-induced xerostomia.

DESIGN, SETTING, AND PARTICIPANTS　A randomized, blinded, 3-arm, placebo-controlled trial was conducted between July 29, 2013, and June 9, 2021. Data analysis was performed from March 9, 2022, through May 17, 2023. Patients reporting grade 2 or 3 radiation-induced xerostomia 12 months or more postradiotherapy for head and neck cancer were recruited from community-based cancer centers across the US that were part of the Wake Forest National Cancer Institute Community Oncology Research Program Research Base. Participants had received bilateral radiotherapy with no history of xerostomia.

INTERVENTIONS　Participants received SOH and were randomized to TA, SA, or SOH only. Participants in the TA and SA cohorts were treated 2 times per week for 4 weeks. Those experiencing a minor response received another 4 weeks of treatment.

MAIN OUTCOMES AND MEASURES　Patient-reported outcomes for xerostomia (Xerostomia Questionnaire, primary outcome) and quality of life (Functional Assessment of Cancer Therapy-General) were collected at baseline, 4 (primary time point), 8, 12, and 26 weeks. All analyses were intention to treat.

RESULTS　A total of 258 patients (201 men [77.9%]; mean [SD] age, 65.0 [9.16] years), participated from 33 sites across 13 states. Overall, 86 patients were assigned to each study arm. Mean (SD) years from diagnosis was 4.21 (3.74) years, 67.1% (n=173) had stage IV disease. At week 4, Xerostomia Questionnaire scores revealed significant between-group differences, with lower Xerostomia Questionnaire scores with TA vs SOH (TA: 50.6; SOH: 57.3; difference, −6.67; 95% CI, −11.08 to −2.27; P=0.003), and differences between TA and SA (TA: 50.6; SA: 55.0; difference, −4.41; 95% CI, −8.62 to −0.19; P=0.04) yet did not reach statistical significance after adjustment for multiple comparisons. There was no significant difference between

SA and SOH. Group differences in Functional Assessment of Cancer Therapy-General scores revealed statistically significant group differences at week 4, with higher scores with TA vs SOH (TA: 101.6; SOH: 97.7; difference, 3.91; 95% CI, 1.43-6.38; P=0.002) and at week 12, with higher scores with TA vs SA (TA: 102.1; SA: 98.4; difference, 3.64; 95%CI, 1.10-6.18; P=0.005) and TA vs SOH (TA: 102.1; SOH: 97.4; difference, 4.61; 95% CI, 1.99-7.23; P=0.001).

CONCLUSIONS AND RELEVANCE The findings of this trial suggest that TA was more effective in treating chronic radiation-induced xerostomia 1 or more years after the end of radiotherapy than SA or SOH.

2. Expert Comments

Comment 1

At the completion of radiotherapy for head and neck cancer, more than 50% of patients will experience insufficient saliva secretion (xerostomia), significantly impacting their quality of life. Although there is no reliable treatment for acute and chronic radiation-induced xerostomia, some randomized and observational studies have suggested that acupuncture may enhance salivary flow and improve patient prognosis. However, these studies are often limited by factors such as lack of blinding, lack of SA control, or small sample sizes, resulting in lack of high-quality evidence to support the efficacy of acupuncture in the treatment of xerostomia after radiotherapy in patients with head and neck cancer. The authors designed this multicenter, randomized, blinded, three-arm, placebo-controlled phase 3 trial to address these limitations.

In this study, patients with head and neck cancer who received radiotherapy were randomly divided into an TA group, SA group, and SOH group. Acupuncture was performed twice a week for 20 minutes for 4 weeks, and 14 acupoints were selected for the intervention. SA was performed with a non-penetrating, retractable needle device to stimulate areas adjacent to the real acupoints. All patients received standard oral care. The primary outcome measure was a patient-reported xerostomia questionnaire completed at week 4. In this randomized clinical trial of 258 patients with head and neck cancer, acupuncture treatment significantly improved xerostomia symptoms and overall quality of life compared with standard oral hygiene. Although there were indications of a placebo effect from the SA, the efficacy of SA treatment was negligible and not associated with improvement in overall quality of life. Although the mechanism involved in this study is unclear, it has been reported that it may be related to fascia-mediated central nervous system effects, vasodilation, and microcirculation improvement caused by increase in some neuropeptides after acupuncture stimulation.

Comment 2

(1) Study design and process implementation

This study provided a thorough report and interpretation of the six elements of PICOST (Population, Intervention, Comparison, Outcome, Study Design, and Time) in clinical research. The inclusion and exclusion of participants, definition and structure of the control group, explanation of the three-group intervention, definition of outcome indicators, detailed analysis of key links in the study design (eg, randomization, sample size, blinding), and trial cycle are all reflected in the article, enhancing the credibility of the study process and results.

The article provides a clear description of the implementation process, detailing that the trial began in July 2013, transferring its test base in April 2015, and concluding in June 2021. Both the main text and supplementary materials are comprehensively detailed. A randomized, blinded, three-arm, multicenter clinical trial over an 8-year period is rare. The sustainability, dropout, quality control and so on of the trial are facing challenges. The authors wisely present the patient flowchart from enrollment to completion of the trial in Figure 1. The detailed data provided in the flowchart help reduce uncertainties regarding the study's implementation.

The study closely adhered to the consolidated standards of reporting trials (CONSORT), and the entire process of design, implementation, analysis, and interpretation of the results is reported completely and accurately, adding credibility to the study findings.

(2) Selection and application of clinical research methodology and statistical methods

The paper meticulously details the key elements of intervention measures, participants, and trial effects, as well as the fundamentals of randomization, control, and repetition to be followed. In particular, the authors describe or elaborate on the key links that determine the success or failure of the study, such as the dynamic randomization using the adaptive minimization method, selection of the points of the SA group for blinding, measures taken to avoid failure of blinding, determination of the sample size and its basis, and even the needles used in the study, significantly enhancing the readers' confidence in the study's quality.

For the analysis of efficacy indices in this prospective study design with repeated measurements, involving quantitative data, a mixed-effect model without a structured covariance matrix was employed to assess the differences among the three primary indices. The chi-square test was utilized for qualitative variables such as clinical reactions and adverse events. Statistical analysis followed the intention-to-treat principle, and multiple imputations, based on monotonic regression, were used for missing efficacy measures owing to inevitable dropout. Sensitivity analysis of the main outcome was performed, and the results were found to be stable.

(3) Conclusion

This was a high-quality clinical trial study, which confirmed the clinical efficacy and safety of acupuncture in the treatment of radiation xerostomia. In addition to the limitations identified by the author, there remain some problems that should be noted and considered. ①Statistical significance and clinical significance: When calculating the sample size, the article explicitly mentioned that "the difference in XQ score (0-100 scale) between each group is 10 points, which is considered to be clinically significant," "but the modified mean of the XQ score in the main results (Table 2) of the article (after adjusting the baseline XQ score), including the true mean provided in eTable 1 and eTable 2 in the Supplementary Online Content, the mean difference in the XQ scores of the TA, SA, and SOH groups did not reach 10 points. For example, the revised mean of the XQ score on the 4th week was in the order of TA 50.59, SA 54.99, and SOH 57.26, according to the values presented in Appendix eTable 1. Is the difference of approximately 7 points clinically significant? To address this issue, we can start with age, race, occupation, and baseline XQ score and conduct subgroup analysis to explore the potential better beneficiaries of acupuncture treatment. Naturally, considering the comprehensive evaluation of safety and economy, acupuncture remains a good choice. ②Impact of dropout: The dropout rates for the three groups are detailed in the Results section of the article. The dropout rates were 2.4% in the TA group, 10.6% in the SA group, and 23.8% in the SOH group. Why was the dropout rate so high in the SOH group? Might it indirectly reflect better adherence or compliance in the TA group? It is also necessary to evaluate the impact of dropout on the extrapolation of the results from the characteristics of dropouts. For example, the dropout rate is notably high among disabled or incapacitated workers, African Americans, American Indians, or Alaska Natives, and it is high for Native Americans or Pacific Islanders.

Given that the study spanned 8 years and involved multiple centers. it is important to consider whether a central effect might have been present. Specifically, poor quality control at one or more centers could have potentially contributed to the higher dropout rates observed for part of the sample.

Section 4 Introduction and Comments of *Effect of Acupuncture vs Sham Acupuncture on Patients With Poststroke Motor Aphasia: A Randomized Clinical Trial*

1. Introduction

IMPORTANCE Motor aphasia is common among patients with stroke. Acupuncture is recommended as an alternative therapy for poststroke aphasia, but its efficacy remains uncertain.

OBJECTIVE To investigate the effects of acupuncture on language function, neurological function, and quality of life in patients with poststroke motor aphasia.

DESIGN, SETTING, AND PARTICIPANTS This multicenter, sham-controlled, randomized clinical trial was conducted in 3 tertiary hospitals in China from October 21, 2019, to November 13, 2021. Adult patients with poststroke motor aphasia were enrolled. Data analysis was performed from February to April 2023.

INTERVENTIONS Eligible participants were randomly allocated (1∶1) to manual acupuncture (MA) or sham acupuncture (SA) groups. Both groups underwent language training and conventional treatments.

MAIN OUTCOMES AND MEASURES The primary outcomes were the aphasia quotient (AQ) of the Western Aphasia Battery (WAB) and scores on the Chinese Functional Communication Profile (CFCP) at 6 weeks. Secondary outcomes included WAB subitems, Boston Diagnostic Aphasia Examination, National Institutes of Health Stroke Scale, Stroke-Specific Quality of Life Scale, Stroke and Aphasia Quality of Life Scale-39, and Health Scale of Traditional Chinese Medicine scores at 6 weeks and 6 months after onset. All statistical analyses were performed according to the intention-to-treat principle.

RESULTS Among 252 randomized patients (198 men [78.6%]; mean [SD] age, 60.7 [7.5] years), 231 were included in the modified intention-to-treat analysis (115 in the MA group and 116 in the SA group). Compared with the SA group, the MA group had significant increases in AQ (difference, 7.99 points; 95% CI, 3.42-12.55 points; $P=0.001$) and CFCP (difference, 23.51 points; 95% CI, 11.10-35.93 points; $P<0.001$) scores at week 6 and showed significant improvements in AQ (difference, 10.34; 95% CI, 5.75-14.93; $P<0.001$) and CFCP (difference, 27.43; 95% CI, 14.75-40.10; $P<0.001$) scores at the end of follow-up.

CONCLUSIONS AND RELEVANCE In this randomized clinical trial, patients with poststroke motor aphasia who received 6 weeks of MA compared with those who received SA demonstrated statistically significant improvements in language function, quality of life, and neurological impairment from week 6 of treatment to the end of follow-up at 6 months after onset.

2. Expert Comments

Comment 1

This study investigated the therapeutic effect of acupuncture on post-stroke motor aphasia using the WAB and CFCP scores at the end of the intervention (Week 6) as primary outcome measures, which is a standard approach. However, for patients with chronic diseases, sustained efficacy is crucial. In fact, the study's results are convincing not only because of the immediate effect observed at Week 6, but also because the significant improvement persisted to Month 6.

The primary outcomes are key to analyzing the effectiveness of interventions. Assuming that the results are only clinically significant only at Week 6, and that there is no significant difference between groups at a later stage, should we affirm the immediate effectiveness of acupuncture in the treatment of motor aphasia after stroke, or should we deny the clinical significance of the acupuncture intervention because of the lack of a long-term effect? Obviously, it is not reasonable to use Week 6 as the primary outcome.

Symptom improvement in chronic disease may fluctuate; hence, determining a more appropriate follow-up period for the primary outcome measure should involve balancing the benefits, risks, and treatment burden of acupuncture treatment. This can both avoid the total denial of the acupuncture effect because of the lack of "time persistence" in certain chronic diseases and avoid the hasty conclusion that acupuncture is effective because it is only effective in a certain period; the research conclusion will then be more rigorous. Designing clinical trials from the perspective of patients will lead to results that better reflect clinical practice and patient needs, thus better supporting the promotion of trial results, formulation of clinical guidelines, and clinical evidence-based decision-making. Listening to the voice of patients should be an important principle in future clinical research.

Comment 2

(1) Study design and process implementation

This was a multicenter, randomized, single-blind clinical trial. The paper accurately described the six elements of PICOST (Population, Intervention, Comparison, Outcome, Study Design, and Time) in the Materials and Methods section. Detailed information is provided for the inclusion and exclusion of participants, definition and division of control groups, analysis of the intervention programs, definition of outcome indicators, and response of key links in the study design (such as randomization, sample size, blinding), especially for the intervention methods. Details such as the determination of the acupuncture angle, depth, manipulation direction and frequency, and retention time are provided in the Appendix. The definition of effect indicators is also supplied in detail. In addition, the central randomization processor and single-blind implementation process are briefly, but accurately, described in the paper, which improves the credibility of the research process and results.

The article provides a concise yet clear description of the trial implementation process. Figure 1 illustrates the study flowchart from participant enrollment to the completion of the study.

The article is well conceived and adheres to the consolidated standards of reporting trials (CONSORT), and the entire process of design, implementation, analysis, and interpretation of the results is reported completely and accurately, which is very readable.

(2) Selection and application of clinical research methodology and statistical methods

As a randomized controlled trial, this paper provides a concise and accurate description of the three critical elements of intervention measures, participants, and trial effects, as well as adherence to the principles of randomization, control, and repetition. All key design elements are covered, including the completion of random enrollment by the central randomization processor, implementation of the single-blind method, and determination of the sample size and its basis. Importantly, the description of the interventions is very detailed, and a set of standardized operational guidelines increases the readers' and reviewers' confidence in the study's quality.

The efficacy outcomes for repeated measures comprised quantitative data, and the study used repeated measures analysis of variance (ANOVA) to compare the differences in the main indicators between groups. Considering the clinical design, the duration of aphasia may be a confounding factor affecting the efficacy evaluation. In this paper, subgroup analysis (stratification strategy) was used for evaluation, and in previous repeated measures ANOVA investigations, the duration of aphasia at baseline was included as a covariate in the ANOVA model to adjust for the confounding effect, making the conclusion more objective and credible. In addition, the statistical analysis adhered to intention-to-treat principle. For missing data because of dropouts, the study used the multiple imputation method under the assumption of missing at random to conduct a sensitivity analysis.

(3) Conclusion

This high-quality study was the first multicenter, sham acupuncture controlled, randomized clinical trial to evaluate the clinical efficacy of acupuncture in treating post-stroke motor aphasia. There remain several issues worth discussing regarding the statistical methodology. ①Multiplicity problem: Bonferroni correction was used to adjust the P-value for multiple comparisons across different time points. However, it is important to note that there were two primary efficacy measures in this study: The AQ from WAB and CFCP score at Week 6. Then, in hypothesis testing, whether for AQ or CFCP, the significance level should be adjusted to 0.025 rather than to 0.050 to avoid false positive results. ②Missing value imputation in intention-to-treat analysis: The multiple imputation method under the assumption of missing at random was used in this study, which has been increasingly used in clinical research in recent years. However, given the six time windows and scale characteristics of the measurement indicators, traditional imputation methods such as last observation carried forward, baseline observation carried forward, and worst observation carried forward remain viable alternatives. Including these methods in sensitivity analyses could help address potential issues and avoid false positive results.

Section 5　Introduction and Comments of *Effect of Acupuncture for Methadone Reduction: A Randomized Clinical Trial*

1. Introduction

BACKGROUND　Methadone maintenance treatment (MMT) is effective for managing opioid use disorder, but adverse effects mean that optimal therapy occurs with the lowest dose that controls opioid craving.

OBJECTIVE　To assess the efficacy of acupuncture versus sham acupuncture on methadone dose reduction.

DESIGN　Multicenter, 2-group, randomized, sham controlled trial.

SETTING　6 MMT clinics in China.

PARTICIPANTS　Adults aged 65 years or younger with opioid use disorder who attended clinic daily and had been using MMT for at least 6 weeks.

INTERVENTION　Acupuncture or sham acupuncture 3 times a week for 8 weeks.

MEASUREMENTS　The 2 primary outcomes were the proportion of participants who achieved a reduction in methadone dose of 20% or more compared with baseline and opioid craving, which was measured by the change from baseline on a 100-mm Visual Analogue Scale (VAS).

RESULTS　Of 118 eligible participants, 60 were randomly assigned to acupuncture and 58 were randomly assigned to sham acupuncture (2 did not receive acupuncture). At week 8, more patients reduced their methadone dose 20% or more with acupuncture than with sham acupuncture (37 [62%] vs. 16 [29%]; risk difference, 32% [97.5% CI, 13% to 52%]; $P<0.001$). In addition, acupuncture was more effective in decreasing opioid craving than sham acupuncture with a mean difference of −11.7 mm VAS (CI, −18.7 to −4.8 mm; $P<0.001$). No serious adverse events occurred. There were no notable differences between study groups when participants were asked which type of acupuncture they received.

LIMITATION　Fixed acupuncture protocol limited personalization and only 12 weeks of follow-up after stopping acupuncture.

CONCLUSION　Eight weeks of acupuncture were superior to sham acupuncture in reducing methadone dose and decreasing opioid craving.

2. Expert Comments

Comment 1

Opioid addiction is a serious public health concern worldwide, characterized by high mortality rates, a propensity to accelerate the spread of infectious diseases, and the instigation of various criminal activities, thereby undermining social stability and leading to substantial economic burdens. Although MMT can temporarily improve the symptoms of opioid addiction, its side effects are multitudinous. Obviously, non-drug therapy is of great significance to reduce methadone dependence and opioid

Chapter 2   Comments of Clinical Trials of Acupuncture and Moxibustion in SCI Journals

addiction.

Professor XU Nenggui's team from Guangzhou University of traditional Chinese medicine employed acupuncture treatment and conducted a multicenter randomized controlled trial to compare the effects of acupuncture with sham acupuncture (8 weeks, 3 times/week, and follow up for 12 weeks after treatment) on 118 patients receiving MMT, using the distinctive "Jin's Three Needles" technique, pioneered by renowned acupuncturist JIN Rui, targeting specific points such as the "Si Shen Zhen" "Ding Shen Zhen" and "Hand Zhi Zhen". The results showed that acupuncture had superior efficacy over sham acupuncture in reducing the methadone dosage and opioid cravings and contributed to improvement in sleep quality. "Jin's Three Needles" focuses on "regulating the spirit and treating the spirit" and has an exact curative effect on mental diseases. This study used "Jin's Three Needles" for the acupuncture intervention with clear theoretical foundations and well-defined principles. In addition, an independent researcher was appointed to supervise the interactions between participants and physicians, ensuring no discussion occurred regarding the treatment allocation in the study, which benefited the data management and quality control efficiency. Owing to the particularity of acupuncture, sham acupuncture is usually difficult to implement. The team used a self-created non-penetrating device to successfully blind 118 participants, augmenting the quality of this clinical trial.

Comment 2

(1) Research design and process implementation

This was a standard randomized controlled trial. The randomization and blinding were rigorous. Various methods were implemented to maintain blinding. For example, the outcome evaluators, physicians, and nurses in the clinic, as well as the data collectors and statisticians, were not aware of the grouping. During the trial, physicians recorded the methadone dosage every day for 8 weeks, ensuring data accuracy. In addition, in the case of a fixed treatment plan, the qualification requirements and unified training of acupuncturists are important to ensuring high-quality research and is worth advocating. ①Considerations regarding the description of the sample size: The sample size estimation required 84 patients in both groups. Because of the pandemic, it was expected that the dropout rate would increase from the initial estimate of 15% to 30%, which was understandable during the outbreak. Therefore, the actual subject recruitment was raised to 120, and 116 patients were enrolled. In total, 105 patients completed the 8-week treatment course and 20-week follow up, and the dropout rate was 12.5%. This case shows that the sample size estimation is a range, and minor adjustments may not affect the actual study results. ②Regarding the accuracy measurement and quality control of the main outcome measures: A primary outcome of the trial was the proportion of patients who achieved a 20% or greater reduction in methadone dosage compared to baseline after 8 weeks of intervention, which is a crucial measure. All enrolled patients were required to attend the clinic daily and ingest methadone administered by the clinic physician once daily. Independent observers obtained the daily methadone consumption data from the physicians to record the methadone doses. The results showed that the proportion of patients with a 20% or greater reduction in methadone dose in the acupuncture group was 62%, much higher than the 29% in the control group.

(2) Selection and application of the clinical research methodology and statistical methods

The statistical analyses and presentation of charts in this study were both rigorous and advanced, serving as an exemplary case for presenting and reporting longitudinal study and continuous measurement results. The detailed description of the statistical methods provided a valuable learning reference for peers.

Regarding the further analysis in the Discussion, it was mentioned that a 5% reduction in the methadone dosage every two weeks was considered effective according to the criteria and clinical guidelines of MMT in the United States and Canada. However, the dosage and rate of methadone reduction every two weeks in the acupuncture group were not provided in the results and discussion, which is a limitation of the study.

3. Author's Talk

Since China began to crack down on drug abuse and trafficking, and strictly managing opioids, there have been very few new opioid addicts; however, community methadone clinics are still providing methadone substitution therapy for voluntary drug addicts, which shows that opioid dependence has not been solved completely. Our original intention was to achieve withdrawal of opioids through acupuncture, enabling MMT patients to completely overcome drug dependence and reintegrate into society.

In the process of the trial, the choice of intervention in the control group was the focus of repeated discussion in the team. The particularity of acupuncture determines that only the patients can be blinded. In previous clinical studies of acupuncture, the control group could choose "non-meridian and non-acupoint" or "shallow acupoint needling" as the intervention, while the participants in this trial were long-time methadone users, characterized by suspicion and lack of security. Therefore, we developed an auxiliary device with the same appearance, which was used in the acupuncture group and the sham acupuncture group based on differences in the design (bottom opening). This was both to ensure blinding and to avoid patient resistance, helping patients fully trust the researchers and cooperate with the treatment. This blinding could minimize the interference of various confounding factors, such as mental stress caused by psychological effects.

In addition, owing to the unique nature of addiction diseases and varying degrees of opioid regulation across countries and regions, our findings may have varying implications for public health in various regional journals and could even influence health policies. This impact is uncommon in the existing literature.

XU Nenggui
Guangzhou University of Traditional Chinese Medicine

Section 6   Introduction and Comments of *Effect of Acupuncture on Neurogenic Claudication Among Patients With Degenerative Lumbar Spinal Stenosis: A Randomized Clinical Trial*

1. Introduction

BACKGROUND   Acupuncture may improve degenerative lumbar spinal stenosis (DLSS), but evidence is insufficient.

OBJECTIVE   To investigate the effect of acupuncture for DLSS.

DESIGN   Multicenter randomized clinical trial.

SETTING   5 hospitals in China.

PARTICIPANTS   Patients with DLSS and predominantly neurogenic claudication pain symptoms.

INTERVENTION   18 sessions of acupuncture or sham acupuncture (SA) over 6 weeks, with 24-week followup after treatment.

MEASUREMENTS   The primary outcome was change from baseline in the modified Roland-Morris Disability Questionnaire ([RMDQ] score range, 0 to 24; minimal clinically important difference [MCID], 2 to 3). Secondary outcomes were the proportion of participants achieving minimal (30% reduction from baseline) and substantial (50% reduction from baseline) clinically meaningful improvement per the modified RMDQ.

RESULTS   A total of 196 participants (98 in each group) were enrolled. The mean modified RMDQ score was 12.6 (95% CI, 11.8 to 13.4) in the acupuncture group and 12.7 (CI, 12.0 to 13.3) in the SA group at baseline, and decreased to 8.1 (CI, 7.1 to 9.1) and 9.5 (CI, 8.6 to 10.4) at 6 weeks, with an adjusted difference in mean change of −1.3 (CI, −2.6 to −0.03; P=0.044), indicating a 43.3% greater improvement compared with SA. The between group difference in the proportion of participants achieving minimal and substantial clinically meaningful improvement was 16.0% (CI, 1.6% to 30.4%) and 12.6% (CI, −1.0% to 26.2%) at 6 weeks. Three cases of treatment-related adverse events were reported in the acupuncture group, and 3 were reported in the SA group. All events were mild and transient.

LIMITATION   The SA could produce physiologic effects.

CONCLUSION   Acupuncture may relieve pain-specific disability among patients with DLSS and predominantly neurogenic claudication pain symptoms, although the difference with SA did not reach MCID. The effects may last 24 weeks after 6-week treatment.

2. Expert Comments

Comment 1

As mentioned in the Background, although the guidelines recommend non-pharmacological treatment for patients with DLSS, there is a lack of high-quality evidence-based data. Therefore, this study focused on intermittent claudication in patients with DLSS, with the main outcome being subjective perception. Although from the perspective of superiority testing, the improvement conferred by acupuncture did not reach the minimum clinically important difference and did not attain clinical significance, based on the primary and secondary outcomes, along with follow-up records, it is evident that acupuncture could alleviate pain-related disability in patients with DLSS experiencing neurogenic claudication. This study offers profound insights and valuable guidance for acupuncture research in this field, making it a significant reference for researchers conducting clinical trials in acupuncture.

In this study, a rigorous standardized acupuncture protocol was implemented, with precise records of the angle, depth, and techniques employed in the acupuncture group. Shallow needling at the same acupoint was used in the sham acupuncture group, which inevitably led to a placebo effect stemming from the acupoint. Especially in studies focusing on pain, owing to the different pain thresholds of patients, the placebo effect of sham acupuncture may be greater than that observed when acupuncture is applied for the treatment of other diseases. As mentioned in the Discussion, the authors recommend adopting non-penetrating sham acupuncture in later studies to reduce the impact of the placebo effect. Therefore, the choice of intervention in the control group is particularly important across studies. Considering the disease and acupoints, choosing different interventions in the control group can have a crucial impact on the outcomes.

Comment 2

(1) Study design and process

The study employed a multicenter, randomized, controlled design, characterized by the following features. The study used a sham acupuncture device and dynamic randomized block randomization, which better reduced the predictability of the randomization and achieved random concealment. The detailed description of the intervention, especially in the acupuncture group, included the location, depth, and angle of each acupoint. Shallow needling at the same acupoint was used in the sham acupuncture group, providing the participants with relatively mild stimulation in contrast to the depth and stimulation strength used for the acupuncture group, thereby facilitating participant blinding. However, a piercing sham needle generally has a greater effect (a greater physiological effect in addition to the placebo effect) than a non-piercing sham needle, thereby narrowing the difference with the acupuncture group. The results also confirmed this point, and the authors discussed this issue accordingly (see the Discussion section).

(2) Selection and application of clinical research methodology and statistical methods

Overall, the statistical methods were relatively standardized. ①Sample size estimation: The sample size estimation adjusted the test level α based on two comparisons determined in advance and considered the proportion of non-compliance, dropout rate, and proportion of possible contamination, but there was no information on the numbers of cases based on the above considerations. ②Statistical analysis: The statistical analysis was mainly based on the multi-factor analysis method, fully considering the possible factors in the study and comprehensively reporting the analysis details, specific covariates, and relevant parameters in the model. Imputation of missing data is a key aspect in statistical analysis. The study used a mixed effects model to analyze missing data, which could handle them without need for filling in missing data. Meanwhile, to assess the robustness of the results, the study used multiple imputations for the sensitivity analysis, a methodological approach of considerable value.

3. Author's Talk

DLSS is prevalent among the elderly, and intermittent claudication is the main cause of disability. Drug therapy offers limited efficacy and lacks robust evidence. Complications and failed back surgery syndrome occur in 10% to 40% of patients undergoing surgery. Current guidelines recommend non-pharmacological interventions, such as individualized training and comprehensive manipulation, as first-line treatments, but their efficacy is limited. Acupuncture is effective in the treatment of lower back pain and recommended by guidelines; however, insufficient evidence of its efficacy in the treatment of neuroischemic pain and intermittent claudication caused by DLSS exists. Preliminary trials and the extensive clinical experience of researchers showed that deep needling of Dachangshu had better curative effects. Based on this, we hypothesized that acupuncture can effectively relieve painful intermittent claudication in patients with DLSS. We thus designed a multicenter randomized trial using a sham acupuncture control to evaluate the efficacy of acupuncture, with the main indicators being the change from baseline in modified RMDQ scores and the difference from sham acupuncture based on the MCID. A six-month follow-up will be conducted post-treatment to evaluate the clinical value and advantages of acupuncture therapy.

The main challenges experienced during implementation of the clinical trial were ensuring compliance with the acupuncture protocol and maintaining data reliability. Each subcenter conducted 2-3 on-site inspections, with all patient data having undergone traceability and verification checks.

The main challenge lies in interpreting the results. Although data of the primary group reached statistical significance, they did not achieve the MCID. Therefore, we cautiously conclude that acupuncture can alleviate intermittent neurogenic claudication. While the between-group differences did not reach the MCID, improvements within each group from baseline exceeded it. To ensure effective blinding, the sham acupuncture group received micro-acupuncture at acupoints, which exhibited a substantial nonspecific effect while also showing a certain degree of a specific effect, thereby diminishing the specific effect value of true acupuncture. Secondary outcomes, such as hip and leg pain scores, symptoms of lumbar spinal stenosis, and physical function scores, all indicate that acupuncture was more effective than sham acupuncture. No specific treatment is available for intermittent claudication due to lumbar spinal stenosis.

LIU Zhishun
Guang'anmen Hospital, China Academy of Chinese Medicine Sciences

Section 7　Introduction and Comments of *Effect of Acupuncture for Temporomandibular Disorders: A Randomized Clinical Trial*

1. Introduction

BACKGROUND Temporomandibular disorders (TMD) are the leading cause of pain and disability among frequently occurring facial pain and the second leading cause of musculoskeletal conditions.

AIM We examined whether acupuncture could alleviate pain intensity in patients with TMD.

DESIGN AND METHODS Sixty participants with TMD were randomly assigned (ratio 1 : 1) to receive three acupuncture or sham acupuncture sessions weekly for 4 weeks. The primary outcome was the change in the mean weekly pain intensity from baseline to week 4. Secondary and exploratory outcomes included proportion of participants with ⩾30% or ⩾50% reduction in pain intensity, change in jaw opening and movement, Graded Chronic Pain Scale (GCPS), Jaw Functional Limitations Scale-20-Item (JFLS-20), Depression Anxiety and Stress Scales-21 (DASS-21), Pittsburgh Sleep Quality Index (PSQI) at week 4 and 8, and the pressure pain threshold and surface electromyography at week 4.

RESULTS AND CONCLUSION The acupuncture group showed significantly reduced pain intensity compared to the sham group at week 4 (−1.49, 95% confidence interval [CI]: −2.32 to −0.65; $P<0.001$) and week 8 (−1.23, 95% CI: −2.11 to −0.54; $P=0.001$). Acupuncture's effectiveness surpassed sham's at 4 weeks and lasted 8 weeks. Participants in the acupuncture group experienced significantly greater improvements in the 30% and 50% response rate, jaw opening and movement, GCPS, JFLS-20, DASS-21 and PSQI than those in the sham acupuncture group. There were no significant between-group differences in pressure pain threshold (PPT) and surface electromyography (sEMG). In summary, acupuncture provided marked pain relief and improvement in physical and emotional function for patients with TMD compared with sham acupuncture.

2. Expert Comments

Comment 1

TMD is a common and difficult disease to treat. This important randomized controlled trial explored the effect of acupuncture on relieving pain and improving joint function in TMD.

The study focused on the difficult and prominent issues in the treatment of TMD and highlighted critical clinical questions, ie, how to relieve pain and improve the joint function of patients with TMD through non-drug treatment. Presently, although there are many treatments for TMD, their efficacy and safety remain controversial, and there is lack of high-quality randomized controlled trials.

Sixty patients with TMD were randomly divided into an acupuncture group and a sham acupuncture group, with 30 patients in each group. The treatment was administered three times a week for 4 weeks. The selected acupoints included the LI4 (Hegu), GB34 (Yanglingquan) on the bilateral sides and SI19 (Tinggong), ST6 (Jiache) and ST7 (Xiaguan) on the affected side. The selection of the acupoints and manipulation were based on classical literature and contemporary research, ensuring a rational and scientific treatment. During the operation, attention was paid to obtain qi. Non-invasive acupuncture was applied to the sham acupuncture group, and the operation was simulated by a special sham acupuncture device to ensure participant blinding.

The results showed that pain intensity in the acupuncture group was significantly lower than that in the sham acupuncture group at the 4th and 8th weeks, and there were significant improvements in mandibular opening and movement, the functional limitation scale score, and emotional function. The response rate and patient satisfaction were also significantly higher in the acupuncture group than in the sham acupuncture group, and no difference in safety was found between the groups. The paper emphasized the value of acupuncture as an effective non-drug treatment for TMD.

Comment 2

(1) Study design and process

The study protocol was prospectively registered on an international platform, increasing the transparency of the program. The inclusion criteria required that TMD pain persist for at least 3 months, reducing the impact of self-healing on the outcome. Patients who had received other treatments in the month prior to screening were excluded to avoid the influence of delayed effects. The reliability of randomization, allocation concealment, and blinding could be boosted by using a network-based interactive system for compartmentalized random grouping. Blinding the patients based on the Park needle device could effectively reduce the rate of breaking blindness during the operation, thereby guaranteeing the compliance of the patients in the control group and eliminating the influence of the placebo effect. The primary outcome was the Visual Analogue Scale score, which effectively measured the pain intensity of TMD, but the minimally clinically important difference of the scale was not reported, which makes the analysis results lack an important reference.

(2) Selection and application of clinical research methodology and statistical methods

The common standard deviation between groups was not defined in the calculation of the sample size, which made it impossible to repeat it. The statistical analysis was based on the intention-to-treat principle, under which the results were relatively conservative; that is, more stringent criteria were used to verify the efficacy of acupuncture. Sensitivity analysis using the per protocol set can test the stability of the main results; however, the definition of the per protocol set was not clear in the paper, and "significant protocol deviation" should be clarified. For the missing values, the multiple interpolation method was used for multiple interpolations, and the average value of the results from each interpolated dataset was considered as the final result, which can reduce the influence of accidental factors on the results in the interpolation. The influence of multiplicity on the conclusion was avoided by setting the measurement obtained at one time point as the main outcome.

Section 8 Introduction and Comments of *Self-Administered Acupressure for Probable Knee Osteoarthritis in Middle-Aged and Older Adults: A Randomized Clinical Trial*

1. Introduction

IMPORTANCE The effects of self-administered acupressure (SAA) on knee osteoarthritis (OA) pain remain unclear.

OBJECTIVE To evaluate the effectiveness of SAA taught via a short training course on reducing knee OA pain in middle-aged and older adults.

DESIGN, SETTING, AND PARTICIPANTS This randomized clinical trial was conducted among community-dwelling individuals in Hong Kong who were aged 50 years or older with probable knee OA from September 2019 to May 2022.

INTERVENTIONS The intervention included 2 training sessions for SAA with a brief knee health education (KHE) session, in which participants practiced acupressure twice daily for 12 weeks. The control group (KHE only) received only education about maintaining knee health on the same schedule and duration.

MAIN OUTCOMES AND MEASURES The primary outcome was the numerical rating scale (NRS) pain score at 12 weeks. Other outcomes included Western Ontario and McMaster University Osteoarthritis Index, Short Form 6 Dimensions (SF-6D), Timed Up and Go, and Fast Gait Speed tests.

RESULTS A total of 314 participants (mean [SD] age, 62.7 [4.5] years; 246 [78.3%] female; mean [SD] knee pain duration, 7.3 [7.6] years) were randomized into intervention and KHE-only groups (each 157). At week 12, compared with the KHE-only group, the intervention group had a significantly greater reduction in NRS pain score (mean difference [MD], −0.54 points; 95% CI, −0.97 to −0.10 points; P=0.02) and higher enhancement in SF-6D utility score (MD, 0.03 points; 95% CI, 0.003 to 0.01 points; P=0.03) but did not have significant differences in other outcome measures. The costeffectiveness acceptability curve demonstrated a greater than 90% probability that the intervention is cost-effective at a willingness to pay threshold of 1 GDP per capita.

CONCLUSIONS AND RELEVANCE In this randomized clinical trial, SAA with a brief KHE program was efficacious and cost-effective in relieving knee pain and improving mobility in middle-aged and older adults with probable knee OA.

2. Expert Comments

Comment 1

(1) Topic selection

How to focus on solving the difficult and prominent issues in clinical practice, analyze the refinement and construction of key clinical issues, and reflect their value and significance.

This study addressed the prevalent and challenging issue of knee OA, particularly affecting individuals over the age of 50 years. In this paper, SAA was proposed as a potential solution, which can avoid the side effects of drugs and enhance the compliance of patients. The study aligned well with actual clinical needs and filled gaps in the existing literature, especially regarding the rigor of the research design, accuracy of acupoint selection, universality of clinical practice, and scientificity of evaluation. The short-term and mid-term effects of SAA were systematically assessed through the formulation of key clinical questions, while a comprehensive health economics analysis was conducted to evaluate the feasibility and cost-effectiveness of this treatment from multiple perspectives. These results not only offer new evidence for the clinical management of knee OA but also establish a robust foundation for future relevant research, demonstrating vital clinical value.

(2) Acupuncture intervention

The implementation of acupuncture was analyzed, such as the rationality of acupuncture treatment, details of acupuncture, treatment plan, auxiliary measures, background of the therapist, and setting of the control group.

The design of intervention in this study was reasonable, fully considering the clinical characteristics of middle-aged and older patients with knee OA, such as the long disease course and recovery difficulty. The therapeutic schedule of the treatment group was full of multi levels, including multi-level operations such as warming up, acupoint pressing, kneading the knee, and moving the knee. The selection of acupoints was based on the meridian theory of traditional Chinese medicine, involving the stomach, spleen, and gallbladder meridians, which are closely related to the function of the knee joint. The precise manipulation of each acupoint was meticulously designed, integrating various finger and thenar strengths and techniques. The study sufficiently reflected the principles of traditional Chinese medicine treatment and strictly controlled the method and time of operation. The study also imposed stringent criteria on the qualifications and professional training of the personnel overseeing patient treatment, ensuring the intervention's suitability and precision. The treatment group was treated with SAA combined with KHE, while the control group was only treated with KHE, which ensured the scientific and comparative validity of the study and enabled the researcher to evaluate the independent effect of SAA in the treatment of knee OA. Designing the study to compare SAA combined with KHE vs sham-SAA combined with KHE could further eliminate the placebo effect and offer a more precise evaluation of the specific therapeutic efficacy of SAA.

Comment 2

(1) Research design and protocol implementation

The study provides a complete protocol in the accompanied attachment, which increases its transparency. By recruiting a larger sample size, the study population's representativeness was improved. Participants were required to have a history of knee pain for at least three months and an NRS score of 3 or above, which effectively avoided the overestimation of efficacy due to self-healing factors and increased the sensitivity of outcome measures. Exclusion of subjects with prior treatment histories minimized the potential impact that other interventions had on the efficacy assessment. The study employed a random sequence of 4- or 6-length mixed blocks with sealed opaque envelopes for allocation concealment. As blinding was not feasible for participants and intervention providers, the mixed block randomization helped prevent group assignment predictions for the last participant in each block. Blinding the assessors reduced the measurement bias caused by subjective factors.

(2) Selection and application of clinical research methodology and statistical methods

The primary analysis adhered to the intention-to-treat principle, providing more conservative estimates of treatment effects and enhancing the rigor of the evaluation. Linear mixed models were used to compare between-group effects, reducing the impact that confounders had on the results. However, the study did not specify the adjusted-fixed or random-effect covariates, which limited transparency of the statistical analysis. A high rate of loss to follow-up was reported; however, the handling of missing data was not clearly described, where statistical efficacy of the missing data may have impacted the results. Additionally, the lack of multiplicity correction for multiple measurements of the primary outcome suggests that the statistical inferences might have been influenced by multiplicity. No sensitivity analysis based on the per-protocol set was conducted for the efficacy analysis, resulting in a lack of further validation of the robustness of the primary analysis results. Nonetheless, 5 000 bootstrap samples were used in the cost-benefit analysis, which improved the robustness of those results.

Section 9 Introduction and Comments of *Efficacy of Acupuncture for Chronic Spontaneous Urticaria: A Randomized Controlled Trial*

1. Introduction

BACKGROUND The effectiveness of acupuncture for patients with chronic spontaneous urticaria (CSU), reported in a few smallscale studies, is not convincing.

OBJECTIVE To investigate whether acupuncture leads to better effects on CSU than sham acupuncture or waitlist control.

DESIGN A multicenter, randomized, sham-controlled trial.

SETTING Three teaching hospitals in China from 27 May 2019 to 30 July 2022.

PARTICIPANTS 330 participants diagnosed with CSU.

INTERVENTION Participants were randomly assigned in a 1∶1∶1 ratio to receive acupuncture, sham acupuncture, or waitlist control over an 8-week study period (4 weeks for treatment and another 4 weeks for follow-up).

MEASUREMENTS The primary outcome was the mean change from baseline in the Weekly Urticaria Activity Score (UAS7) at week 4. Secondary outcomes included itch severity scores, self-rated improvement, and Dermatology Life Quality Index scores.

RESULTS The mean change in UAS7 (range, 0 to 42) for acupuncture from baseline (mean score, 23.5 [95% CI, 21.8 to 25.2]) to week 4 (mean score, 15.3 [CI, 13.6 to 16.9]) was −8.2 (CI, −9.9 to −6.6). The mean changes in UAS7 for sham acupuncture and waitlist control from baseline (mean scores, 21.9 [CI, 20.2 to 23.6] and 22.1 [CI, 20.4 to 23.8], respectively) to week 4 (mean scores, 17.8 [CI, 16.1 to 19.5] and 20.0 [CI, 18.3 to 21.6], respectively) were −4.1 (CI, −5.8 to −2.4) and −2.2 (CI, −3.8 to −0.5), respectively. The mean differences between acupuncture and sham acupuncture and waitlist control were −4.1 (CI, −6.5 to −1.8) and −6.1 (CI, −8.4 to −3.7), respectively, which did not meet the threshold for minimal clinically important difference. Fifteen participants (13.6%) in the acupuncture group and none in the other groups reported adverse events. Adverse events were mild or transient.

LIMITATION Lack of complete blinding, self-reported outcomes, limited generalizability because antihistamine use was disallowed, and short follow-up period.

CONCLUSION Compared with sham acupuncture and waitlist control, acupuncture produced a greater improvement in UAS7, although the difference from control was not clinically significant. Increased adverse events were mild or transient.

2. Expert Comments

Comment 1

(1) Analysis of topics

Chronic urticaria is an allergic disease commonly encountered in the clinic, and acupuncture is effective in treating it, but there is lack of high-quality clinical research evidence. This study examined CSU and confirmed that acupuncture was beneficial for the treatment of this disease using a randomized controlled trial design encompassing three centers, which helped expand the scope of the clinical application of acupuncture. The topic bears important academic value and clinical significance.

(2) Implementation of acupuncture intervention

The study was closely associated with an acupuncture clinic, and the study protocol was registered in the China Clinical Trial Registration Center (ChiCTR1900022994). The participants were divided into an acupuncture group, a sham acupuncture group, and a waiting treatment group; a non-acupoint and non-puncturing approach was adopted for the sham acupuncture group; the selected acupoints LI11 (Quchi), SP10 (Xuehai), ST36 (Zusanli), ST25 (Tianshu), SP6 (Sanyinjiao), HT7 (Shenmen), and CV12 (Zhongwan) are considered strong candidates for treating this disease; in terms of the frequency and course of treatment, antihistamines are generally used regularly for 3 to 6 months, and drug control of the disease takes approximately 2 to 4 weeks. In clinical practice, acupuncture treatment generally requires a longer course of treatment to improve symptoms and control the disease. Although the 4-week course of treatment in this study was short, it significantly improved the feasibility of the study. In addition, 16 sessions of high-frequency treatment in 4 weeks may also make up for the shortage of short course of treatment. In view of the characteristics of CSU, the UAS7 scale recommended by the joint initiative of Dermatological Societies was used as the main efficacy index to evaluate the efficacy of acupuncture CSU treatment. For auxiliary interventions, only the prescribed dose of antihistamines was allowed to be taken in emergency situations. Acupuncture and sham acupuncture were performed by acupuncturists who had received training and had passed the examination. The research process was standardized and the results were highly credible.

Comment 2

(1) Study design and implementation

This multicenter, randomized, sham-controlled trial of acupuncture for the treatment of CSU demonstrated strict clinical research standards and meticulous process control.

First, the study selected tertiary hospitals in three cities as research centers, which ensured the diversity of patient samples and generalizability of the results, enhanced the external validity of the results, and made them more widely applicable to different regions and populations.

Secondly, the study used a 1 : 1 : 1 random allocation method to ensure balance across the acupuncture group, sham acupuncture group, and waiting treatment group. The online response system used in the study generated random sequences and allocated groups through mobile phone text messages, which effectively prevented human intervention and bias in the randomization process and demonstrated the rigor of the research team in the process of randomization and allocation of concealment.

The implementation of blinding in this study is also quite rigorous. Patients, outcome assessors and statisticians were all unaware of the allocation situation, and the research team conducted a blind credibility assessment at the end of the intervention to ensure the effectiveness of the blind method.

(2) Selection and application of clinical research methodology and statistical methods

In this study, various suitable statistical methods were used, providing strong support for the reliability and scientificity of the results.

Linear regression models were used for the primary outcome measure and some of the secondary outcome measures, providing a clear quantitative assessment of the primary outcome. In addition, the research team performed *Bonferroni* adjustments in the analysis to reduce the risk of type I errors from multiple comparisons. Simultaneously, the study set the minimum clinically important difference for UAS7 at 10, allowing a clear assessment of the difference in clinical effect between treatment groups, not just statistical significance.

The chain equation multiple imputation method was used to handle missing data, which is effective and can minimize the associated bias.

Importantly, the study also performed two subgroup analyses to explore treatment effects in different patient populations. This stratified analysis provided a more detailed assessment of the effect for different patient subgroups, facilitating the development of individualized treatment plans.

In summary, the study showed a very rigorous attitude in the application of clinical research methods and selection of statistical methods. Reasonable research design and rigorous statistical methods ensure the value of the results and their clinical application. However, although the study considered and adjusted for multiple potential sources of bias, future studies could further validate the reliability and long-term effects of the results by increasing the sample size and extending the duration of the acupuncture intervention.

Section 10 Introduction and Comments of *Acupuncture and Doxylamine-Pyridoxine for Nausea and Vomiting in Pregnancy: A Randomized, Controlled, 2×2 Factorial Trial*

1. Introduction

BACKGROUND An effective and safe treatment for nausea and vomiting of pregnancy (NVP) is lacking.

OBJECTIVE To assess the efficacy and safety of acupuncture, doxylamine-pyridoxine, and a combination of both in women with moderate to severe NVP.

DESIGN Multicenter, randomized, double-blind, placebocontrolled, 2×2 factorial trial.

SETTING 13 tertiary hospitals in mainland China from 21 June 2020 to 2 February 2022.

PARTICIPANTS 352 women in early pregnancy with moderate to severe NVP.

INTERVENTION Participants received daily active or sham acupuncture for 30 minutes and doxylamine-pyridoxine or placebo for 14 days.

MEASUREMENTS The primary outcome was the reduction in Pregnancy-Unique Quantification of Emesis (PUQE) score at the end of the intervention at day 15 relative to baseline. Secondary outcomes included quality of life, adverse events, and maternal and perinatal complications.

RESULTS No significant interaction was detected between the interventions (*P*=0.69). Participants receiving acupuncture (mean difference [MD], −0.7 [95% CI, −1.3 to −0.1]), doxylamine-pyridoxine (MD, −1.0 [CI, −1.6 to −0.4]), and the combination of both (MD, −1.6 [CI, −2.2 to −0.9]) had a larger reduction in PUQE score over the treatment course than their respective control groups (sham acupuncture, placebo, and sham acupuncture plus placebo). Compared with placebo, a higher risk for births with children who were small for gestational age was observed with doxylamine-pyridoxine (odds ratio, 3.8 [CI, 1.0 to 14.1]).

LIMITATION The placebo effects of the interventions and natural regression of the disease were not evaluated.

CONCLUSION Both acupuncture and doxylamine-pyridoxine alone are efficacious for moderate and severe NVP. However, the clinical importance of this effect is uncertain because of its modest magnitude. The combination of acupuncture and doxylamine-pyridoxine may yield a potentially larger benefit than each treatment alone.

2. Expert Comments

Comment 1

Moderate and severe NVP not only affects the quality of life of pregnant women, but pregnant women may terminate their pregnancies due to the intolerable conditions. Acupuncture is widely used in the treatment of NVP in China, but the existing treatments for moderate-to-severe NVP are insufficient, as there is lack of evidence for the treatment's effectiveness and of individual treatment needs. This study provided high-quality clinical evidence on the efficacy and safety of acupuncture in the treatment of moderate-to-severe NVP, which may provide individualized treatment options for NVP.

This was a multicenter, randomized, 2×2 factorial design, large-sample clinical study of acupuncture in 13 tertiary hospitals nationwide, aiming to investigate the efficacy and safety of acupuncture combined with the extended-release antihistamine doxylamine-pyridoxine in the treatment of moderate-to-severe NVP. After a 2-week intervention, patients in each group were treated with acupuncture+antiemetic, sham acupuncture+antiemetic, acupuncture+placebo, and sham acupuncture+placebo, respectively. ST36 (Zusanli) and PC6 (Neiguan) were selected as the classic points for regulating the stomach and stopping vomiting, combined with individualized reasonable acupoint matching for patients with stomach deficiency, liver heat, phlegm-dampness, and other syndromes. Placebo or sham acupuncture was selected as a reasonable control, the design of the trial was scientifically sound and rigorous, and finally 284 patients completed the intervention. The results of the intervention showed that the reduction in the severity score of pregnancy vomiting was greater than that of their respective control groups, regardless of whether the treatment included acupuncture alone, antiemetic drugs, or a combination of the two, and that the combined treatment was better and could reduce the dosage of antiemetic drugs. The study demonstrated a high degree of professionalism and innovation in the selection of the topic, refinement of the clinical problem, design of the treatment plan, and implementation of the acupuncture intervention, and generated high-level evidence-based medical data, providing new insights and methods for the future development of comprehensive treatment and guidelines for vomiting during pregnancy.

Comment 2

(1) Study design and process implementation

This was a multicenter, double-blind, placebo-controlled trial designed to analyze the efficacy and safety of acupuncture in patients with moderate-to-severe nausea and vomiting during pregnancy. It is worth recognizing that the study was well structured and executed, with high quality in terms of research design and process implementation.

First, the study had a multicenter design, covering 13 hospitals nationwide. This large multicenter design increased the generalizability of the results, reduced the bias of individual hospitals, and enhanced the representation of the target population, which helped improve the external validity of the study conclusions.

Second, the study used a double-blind design, which can effectively reduce the influence of observer bias and expectation effect and ensure the objectivity and accuracy of the test results. In addition, randomization was performed via computer generation and the PLAN program of the SAS system, and the pre-printing and distribution of the randomization scheme further ensured the effectiveness of the blinding method.

In addition, the study used strict inclusion and exclusion criteria, such as age, gestational age, and weight loss, which ensured the homogeneity of the participants and reduced potential confounders. This helped improve the internal validity of the findings, that is, the causal relationship between the findings and the intervention. The standardized assessment of the severity of NVP using the PUQE score made the comparison of outcomes more objective and consistent.

(2) Selection and application of clinical research methodology and statistical methods

The study adopted the principle of intention-to-treat

analysis, effectively reducing the bias caused by trial withdrawal or violation of the trial protocol. The use of chain multiple imputations to handle missing data also reduced the bias caused by missing data to some extent.

The study effectively dealt with interactions between multiple interventions using a factor analysis of variance approach, providing a detailed analysis of the independent effects of different treatment combinations. In addition, a repeated measures linear mixed model was used to evaluate the treatment effect in time series data, making full use of the advantages of longitudinal data and improving statistical efficiency.

For the treatment of binary variables, the study applied a modified Poisson regression model, which can effectively handle the abnormal variance of binomial distribution data and provide accurate estimates.

To sum up, this study was characterized by a high degree of scientificity and rigor in terms of the research design, methodology selection, statistical analysis, and execution. However, future studies can further enhance the sample size calculation of complex interaction effects and consider the correction method of multiple comparisons to improve the robustness of the results and reliability of interpretation. In future studies, multiple testing correction methods can be considered to enhance the robustness of secondary results to reduce the impact of type Ⅰ errors.

Section 11　Introduction and Comments of *Electroacupuncture vs Sham Electroacupuncture in the Treatment of Postoperative Ileus After Laparoscopic Surgery for Colorectal Cancer: A Multicenter, Randomized Clinical Trial*

1. Introduction

IMPORTANCE　Despite the adoption of the optimized Enhanced Recovery After Surgery (ERAS) protocol, postoperative ileus (POI) severely impairs recovery after colorectal resection and increases the burden on the health care system.

OBJECTIVE　To assess the efficacy of electroacupuncture (EA) in reducing the duration of POI with the ERAS protocol.

DESIGN, SETTING, AND PARTICIPANTS　This multicenter, randomized, sham-controlled trial was conducted in China from October 12, 2020, through October 17, 2021. There was a 1∶1 allocation using the dynamic block random method, and analyses were by intention to treat. Patients 18 years or older undergoing laparoscopic resection of colorectal cancer for the first time were randomly assigned to treatment group by a central system.

INTERVENTIONS　Patients were randomly assigned to 4 sessions of EA or sham electroacupuncture (SA) after surgery. All patients were treated within the ERAS protocol.

MAIN OUTCOMES AND MEASURES　The primary outcome was the time to first defecation. Secondary outcomes included other patient-reported outcome measures, length of postoperative hospital stay, readmission rate within 30 days, and incidence of postoperative complications and adverse events.

RESULTS　A total of 249 patients were randomly assigned to treatment groups. After the exclusion of 1 patient because of a diagnosis of intestinal tuberculosis, 248 patients (mean [SD] age, 60.2 [11.4] years; 153 men [61.7%]) were included in the analyses. The median (IQR) time to first defecation was 76.4 (67.6-96.8) hours in the EA group and 90.0 (73.6-100.3) hours in the SA group (mean difference, −8.76; 95% CI, −15.80 to −1.73; P=0.003). In the EA group compared with the SA group, the time to first flatus (median [IQR], 44.3 [37.0-58.2] hours vs 58.9 [48.2-67.4] hours; P<0.001) and the tolerability of semiliquid diet (median [IQR], 105.8 [87.0-120.3] hours vs 116.5 [92.0-137.0] hours; P=0.01) and solid food (median [IQR], 181.8 [149.5-211.4] hours vs 190.3 [165.0-228.5] hours; P=0.01) were significantly decreased. Prolonged POI occurred in 13 of 125 patients (10%) in the EA group vs 25 of 123 patients (20%) in the SA group (risk ratio [RR], 0.51; 95% CI, 0.27-0.95; P=0.03). Other secondary outcomes were not different between groups. There were no severe adverse events.

CONCLUSIONS AND RELEVANCE　Results of this randomized clinical trial demonstrated that in patients undergoing laparoscopic surgery for colorectal cancer with the ERAS protocol, EA shortened the duration of POI and decreased the risk for prolonged POI compared with SA. EA may be considered as an adjunct to the ERAS protocol to promote gastrointestinal function recovery and prevent prolonged POI after surgery.

2. Expert Comments

Comment 1

ERAS has been widely used in the treatment

of colorectal cancer, but POI remains an inevitable complication, lacking specific treatment. The inflammatory response triggered by surgical trauma and intestinal manipulation is a key pathological mechanism leading to POI-related gastrointestinal motility disorders. EA attenuates inflammation by activating the vago-adrenal pathway and may protect smooth muscle cells by reducing local intestinal muscle inflammation in the POI, thereby improving the peristaltic function of the gastrointestinal tract. These mechanisms may be an important reason for EA as a potential option for the treatment of postoperative POI and gastrointestinal dysfunction. The researchers' preliminary trial showed that EA treatment shortened the time to first postoperative bowel movement by up to 12 hours compared to sham EA in patients undergoing laparoscopic colorectal cancer surgery and alleviated related gastrointestinal dysfunction symptoms. Based on the previous study, the scientific mechanism of EA in promoting the recovery of gastrointestinal function after operation, and the results of the pilot test, it is reasonable and clinically significant to propose the hypothesis that EA can effectively treat postoperative intestinal obstruction. The intervention program implemented coordination of the gastrointestinal and mu-meridian acupoints, comprising an optimized design under the guidance of the classical theory of acupuncture. The primary outcome measures were objective, and the secondary outcome measures supported the validity of the primary outcome. The sham EA control could confirm the specific promoting effect of EA on gastrointestinal function. The results of the study showed that EA, as a powerful adjunct to the fast-track surgery program, can effectively promote the recovery of gastrointestinal function in patients after laparoscopic colorectal cancer surgery, supported by strong evidence. The weakness of the study is that there was no current output for sham EA, which may have affected the blinding effect of patients, but this bias was minimized owing to the objectivity of the primary outcome measure and the successful implementation of the blinding.

Comment 2

This study was a multicenter randomized controlled trial with acupuncture treatment as the intervention. The article clearly described the requirements of the acupuncture practitioner, introduced the acupuncture administration to the EA group and SA groups, and the design of acupoints and non-acupoints. Participants were randomized using dynamic blocks, and the patients, practitioners, and observers were blinded. Based on the results of the pilot test, the sample size of the study was estimated, and the study power was set at 80%. Results were reported in the order of comparability analysis, efficacy comparison, and safety evaluation of randomized controlled trials. The baseline data of the two groups were first described and compared. intention-to-treat analysis was used for the analysis of efficacy indicators. In the methodology, it is mentioned that the sensitivity analysis of the missing values of the main indicators was carried out by filling in the best and worst values, but data for the secondary outcomes were not filled in. Although there were some differences between the before and after descriptions (all the intentionality analyses mentioned above were used, but data for the secondary indicators were not filled in), this had little impact on the main conclusions. The description of the statistical methods outlined the principle basis for the method selection, but it would have been clearer to be more specific, such as explaining the use of independent t-tests for normally distributed data and Mann-Whitney U tests for skewed data, and specifying which indicators were analyzed with t-tests and which with use of non-parametric tests. This study was a multicenter randomized controlled trial, but the data composition of each center and whether there was a center effect were not reported.

Overall, this study was a multicenter randomized controlled trial with a reasonable design, standardized reporting, and simple, clear, and intuitive statistical description and inferences.

Section 12 Introduction and Comments of *Electroacupuncture for Motor Dysfunction and Constipation in Patients With Parkinson's Disease: A Randomised Controlled Multi-centre trial*

1. Introduction

BACKGROUND Motor disturbances and non-motor disturbances such as constipation are the main factors affecting the quality of life in patients with Parkinson's disease (PD). We investigated the efficacy and safety of electroacupuncture combined with conventional pharmacological treatment on motor dysfunction and constipation in PD.

METHODS In this multi-center randomised controlled trial, we enrolled 166 eligible participants between September 19, 2018 and September 25, 2019 in four hospitals in China. Participants were randomly assigned (1 : 1) to the electroacupuncture (EA) group and the waitlist control group. Each participant in both groups received the conventional pharmacological treatment, EA group received 3 sessions of electroacupuncture per week for 12 weeks. The primary outcome was the change in the Unified Parkinson's Disease Rating Scale (UPDRS) score from baseline to week 12. The secondary outcomes included the evaluation of functional disability in motor symptoms and constipation, the adherence and adverse events were also recorded. Registered with Chictr. org. cn, ChiCTR1800019517.

FINDINGS At week 12, the change in the UPDRS score of the EA group was significantly higher than that of the control group, with a difference of −9.1 points (95% CI, −11.8 to −6.4), and this difference continued into weeks 16 and 24. From baseline to week 12, the 39-item Parkinson Disease Question (PDQ-39) decreased by 10 points (interquartile range, IQR −26.0 to 0.0) in the EA group and 2.5 points (IQR: −11.0 to 4.0) in the control group, the difference was statistically significant. The time and steps for the 20-m walk at week 12, as well as the changes from baseline in the EA group, were comparable with that in the control group. But the EA group had a greater decrease than the control group from baseline in the times for 20-m walks at weeks 16 and 24. From week 4 to week 24, the median values of pontaneous bowel movements (SBMs) per week in the EA group were higher than that in the control group, the differences were all statistically significant. The incidence of EA-related adverse events during treatment was low, and they are mild and transient.

INTERPRETATION The findings of our study suggested that compared with conventional pharmacological treatment, conventional pharmacological treatment combined with electroacupuncture significantly enhances motor function and increased bowel movements in patients with PD, electroacupuncture is a safe and effective treatment for PD.

2. Expert Comments

Comment 1

This study focused on the motor dysfunction and constipation of patients with PD, which seriously affect patient quality of life, and accurately addressed difficult and prominent issues in the treatment of PD. By exploring the improvement effect of EA on motor function and constipation of patients with PD, it provided a new perspective for the comprehensive treatment of PD, reflected on the potential value and application prospects of acupuncture of traditional Chinese medicine, and has high clinical practicability, which is of great importance for improving the quality of life of patients with PD.

In the implementation of the acupuncture intervention, the overall design was scientifically sound and reasonable. The acupuncture operation was carried out by experienced acupuncturists with at least 2 years of work experience and followed a standardized process to ensure the consistency and safety of the treatment. Concurrently, the acupuncture process paid attention to the sense of deqi and stimulation through the EA instrument. Presenting these details enhanced the quality of the report. However, the study could be further improved. First, the study observed the effect of 12 weeks of treatment, but the long-term effect of EA treatment (such as the effect in more than half a year) was not discussed, which limited the general applicability of the study conclusions and their guiding value for long-term application. Second, the use of a waiting treatment control group controlled the variables to some extent but could not eliminate the influence of the placebo effect. Future studies may consider adding a sham acupuncture group to more accurately assess the true effect of EA treatment. Finally, given the long duration of the study, different research centers may have different evaluation criteria, which would have affected the consistency of the results, and moreover, there may have been bias because the study could not ensure blinding.

Comment 2

This study was a multicenter, randomized, controlled, single-blind clinical trial conducted in four tertiary hospitals in China from September 19, 2018, to September 25, 2019. The purpose of this study was to evaluate the safety and efficacy of EA combined with conventional drugs in the treatment of PD. The intervention group received EA combined with conventional drug treatment, and the control group received conventional drug treatment. The primary outcome measure was change in the UPDRS score from baseline to 12 weeks after treatment. Based on the sample size estimates from the pilot results, a minimum of 57 patients per group would be required to identify a difference in the UPDRS score of 7.4 between the two groups with 90% confidence at the 0.05 test level. Considering an exit rate of 20%, the total sample size increased to 144. To compensate for the center effect and prespecified subgroup analysis, the sample size was again increased to 166. Patients were stratified and randomized at a 1 : 1 ratio. Stratification factors included the study center and constipation. Missing data for the primary outcome

Chapter 2 Comments of Clinical Trials of Acupuncture and Moxibustion in SCI Journals

were assumed to be missing at random and were imputed using multiple imputations. A generalized linear model was used to evaluate the difference in the UPDRS score change between the groups. The baseline UPDRS score was included as a covariate and adjusted. The study protocol was approved by the ethics committees of the four hospitals and registered in the China Clinical Trial Registry. The study was conducted, and the results were reported, in accordance with the Guidelines for the consolidated standards of reporting trials (CONSORT) and the standards for reporting of interventions in clinical trials of acupuncture (STRICTA).

The baseline data of the two groups were balanced and comparable. In the intentionality analysis, the baseline UPDRS scores of the intervention and control groups were 36.1±16.6 and 32.2±16.5, respectively. After 12 weeks of treatment, the UPDRS scores of the two groups were 30.9 (95% CI, 27.3 to 34.4) and 36.1 (95% CI, 32.2 to 39.9), respectively. The change in the UPDRS score was −5.3 (95% CI, −6.9 to −3.6) and 3.9 (95% CI, 1.7 to 6.1) in the two groups, respectively, and the difference was −9.1 (95% CI, −11.8 to −6.4), which was statistically significant ($P<0.001$). In the per-protocol analysis, the primary outcome was similar between the groups, indicating the robustness of the primary outcome analysis.

Section 13 Introduction and Comments of *Effects of Electroacupuncture for Opioid-Induced Constipation in Patients With Cancer in China: A Randomized Clinical Trial*

1. Introduction

IMPORTANCE Opioid-induced constipation (OIC) is prevalent among patients treated with opioids for cancer pain. Safe and effective therapies for OIC in patients with cancer remain an unmet need.

OBJECTIVE To determine the efficacy of electroacupuncture (EA) for OIC in patients with cancer.

DESIGN, SETTING, AND PARTICIPANTS This randomized clinical trial was conducted at 6 tertiary hospitals in China among 100 adult patients with cancer who were screened for OIC and enrolled between May 1, 2019, and December 11, 2021.

INTERVENTIONS Patients were randomized to receive 24 sessions of EA or sham electroacupuncture (SA) over 8 weeks and then were followed up for 8 weeks after treatment.

MAIN OUTCOMES AND MEASURES The primary outcome was the proportion of overall responders, defined as patients who had at least 3 spontaneous bowel movements (SBM) per week and an increase of at least 1 SBM from baseline in the same week for at least 6 of the 8 weeks of the treatment period. All statistical analyses were based on the intention-to-treat principle.

RESULTS A total of 100 patients (mean [SD] age, 64.4 [10.5] years; 56 men [56.0%]) underwent randomization; 50 were randomly assigned to each group. Among them, 44 of 50 patients (88.0%) in the EA group and 42 of 50 patients (84.0%) in the SA group received at least 20 (≥83.3%) sessions of treatment. The proportion of overall responders at week 8 was 40.1% (95% CI, 26.1%-54.1%) in the EA group and 9.0% (95% CI, 0.5%-17.4%) in the SA group (difference between groups, 31.1 percentage points [95% CI, 14.8-47.6 percentage points]; $P<0.001$). Compared with SA, EA provided greater relief for most OIC symptoms and improved quality of life among patients with OIC. Electroacupuncture had no effects on cancer pain and its opioid treatment dosage. Electroacupuncture-related adverse events were rare, and, if any, all were mild and transient.

CONCLUSIONS AND RELEVANCE This randomized clinical trial found that 8-week EA treatment could increase weekly SBM with a good safety profile and improve quality of life for the treatment of OIC. Electroacupuncture thus provided an alternative option for OIC in adult patients with cancer.

2. Expert Comments

Comment 1

This study focused on solving the problem of OIC in patients with cancer, which affects the quality of life of most cancer-related opioid users and is an urgent clinical problem to be solved. The work investigated the efficacy of EA in treating OIC, aiming to both provide a safe and effective therapeutic option for clinical use and to mitigate the side effects of opioids, thereby offering considerable clinical value and significance.

The details of the acupuncture intervention were reported in detail in the paper, including the parameters of EA and the depth of acupuncture. These details are essential for the repeatability of the implementation. The study used an 8-week, 24-session EA regimen, which was designed to help assess the long-term efficacy and safety of EA. During the implementation of the trial, the participants were not encouraged to accept other interventions, but emergency medication was set up to ensure the objective evaluation of the efficacy of EA and the safety of the participants. The study also established stringent qualifications for the acupuncture therapists and standardized training to minimize operator variability and enhance the consistency of acupuncture administration. The use of shallow needling at non-acupoints as a sham EA control, application of a centralized randomization method, and blinded assessment procedures ensured the scientific rigor and validity of the study.

In summary, this study addressed a critical issue in clinical practice by providing a safe and effective approach for managing OIC through a comprehensive treatment plan and rigorous, scientifically sound methodology. The findings contribute to improving the quality of life of patients with cancer.

Comment 2

(1) Study design and process implementation

The trial employed a multicenter design to minimize selection bias that might arise from recruiting patients from a single center, thereby making the patient population more representative. An EA group and a SA group were established to eliminate the potential impact of the placebo effect on the outcomes. Strict inclusion and exclusion criteria were applied to ensure consistency in patient characteristics and to mitigate the influence of potential confounding factors on the results. Patients included in the study were required to have a life expectancy of at least 6 months to prevent data loss due to mortality. While the acupuncturists were not blinded, the patients, outcome assessors, data managers, and statisticians were blinded to maintain the integrity of the blinding process as much as possible. The success rate of the blinding was also evaluated to ensure it adhered to objective standards and to minimize information bias.

(2) Selection and application of clinical research methodology and statistical methods

The trial used the central randomization method, which improved the efficiency of randomized grouping and reduced the risk of grouping information being leaked. A primary outcome measure was set up to avoid the problem of multiplicity caused by multiple primary outcome measures. This is a composite measure that converts quantitative data into qualitative data. The criteria were strict. It was considered necessary to meet the requirements of at least three bowel movements per week for at least 6 weeks during 8 weeks of treatment and at least one increase in the number of bowel movements per week compared with baseline. The sample size estimate was also consistent with the primary outcome measure. The principle of intentionality analysis was used to ensure consistency between the data analysis population and randomized population as far as possible. Multiple imputations were performed for missing primary efficacy measures to minimize the impact of missing data on the results. Additionally, four sensitivity analyses were conducted to assess the robustness of the results, thereby enhancing their credibility.

Section 14   Introduction and Comments of *Acupuncture vs Massage for Pain in Patients Living With Advanced Cancer: The IMPACT Randomized Clinical Trial*

1. Introduction

IMPORTANCE Pain is challenging for patients with advanced cancer. While recent guidelines recommend acupuncture and massage for cancer pain, their comparative effectiveness is unknown.

OBJECTIVE To compare the effects of acupuncture and massage on musculoskeletal pain among patients with advanced cancer.

DESIGN, SETTING, AND PARTICIPANTS A multicenter pragmatic randomized clinical trial was conducted at US cancer care centers consisting of a northeastern comprehensive cancer center and a southeastern cancer institute from September 19, 2019, through February 23, 2022. The principal investigator and study statisticians were blinded to treatment assignments. The duration of follow-up was 26 weeks. Intention-to-treat analyses were performed (linear mixed models). Participants included patients with advanced cancer with moderate to severe pain and clinicianestimated life expectancy of 6 months or more. Patient recruitment strategy was multipronged (eg, patient database queries, mailings, referrals, community outreach). Eligible patients had English or Spanish as their first language, were older than 18 years, and had a Karnofsky score greater than or equal to 60 (range, 0-100; higher scores indicating less functional impairment).

INTERVENTIONS Weekly acupuncture or massage for 10 weeks with monthly booster sessions up to 26 weeks.

MAIN OUTCOMES AND MEASURES The primary end point was the change in worst pain intensity score from baseline to 26 weeks. The secondary outcomes included fatigue, insomnia, and quality of life. The Brief Pain Inventory (range, 0-10; higher numbers indicate worse pain intensity or interference) was used to measure the primary outcome. The secondary outcomes included fatigue, insomnia, and quality of life.

RESULTS A total of 298 participants were enrolled (mean [SD] age, 58.7 [14.1] years, 200 [67.1%] were women, 33 [11.1%] Black, 220 [74.1%] White, 46 [15.4%] Hispanic, and 78.5% with solid tumors). The mean (SD) baseline worst pain score was 6.9 (1.5). During 26 weeks, acupuncture reduced the worst pain score, with a mean change of −2.53 (95% CI, −2.92 to −2.15) points, and massage reduced the Brief Pain Inventory worst pain score, with a mean change of −3.01 (95% CI, −3.38 to −2.63) points; the between-group difference was not significant (−0.48; 95% CI, −0.98 to 0.03; P=0.07). Both treatments also improved fatigue, insomnia, and quality of life without significant between-group differences. Adverse events were mild and included bruising (6.5% of patients receiving acupuncture) and transient soreness (15.1% patients receiving massage).

CONCLUSIONS AND RELEVANCE In this randomized clinical trial among patients with advanced cancer, both acupuncture and massage were associated with pain reduction and improved fatigue, insomnia, and quality of life over 26 weeks; however, there was no significant different between the treatments. More research is needed to evaluate how best to integrate these approaches into pain treatment to optimize symptom management for the growing population of people living with advanced cancer.

2. Expert Comments

Comment 1

The pain management of patients with advanced cancer is a difficult and prominent issue in clinical treatment. The integrative medicine for pain in patients with advanced cancer trial (IMPACT) addressed this issue by comparing two non-drug therapies, acupuncture and massage, to explore their effectiveness in relieving pain in patients with advanced cancer. The study not only focused on pain itself, but also covered pain-related symptoms such as fatigue and insomnia, which have a significant impact on the quality of life of patients. The research topic reflects the profound understanding of clinical needs and the pursuit of improving the quality of life of patients, which has important clinical value and social significance.

In this study, the treatment was administered by acupuncturists or massage therapists with oncology experience, who received uniform training and followed a strict treatment protocol. The treatment included acupuncture in the most painful area of the patient's body and selection of acupoints according to the patient's combined symptoms, but the depth of acupuncture, specific acupoints and other details should have been further clarified. The study considered the individual differences among the participants and made individualized adjustments to the intervention plan to ensure the safety and effectiveness of the treatment. The control group was treated with massage therapy, and the implementation process, location, and manipulation were described in detail. The study was not blinded owing to the specificity of the treatment.

The results showed that both acupuncture and massage had a positive effect on reducing pain and improving related symptoms in patients with advanced cancer, and there was no significant difference between the two therapies. This finding provides new perspectives and options for pain management in patients with advanced cancer, emphasizing the importance of non-pharmacological therapies in comprehensive treatment. Concurrently, the study also suggested that these non-drug therapies should be integrated into clinical treatment strategies in the future to achieve the necessity of comprehensive symptom management.

Comment 2

(1) Study design and process implementation

The study published the trial protocol, which improved its transparency. The multicenter recruitment of patients ensured the diversity of the sample, which is conducive to improving the extrapolation of the conclusions. The patients' baseline Karnofsky score was not less than 60 points, and the life expectancy was not less than 6 months to ensure that the patients could successfully complete the trial. The patients' baseline pain level was moderate to severe, and the primary outcome measure was the most severe rather than the average pain level in the past week. These design elements can more objectively reflect patient pain improvement. The two intervention types, ie, acupuncture and massage, precluded blinding of the physicians and patients, but the principal investigator and statistician were blinded, in line with clinical practice. A stratified block randomization approach was used to avoid the effects of baseline opioid use and central factors on outcomes.

(2) Selection and application of clinical research methodology and statistical methods

The principle of intention-to-treat analysis was adopted to ensure as much consistency as possible between the data analysis population and the randomized population. Linear mixed models were used to analyze the primary outcome measures. These models allow for the explicit modeling of correlation structures in the data, considering both fixed and random effects, thereby improving the handling of missing data and providing more accurate estimates. In the linear mixed model, a common baseline mean was set for different groups, known as the constrained longitudinal data analysis model. Compared with the traditional model that uses the baseline as a covariate, this model provides more appropriate variance and confidence interval estimates for the adjusted mean. For exploratory analysis purposes, the analysis of secondary efficacy measures does not need to account for multiplicity issues.

Section 15 Introduction and Comments of *Efficacy and Safety of Auricular Acupuncture for Depression: A Randomized Clinical Trial*

1. Introduction

IMPORTANCE Depression is a leading cause of disability worldwide, and there is increasing interest in nonpharmacological treatments. Auricular acupuncture (AA) is a simple, low-cost, and well-tolerated option, but further studies are needed to establish its efficacy and safety.

OBJECTIVE To estimate the efficacy and safety of auricular acupuncture as a treatment for depression.

DESIGN, SETTING, AND PARTICIPANTS This randomized clinical trial was conducted at 4 university research centers in Brazil, from March to July 2023. Eligible patients were adults aged 18 to 50 years whose score on the Patient Health Questionnaire-9 (PHQ-9) indicated moderate depression (score 10-14) or moderately severe depression (score 15-19). Exclusion criteria included previous application of AA, risk of suicidal ideation, or severe depression (PHQ-9 score >20). An intent-to-treat analysis and modified intent-to-treat analysis were conducted.

INTERVENTION Participants were randomized into 2 treatment groups, which included specific AA (SA) and nonspecific AA (NSA). Both groups received 12 sessions of AA with semipermanent needles with daily stimulation twice a week over 6 weeks and were followed-up for 3 months. All participants continued with their usual care for ethical reasons. The SA group's treatment protocol consisted of 6 acupuncture points on the auricular pavilion chosen according to the diagnosis of depression by traditional Chinese medicine (Shenmen, subcortex, heart, lung, liver, and kidney). The NSA group's acupuncture points were the external ear, the cheek and face area, and 4 nonspecific points in the helix region unassociated with mental health symptoms. A locator device was used to confirm which areas had neuroreactive points.

MAIN OUTCOMES AND MEASURES The primary outcome was a reduction of at least 50% in the PHQ-9 score (ie, depression recovery) at 3 months. Secondary outcomes included depression recovery at 4 and 6 weeks; depression remission (PHQ-9 score <5) at 4 weeks, 6 weeks, and 3 months); and adverse events.

RESULTS A total of 304 participants were screened, and 74 participants (62 women [84%]; median [IQR] age, 29 [23-27] years) were included in the intention-to-treat analysis, with 37 participants randomized to each group (SA and NSA). A total of 47 participants (64%) were followed-up through 3 months. The results showed no statistically significant difference in depressive recovery between the groups at 3 months (14 of 24 participants in the SA group [58%] vs 10 of 23 participants in the NSA group [43%]; risk ratio [RR], 1.34; 95% CI, 0.76-2.45; P=0.38). The proportions of depression recovery and remission at 4 and 6 weeks based on the PHQ-9 were higher in the SA group (except for depression recovery at 6 weeks) with no statistically significant differences. However, a statistically significant difference was observed in symptom remission at 3 months (11 of 24 participants in the SA group [46%] vs 3 of 23 participants in the NSA group [13%]; RR, 1.99; 95% CI, 1.16-3.34; P=0.02) in favor of SA. There were no significant differences in adverse event rates between the groups, evidencing the intervention's safety. Most participants reported mild pain at the needle application site (33 patients [94%] in the SA group vs 32 patients [91%] in the NSA group). Five participants dropped out of the study due to adverse events.

CONCLUSIONS AND RELEVANCE The results of this randomized clinical trial suggest that SA over 6 weeks is safe. Although there was no statistically significant difference between groups for the primary

Chapter 2 Comments of Clinical Trials of Acupuncture and Moxibustion in SCI Journals

efficacy outcome, patients receiving SA did experience greater symptom remission at 3 months. A larger sample size and longer intervention are needed to further evaluate the efficacy of SA for depression.

2. Expert Comments

Comment 1

This study focused on the global issue of depression, especially in Brazil, a country with a high prevalence of depression, and explored the potential value of AA in the treatment of this condition. The topic was closely related to clinical difficulties and prominent issues, with marked practical significance and scientific research value. Depression is one of the main causes of global disability, and its poor treatment compliance and unstable efficacy have always challenged clinicians. The purpose of this study was to evaluate the efficacy and safety of AA in the treatment of depression through a randomized controlled trial design and to provide a new treatment option for use in clinical practice.

This study followed strict scientific norms in research methods, was approved by the appropriate ethics committee, and followed the consolidated standards of reporting trials (CONSORT) and the standards for reporting of interventions in clinical trials of acupuncture (STRICTA) reporting standards to ensure a scientifically sound and transparent workflow. The use of randomization and blinding reduced bias and increased the reliability of the findings.

Regarding the implementation of AA treatment, the article describes the treatment process in detail, including the selection of auricular points, AA specifications, and acupuncture depth and stimulation methods, fully demonstrating the rationality and operability of AA treatment. TF4 (Shen Men), AT4 (Subcortical), CO15 (Heart), CO14 (Lung), CO12 (Liver), and CO10 (Kidney) are common auricular points for the treatment of depression. Although a treatment frequency of twice a week is lower than that in China, it is reasonable considering the compliance and economic cost incurred by foreign patients. Simultaneously, the researchers set up a control group of shallow needling of non-specific acupoints, avoiding nerve reaction points to the extent possible, to further verify the specific efficacy of AA treatment. In addition, special attention was paid to the background of experienced acupuncturists, who received standardized training to ensure the standardization and consistency of the AA treatment.

The results showed that while there was no significant difference between the SA group and NSA group in the primary outcome (depression recovery rate), the SA group showed a clear advantage in the secondary outcome (depression remission rate). Depression remission is essential for patients, contributing to improved psychosocial functioning and long-term outcomes, not just symptom relief. This finding suggests that AA may have potential efficacy in improving depressive symptoms, but further studies are needed to confirm its long-term efficacy and stability.

In the discussion section, the authors thoroughly analyzed factors that may have influenced the study's results, such as the small sample size, short treatment duration, and high follow-up loss rate, and proposed directions for future research improvements. Additionally, the authors explored the potential mechanisms of AA in treating depression, including vagus nerve activation and hypothalamus-pituitary-adrenal axis regulation, offering insights into the biological basis of AA for depression treatment.

In summary, this study provided preliminary evidence for the efficacy and safety of AA in the treatment of depression. Although there was no statistically significant difference in the primary outcome, the positive findings for the secondary outcome were encouraging. Future studies should further expand the sample size, extend the treatment cycle and follow-up period, and use more objective evaluation tools to verify the long-term effect and stability of AA treatment. Additionally, the specific mechanism of AA in the treatment of depression should be further explored to provide a more scientifically sound and reasonable basis for clinical treatment.

Comment 2

This was a multicenter, randomized, double-blind clinical trial that enrolled community-based patients at four university research centers in the state of Santa Catarina, Brazil, from March to April 2023. The objective of this study was to evaluate the efficacy and safety of semi-permanent acupuncture in the treatment of depression. The experimental group received semi-permanent acupuncture along with conventional treatment, while the control group received sham acupuncture and conventional treatment. Depressive symptoms were assessed using the PHQ-9. The primary outcome measure was the proportion of participants with a PHQ-9 score improvement of 50% or higher (indicating recovery from depression) 3 months post-treatment. The sample size was estimated assuming a 30% difference in the depression recovery rates between the groups (60% in the experimental group and 30% in the control group) ; with a power of 80%, and a significance level of 0.05, at least 36 participants were required per group. To account for potential attrition, an additional 10% was added, resulting in a total of 40 participants per group, or 80 participants overall. Block randomization was conducted in a 1 : 1 ratio, with block sizes randomly assigned as 4, 6, or 8. Intention-to-treat analysis and modified intention-to-treat analysis were performed to compare the proportion of depression recovery between the groups using Fisher's exact test. The study was conducted, and the results reported, in accordance with the CONSORT guidelines and the STRICTA guidelines, ensuring methodological rigor.

Of 304 volunteers, 74 were selected for randomization. The intention-to-treat analysis included 37 patients in the experimental group and 37 in the control group. At the 3-month assessment of the primary outcome, 27 patients (36%) were lost to follow-up. Based on the observed data, the depression recovery rate was 58% among 24 patients in the experimental group, and 43% among 23 patients in the control group. The difference between the groups was not statistically significant (P=0.38). Among all secondary outcome analyses, only the proportion of PHQ-9 scores below 5 (indicating depression cured) at 3 months showed a statistically significant difference between the groups (46% in the experimental group and 13% in the control group, P=0.02). The results of the modified intention-to-treat and sensitivity analyses were similar. There was no statistically significant difference in adverse reactions and adverse events between the groups. In this study, the depression recovery rate in the control group (43%) was higher than the expected value estimated via the sample size calculation (30%), suggesting a placebo effect. The difference between the groups was overestimated during the sample size estimation, leading to an underestimation of the required sample size. Additionally, the actual loss to follow-up rate was higher than expected. Ultimately, the insufficiently effective sample size for the entire study may have been the primary reason for not observing statistically significant results.

Section 16   Introduction and Comments of *Effect of Acupuncture on Postoperative Ileus After Laparoscopic Elective Colorectal Surgery: A Prospective, Randomised, Controlled Trial*

1. Introduction

BACKGROUND   Postoperative ileus (POI) after colorectal surgery is a frequent problem that significantly delays recovery, increases perioperative costs, and negatively impacts on daily life, physical and psychosocial functioning, and wellbeing. We investigated the effect of acupuncture at different single acupoint combined with standard care on postoperative ileus.

METHODS   In this single-center, three-arm, prospective, randomised trial, we enrolled patients with primary colorectal cancer undergoing elective colorectal resection at Cancer Hospital Chinese Academy of Medical Science in Beijing, China. Patients were randomly assigned (1 : 1 : 1) to receive either electroacupuncture (EA) at ST36 (Zusanli) or ST25 (Tianshu) combined with standard care (two EA groups) once daily from post-operative days 1-4, or standard care alone (standard care group). The co-primary outcomes were time to first flatus and time to defecation assessed in the intention-to-treat population. This study is registered with Chictr. org. cn, ChiCTR1900027466.

FINDING   Between Nov 15, 2019, and Sep 30, 2020, 129 patients were assessed for eligibility, 105 patients (35 patients per group) were enrolled and included in the intention-to-treat analysis. After receiving EA at ST36, the time to first flatus and defecation were shorter (between-group difference −10.98 [97.5% CI −21.41 to −0.56], P=0.02 for flatus; −25.41 [−47.89 to −2.93], P=0.02 for defecation). However, we did not observe a significant difference in time to first flatus and defecation between the EA at ST25 group and standard care group (between-group difference −5.54 [97.5% CI −15.78 to 4.70], P=0.26 for flatus; −17.69 [−40.33 to 4.95], P=0.08 for defecation). There were no serious adverse events.

INTERPRETATION   Compared with standard care alone, standard care combined with EA at ST36, but not ST25, significantly enhances bowel function recovery in a postoperative setting to patients with colorectal cancer with laparoscopic elective colorectal resection.

2. Expert Comments

Comment 1

POI is a common and challenging issue following laparoscopic colorectal surgery. POI can extend the length of hospital stay, increase healthcare costs and readmission rates, and negatively impact the physical and mental health of patients. While numerous studies have shown that EA can promote the recovery of gastrointestinal motility, its application in the perioperative setting has been limited. This study examined the effect of EA intervention on POI, aiming to provide a safe and effective non-pharmacological treatment option for enhanced recovery after surgery (ERAS). The findings offer important supporting evidence for the integration of acupuncture therapy into modern medical practice.

The objectives of this study were twofold: ① To compare the efficacy of EA at ST36 and ST25 in improving POI; ② to test the hypothesis that EA can promote the recovery of intestinal function after laparoscopic colorectal surgery as part of an ERAS program. Accordingly, the study included three groups: ST36 acupoint EA group, ST25 acupoint EA group, and standard care group. Patients in the EA groups received 30 minutes of EA treatment once daily starting from the first day after surgery and continuing for 4 days or until discharge. The standard care group received only routine management to eliminate other factors that might affect intestinal function recovery. The results indicated that, compared to standard care, the ST36 EA group experienced a significantly shorter time to first postoperative gas passage and defecation, whereas no significant difference was observed between the ST25 EA group and the control group. This suggests that EA at ST36 is more effective in accelerating the recovery of intestinal function. Additionally, the ST36 EA group had a shorter tolerance time for liquid and semi-liquid diets. No serious adverse events were reported during the treatment period.

The results of this study indicate that EA at ST36 can significantly accelerate the recovery of intestinal function after surgery, hinting at important clinical application potential. The study design was rigorous, with a limited number of acupoints selected and clear implementation details for the acupuncture intervention. The findings both confirmed the efficacy of EA at ST36 and provided supporting evidence for the specificity of acupoints.

Comment 2

(1) Study design and process implementation

This study evaluated the efficacy of acupuncture in the treatment of ileus after laparoscopic elective colorectal surgery. This was a single-center, three-arm, prospective, randomized controlled trial of 105 patients undergoing elective surgery for colorectal cancer. The patients were randomly assigned to one of three groups: ST36 acupoint EA group, ST25 acupoint EA group, or control group, which received standard treatment only. The primary study outcome was dual (time to first flatus and bowel movement), and the efficacy was determined only when both outcomes were statistically significant. The results showed that during the recovery period after colorectal cancer surgery, EA at ST36 combined with standard treatment could significantly improve the recovery of intestinal function. The study is characterized by clear conceptualization, a reasonable design, and straightforward methods to determine the outcome indicators and their effectiveness.

(2) Selection and application of clinical research methodology and statistical methods

This was a single-center randomized controlled trial study. After providing informed consent, the patients were randomly divided into an ST36 acupoint EA group, ST25 acupoint EA group, and control group. The size of the block was 6 or 9. The research team balanced the baseline characteristics of the patients between the intervention groups through randomization to ensure that the characteristics of the patients receiving different interventions would be consistent at baseline to facilitate the evaluation of intervention efficacy. Further, the study used block randomization to a certain extent, to ensure the consistency of the sample size across the groups. Because this study was an randomized controlled trial with a three-group design, the α was adjusted to 0.025 for both sides in the sample size estimation. In the evaluation of the primary outcome indicators, the research team used survival analysis to evaluate the outcome indicators, and the t-test results were used as the results of the sensitivity analysis. Moreover, this study also used the principle of intentionality analysis, for reasonable filling in of missing data, ensuring the reliability and stability of the results.

Section 17 Introduction and Comments of *Acupuncture Improves the Symptoms, Intestinal Microbiota, and Inflammation of Patients With Mild to Moderate Crohn's Disease: A Randomized Controlled Trial*

1. Introduction

BACKGROUND The efficacy and mechanisms of acupuncture for Crohn's disease (CD) are not well understood. We investigated its effects on symptoms, intestinal microbiota, and circulating inflammatory markers in CD patients.

METHODS This 48-week, randomized, sham controlled, parallel-group clinical trial was performed at a tertiary outpatient clinic in China. From April 2015 to November 2019, 66 patients (mean age 40.4, 62.1% were male, all were Han Chinese) with mild to moderate active CD and unresponsive to drug treatment were enrolled and randomly assigned equally to an acupuncture group or a sham group. The treatment group received 3 sessions of acupuncture plus moxibustion per week for 12 weeks and a follow-up of 36 weeks.

FINDINGS At week 12, the clinical remission rate (the primary outcome) and clinical response rate of acupuncture group were significantly higher than that of sham group, with a difference of 42.4% (95% CI: 20.1%-64.0%) and 45.5% (95% CI: 24.0%-66.9%), respectively, both of which maintained at week 48. The acupuncture group had significantly lower CD activity index and C-reactive protein level at week 12, which maintained at 36-week follow-up. The CD endoscopic index of severity, histopathological score, and recurrence rate at week 48 were significantly lower in acupuncture group. The number of operational taxonomic unit of intestinal microbiota and relative abundance of Faecalibacterium prausnitzii and Roseburia faecis were increased. Plasma diamine oxidase, lipopolysaccharide, and Th1/Th17 related cytokines were decreased in 12-week after acupuncture.

INTERPRETATION Acupuncture was effective in inducing and maintaining remission in patients with active CD, which was associated with increased abundance of intestinal anti-inflammatory bacteria, enhanced intestinal barrier, and regulation of circulating Th1/Th17-related cytokines.

2. Expert Comments

Comment 1

Drug therapy is conventionally used for the treatment of most diseases, and poor drug efficacy, drug tolerance, and the side effects of the drugs are all possible entry points for acupuncture to play a role. It is necessary to combine the characteristics of acupuncture and moxibustion therapy, analyze and verify the role or advantages of acupuncture and moxibustion in pharmacodynamic substitution, synergy, assistance in drug dosage reduction, and reduction of drug side effects to provide high-level, evidence-based data, clarify the mechanism of acupuncture and moxibustion, and promote the integration of acupuncture and moxibustion into the contemporary medical system.

The focus of this study on mild to moderate active CD not responding well to conventional medical therapy is a good demonstration, and 12 weeks of acupuncture treatment may regulate intestinal microbial composition and Th1/Th17 cell-mediated inflammation to improve disease activity in patients with CD. Studies have found that the effect of acupuncture can be maintained for 9 months after the end of treatment, which is also an important aspect of the advantage of acupuncture therapy; that is, acupuncture works by activating endogenous protective mechanisms, with the effect persisting even after the end of treatment.

The intervention in this study comprised combined acupuncture and moxibustion. At present, most of the clinical evaluation studies of acupuncture and moxibustion published in journals with high impact factors have used electroacupuncture compared with sham electroacupuncture. However, in domestic clinical practice, the combination of acupuncture and moxibustion is very common, and this intervention design has greater guiding significance for clinical practice. The authors used sham acupuncture combined with sham moxibustion to achieve effective control and fully reported the implementation details; this study model is worth studying and promoting.

To conclude, this study conducted high-quality sham-controlled acupuncture efficacy evaluation and mechanism research on the clinical challenges of drug therapy, providing safe and effective treatment for mild to moderate active CD responding poorly to conventional drug treatment.

Comment 2

(1) Study design and process implementation

This study evaluated the efficacy of acupuncture in the treatment of CD and explored its mechanism of action. The research team conducted a multicenter randomized controlled trial, and randomly divided the participants into an acupuncture group and sham acupuncture group in a 1∶1 ratio. Participants received treatment three times per week for 12 consecutive weeks, followed by 36 weeks of follow-up. A blinded design was implemented to ensure that the patients, prescribing physicians, outcome evaluators, and statistical analysts were unaware of group assignments throughout the study. The primary outcome measure was the clinical response rate at the completion of treatment, and the secondary outcome measures included the clinical response rate, C-reactive protein level, and CD endoscopic index of severity score at Weeks 24, 36, and 48. The results showed that acupuncture and moxibustion could effectively contribute to remission and maintenance of remission in patients with active CD, which may be related to the increase of intestinal anti-inflammatory bacteria and enhancement of the intestinal barrier. In this study, the research idea is clear, the design is reasonable, the research content involves curative effect appraisal and mechanism exploration, and the content is comprehensive.

(2) Selection and application of clinical study methodology and statistical methods

This was a multicenter randomized controlled trial study, and a reasonable sample size calculation was used to estimate that at least 33 patients were required in each group. To evaluate the reliability of the blinding method in this study, the researchers and patients were blinded at several stages, and the patients were asked to guess their group allocation at the end of the study. The study strictly adhered to the principle of intentionality analysis, and the statistical analysis was divided into intention to treat and per protocol, with the results of the two analyses confirming each other. This study deeply delved into the mechanism of acupuncture and carried out bioinformatics analysis to explore the regulatory role of related cytokines. The work both evaluated the clinical effect of acupuncture and moxibustion treatment and explored the mechanism of acupuncture and moxibustion efficacy to a certain extent.

3. Author's Talk

This study took seven years to complete, from conception to the final publication, and encountered numerous challenges in topic selection, clinical implementation, and manuscript submission. Firstly, the design and implementation were based on a previous publication by the research team, "*Randomized controlled trial: Moxibustion and acupuncture for the treatment of Crohn's disease*" (*World J Gastroenterol*, 2014). As the prior study had already evaluated the clinical efficacy and safety of acupuncture for active CD, the current study had to reframe its focus to explore a novel perspective.

Secondly, in the clinical implementation phase, the most difficult problem encountered was the slow pace of participant recruitment. A total of 66 patients were included in the study, which took five years to achieve, from the first enrollment to the completion of recruitment; reviewers noted the prolonged enrollment period. This challenge was primarily due to the low incidence of CD. In recent years, although the incidence and prevalence of CD have rapidly risen in China, its overall prevalence remains low. In addition, this study selected a population with poor response to CD medications, which accounts for only 1/3 to 2/3 of patients with CD. In addition, most participants were unfamiliar with acupuncture and moxibustion, and the requirement for three weekly acupuncture sessions further complicated adherence, which undoubtedly increased the difficulty of recruitment and implementation experienced during the study.

Finally, the initial target journal for submission was *Gastroenterology*, a leading journal in the field of gastroenterology. Although the journal's editors recognized the innovation of this study after submission and forwarded it through for external peer review, the three reviewers provided extensive feedback. Unfortunately, due to the limited number of journals published annually, this study was ultimately rejected after careful consideration of the reviewers' comments. Subsequently, Lancet's sub-journal, *eClinicalMedicine*, was chosen as the new target journal, and after multiple rounds of revision, was finally accepted for publication.

Reflecting on the entire research process, it is crucial to devote significant effort into the study design and to find an appropriate angle of inquiry. Moreover, rigorous control of the implementation process, with careful attention to details, should be conducted. In summary, we should be careful and deliberate repeatedly. In a word, standardized research practices are a key factor in producing high-quality outcomes.

WU Huangan
Shanghai Research Institute of Acupuncture and Meridian

Section 18 Introduction and Comments of *Effect of Electroacupuncture on Insomnia in Patients With Depression: A Randomized Clinical Trial*

1. Introduction

IMPORTANCE Electroacupuncture (EA) is a widely recognized therapy for depression and sleep disorders in clinical practice, but its efficacy in the treatment of comorbid insomnia and depression remains uncertain.

OBJECTIVE To assess the efficacy and safety of EA as an alternative therapy in improving sleep quality and mental state for patients with insomnia and depression.

DESIGN, SETTING, AND PARTICIPANTS A 32-week patient-and assessor-blinded, randomized, sham-controlled clinical trial (8-week intervention plus 24-week observational follow-up) was conducted from September 1, 2016, to July 30, 2019, at 3 tertiary hospitals in Shanghai,

China. Patients were randomized to receive EA treatment and standard care, sham acupuncture (SA) treatment and standard care, or standard care only as control. Patients were 18 to 70 years of age, had insomnia, and met the criteria for depression as classified in the *Diagnostic and Statistical Manual of Mental Disorders (Fifth Edition)*. Data were analyzed from May 4 to September 13, 2020.

INTERVENTIONS All patients in the 3 groups were provided with standard care guided by psychiatrists. Patients in the EA and SA groups received real or sham acupuncture treatment, 3 sessions per week for 8 weeks, for a total of 24 sessions.

MAIN OUTCOMES AND MEASURES The primary outcome was change in Pittsburgh Sleep Quality Index (PSQI) from baseline to week 8. Secondary outcomes included PSQI at 12, 20, and 32 weeks of follow-up; sleep parameters recorded in actigraphy; Insomnia Severity Index; 17-item Hamilton Depression Rating Scale score; and Self-rating Anxiety Scale score.

RESULTS Among the 270 patients (194 women [71.9%] and 76 men [28.1%]; mean [SD] age, 50.3 [14.2] years) included in the intention-to-treat analysis, 247 (91.5%) completed all outcome measurements at week 32, and 23 (8.5%) dropped out of the trial. The mean difference in PSQI from baseline to week 8 within the EA group was −6.2 (95% CI, −6.9 to −5.6). At week 8, the difference in PSQI score was −3.6 (95% CI, −4.4 to −2.8; $P<0.001$) between the EA and SA groups and −5.1 (95% CI, −6.0 to −4.2; $P<0.001$) between the EA and control groups. The efficacy of EA in treating insomnia was sustained during the 24-week postintervention follow-up. Significant improvement in the 17-item Hamilton Depression Rating Scale (−10.7 [95% CI, −11.8 to −9.7]), Insomnia Severity Index (−7.6 [95% CI, −8.5 to −6.7]), and Self-rating Anxiety Scale (−2.9 [95% CI, −4.1 to −1.7]) scores and the total sleep time recorded in the actigraphy (29.1 [95% CI, 21.5-36.7] minutes) was observed in the EA group during the 8-week intervention period ($P<0.001$ for all). No between-group differences were found in the frequency of sleep awakenings. No serious adverse events were reported.

CONCLUSIONS AND RELEVANCE In this randomized clinical trial of EA treatment for insomnia in patients with depression, quality of sleep improved significantly in the EA group compared with the SA or control group at week 8 and was sustained at week 32.

2. Expert Comments

Comment 1

Insomnia is a primary symptom of depression, and the two conditions are often comorbid. Their interaction significantly impacts the physical and mental health of patients. While antidepressants, cognitive behavioral therapy for insomnia (CBT-I), and sleeping pills are effective treatments recommended by clinical guidelines, challenges remain including adverse drug reactions, limited access to CBT-I, and the need to improve patient compliance and acceptance. Enhancing treatment efficacy while reducing side effects is a critical challenge for the medical community.

EA has shown potential efficacy in treating both insomnia and depression, but the evidence is currently insufficient, particularly for the comorbidity of these conditions. This trial aimed to evaluate the effects of EA on sleep disorders in patients with comorbid insomnia and depression, with clear objectives and defined entry criteria. The primary outcome measure was the change in the internationally recognized PSQI from baseline, supplemented by objective assessments of sleep quality and evaluations of depression and anxiety through actigraphy, effectively reflecting the improvement in sleep quality due to EA in this patient population.

A sham EA control was implemented to isolate the specific therapeutic effects of EA by excluding nonspecific effects. Standard nursing care served as a comparison to highlight the clinical value of EA therapy. The trial results were reasonably interpreted, showing that 8 weeks of EA was both effective and safe for patients with comorbid depression and insomnia.

However, the study had several limitations.

The baseline data did not include the severity or classification of depression in patients or information on the use of antidepressants, making it difficult to determine whether these factors influenced the efficacy of EA.

The study did not clarify when EA should be used as a standalone treatment and when it should serve as an adjunctive therapy.

The sham EA did not involve electrical stimulation, making it theoretically challenging to maintain patient blinding, especially among Chinese patients with prior acupuncture experience.

Comment 2

In terms of research design and process implementation, the researchers designed a multicenter, patient-evaluator double-blind, 1∶1∶1 randomized controlled trial to evaluate the efficacy of electroacupuncture in the treatment of insomnia in patients with depression, and the sample size was calculated according to the superiority margin, type Ⅰ error, and statistical power set by existing studies.

At the end of the intervention, the Bang Blind Index was used to verify the effectiveness of blinding implementation, which fundamentally determined that the sample size met the requirements and the effectiveness of the trial design, reduced potential bias, improved the reliability of the results, and showed that the underlying design was feasible.

In terms of clinical research methodology and statistical methods, this study applied the principle of "last observation carried forward" to address missing data, which effectively prevented sample size loss. However, to further enhance the robustness of the results, it is recommended to supplement this approach with the more widely accepted multiple imputation method for sensitivity analysis. It is commendable that the study strictly adhered to the intention-to-treat principle in constructing the statistical analysis database, effectively managing potential patient dropouts and protocol deviations during the trial.

Given the multicenter design, repeated measurements, and hierarchical nature of the data, the use of a mixed-effects model was both scientifically sound and appropriate, as it accounts for situations where the assumption of independence is not satisfied. Additionally, the researchers applied *Bonferroni* correction for multiple comparisons, effectively controlling for type I error and further ensuring the authenticity and reliability of the results from a statistical perspective.

Section 19　Introduction and Comments of *Effectiveness of Acupuncture for Anxiety Among Patients With Parkinson Disease: A Randomized Clinical Trial*

1. Introduction

IMPORTANCE　One of the ordinary manifestations of Parkinson disease (PD) is anxiety, which remains untreated. Anxiety is closely associated with the accelerated progression of PD. Efficacy of acupuncture for anxiety has been reported. However, to date, there are no data on acupuncture's effectiveness on anxiety for patients with PD.

OBJECTIVE　To investigate the effect of acupuncture vs sham acupuncture for treating anxiety in patients with PD.

DESIGN, SETTING, AND PARTICIPANTS　This is randomized, double-blinded, clinical trial enrolled patients between June 20, 2021, and February 26, 2022. Final follow-up was April 15, 2022. Patients with Parkinson disease and anxiety were allocated randomly (1∶1) to receive acupuncture or sham acupuncture for 8 weeks. Acupuncture operators, outcome measures evaluators, and statistical analysts were blinded to the grouping of patients. Patients were blinded to their own grouping during the study. This study took place in the Parkinson clinic of a hospital in China.

INTERVENTIONS　Real acupuncture or sham acupuncture for 8 weeks.

MAIN OUTCOMES AND MEASURES　Primary outcome was Hamilton Anxiety Scale (HAM-A) score. Secondary outcomes were scores on the Unified Parkinson Disease Rating Scale (UPDRS), 39-item Parkinson Disease Questionnaire (PDQ-39), and serum levels of the adrenocorticotropic hormone (ACTH) and cortisol (CORT).

RESULTS　Seventy eligible patients were enrolled, including 34 women (48.5%) and 36 men (51.4%). Sixty-four patients (91%) completed the intervention and the 8-week follow-up, including 30 women (46.9%) and 34 men (53.1%) with a mean (SD) age of 61.84 (8.47) years. At the end of treatment, the variation of HAM-A score was 0.22 (95% CI, −0.63 to 1.07; $P=0.62$) between the real acupuncture and sham acupuncture groups. At the end of follow-up, the real acupuncture group had a significant 7.03-point greater (95% CI, 6.18 to 7.88; $P<0.001$) reduction in HAM-A score compared with the sham acupuncture group. Four mild adverse reactions occurred during the study.

CONCLUSIONS AND RELEVANCE　This study found acupuncture to be an effective treatment for anxiety in patients with PD. These findings suggest that acupuncture may enhance the wellbeing of patients who have PD and anxiety.

2. Expert Comments

Comment 1

As a neurodegenerative disease, PD is accompanied by a series of related symptoms, which severely impact the quality of life of patients and promote the progression of the disease. Effectively utilizing the benefits of acupuncture and moxibustion to treat these complications holds great significance and is deserving of broader recognition and adoption within the medical field. In this regard, the acupuncture and moxibustion research team of Guangzhou University of traditional Chinese medicine has made remarkable progress.

The team's research addressed challenges in modern medical treatment, such as the high incidence of PD complications and the uncertain efficacy of drug therapies, while focusing on the potential effectiveness of acupuncture and moxibustion. Initially, no data confirmed their efficacy. Using the standard model of modern medical research, the study employed standardized acupuncture stimulation and internationally recognized scales as outcome measures to verify that acupuncture can reduce anxiety in patients with anxiety disorders complicated by PD. Additionally, the study demonstrated that acupuncture can lower elevated stress hormone levels, thereby alleviating anxiety. The research design was clear and well-structured. The study adhered to the principles of traditional Chinese medicine for acupuncture and moxibustion diagnosis and treatment, with selection of acupoints based on traditional Chinese medicine theory and prior clinical practice. For example, all patients were clinically monitored, special devices were used to insert needles by the study operators, and patients in both groups were blinded to group assignment and intervention methods. Additionally, all patients were evaluated by psychologists who were unaware of the study design and patient grouping. The results are credible, and the conclusions reliable, making this paper a strong candidate for publication in top-tier journals, serving as a model for clinical research on acupuncture and moxibustion.

This study also highlighted some common problems in current acupuncture and moxibustion research, such as completely replicating the Western medicine model, which makes it challenging to showcase the individualized treatment approach of traditional Chinese medicine, and it is difficult to reflect the syndrome differentiation of traditional Chinese medicinein research, among other issues. Similar problems should be noted and considered by the industry.

Comment 2

In terms of study design and process implementation, the study employed a single-center, randomized, double-blind design to evaluate the effectiveness of real acupuncture compared with sham acupuncture in alleviating anxiety symptoms in patients with PD. The sample size was calculated based on evidence from a pilot study, and the sample size met the necessary requirements and supported the validity of the experimental design, ensuring the feasibility of the study. The reporting process followed both the consolidated standards of reporting trials (CONSORT) guidelines and the standards for reporting of interventions in clinical trials of acupuncture (STRICTA) specifications to ensure the reliability of the findings.

In terms of the selection and application of clinical research methodologies and statistical methods, the main outcome was the difference between the real acupuncture group and the sham acupuncture group in the change in HAM-A scores--a quantitative variable after treatment and during follow up. Regarding the analysis strategy, the study constructed a generalized linear regression model and introduced an interaction term between group and follow-up time to test whether there was a difference between the groups in the change in HAM-A scores at different periods compared to baseline. This statistical method was feasible and effective. Additionally, besides reporting the traditional between-group mean difference, the study also reported Cohen's d and other indicators to quantify between-group differences, providing double assurance for the reliability of the results at the level of indicator calculation.

Section 20 Introduction and Comments of *Effectiveness of Acupuncture for Pain Control After Cesarean Delivery: A Randomized Clinical Trial*

1. Introduction

IMPORTANCE A pharmacological approach to pain control after cesarean delivery is often insufficient on its own. Acupuncture is a promising method for mitigating postoperative pain and reducing postoperative opioid requirements.

OBJECTIVE To evaluate the efficacy and effectiveness of acupuncture as an adjunctive therapy for pain control after cesarean delivery, compared with a placebo intervention and standard care alone.

DESIGN, SETTING, AND PARTICIPANTS This single-center, placebo-controlled, patient-and assessor-blinded randomized clinical trial was conducted from January 13, 2015, to June 27, 2018, at a tertiary university hospital in Greifswald, Germany. Participants were women who were scheduled for elective cesarean delivery under spinal anesthesia and were randomized to either the acupuncture group (n=60) or placebo group (n=60). Another 60 consecutive patients who met the eligibility criteria and received the standard postoperative analgesia were selected to form a nonrandomized standard care group. The intention-to-treat analysis was performed from August 19, 2019, to September 13, 2019.

INTERVENTIONS In addition to standard pain treatment, each patient in the acupuncture group received auricular and body acupuncture with indwelling intradermal needles, whereas patients in the placebo group were treated with nonpenetrating placebo needles.

MAIN OUTCOMES AND MEASURES The primary outcome was pain intensity on movement, which was measured using an 11-item verbal rating scale. Secondary outcomes were analgesia-related adverse effects, analgesics consumption, time to mobilization and Foley catheter removal, quality of patient blinding to randomization, and patient satisfaction with treatment of pain.

RESULTS A total of 180 female patients (mean [SD] age, 31 [5] years) were included in the intentionto-treat analysis. The mean pain intensity on movement in the acupuncture group on the first postoperative day was lower than in the placebo group (4.7 [1.8] vs 6.0 [2.0] points; Cohen d, 0.73; 95% CI, 0.31-1.01; P=0.001) and the standard care group (6.3 [1.3] points; Cohen d, 1.01; 95% CI, 0.63-1.40; P<0.001). On the first postoperative day, 59 patients (98%) in the acupuncture group were fully mobilized vs 49 patients (83%) in the placebo group (relative risk [RR], 1.18; 95% CI, 1.06-1.33; P=0.01) and 35 patients (58%) in the standard care group (RR, 1.69; 95% CI, 1.36-2.09; P<0.001). The Foley catheter was removed in a total of 57 patients (93%) from the acupuncture group vs 43 patients (72%) from the placebo group (RR, 1.33; 95% CI, 1.12-1.57; P=0.003) and 42 patients (70%) from the standard care group (RR, 1.37; 95% CI, 1.14-1.62; P=0.002). Other parameters were comparable across the 3 study groups.

CONCLUSIONS AND RELEVANCE Results of this trial showed that acupuncture was safe and effective in reducing pain and accelerating mobilization of patients after cesarean delivery. With consideration for personnel and time expenditures, acupuncture can be recommended as routine, supplemental therapy for pain control in patients after elective cesarean delivery.

2. Expert Comments

Comment 1

Pain management after cesarean delivery has become a key issue to be solved in clinical practice because of its far-reaching impact on the rehabilitation process, quality of life, and utilization efficiency of medical resource of parturients. The implementation of effective pain management strategies is of great significance for promoting the rapid recovery of parturients, improving their quality of life and optimizing the allocation of medical resources. In view of the strict restrictions on the use of analgesic medications, it is particularly important to seek non-drug analgesic means.

As a non-drug and low-risk means of analgesia, the unique advantage of acupuncture is that it can reduce drug dependence, reduce side effects, and promote the body's ability to regulate itself. In recent years, various clinical studies on the application of acupuncture and moxibustion therapy in perioperative analgesia have emerged in an endless stream, and the efficacy of acupuncture and moxibustion analgesia has been widely recognized worldwide and has gradually become an important part of postoperative pain management. Its non-drug characteristics are especially suitable for pregnant women who have strict restrictions or preferences on drug use, thus exhibiting unique advantages and high rationality in the field of pain management after cesarean delivery.

In clinical research of acupuncture and moxibustion therapy, the reasonality of the placebo group is a key link to ensure the scientificity and accuracy of the research results. Given the complexity and diversity of acupuncture and moxibustion, researchers should comprehensively consider the operability, safety, difficulty of blinding implementation, and minimization of therapeutic effect of placebo acupuncture. This study used auricular acupuncture combined with intradermal acupuncture, including a simple operation process, high safety and continued stability stimulation, to achieve the standardization of the intervention and effective implementation of the blinding method. Furthermore, the placebo effect was enhanced by using tools to make the participants feel real pain before the placebo acupuncture operation, which ensured the successful implementation of the blinding method, to more accurately evaluate the efficacy of acupuncture.

Comment 2

(1) Study design and setting

The study used a single-center, placebo-controlled, patient and assessor double-blind design with an additional non-randomized control group to ensure the reliability and reproducibility of the results, and to provide a baseline comparison for the effects of conventional care. The study used a sealed envelope for randomization, and the randomization and intervention were conducted by three skilled physicians. This design ensures the concealment of randomization and blind evaluation of the results and reduces selection and information biases. The placebo effect was effectively controlled given the rigorous intervention design for the acupuncture and placebo groups. During the intervention, sham acupuncture needles and nerve pens were used to ensure consistency in the sensory experience between the control and experimental groups.

(2) Selection and application of clinical research methodology and statistical methods

The primary endpoint outcome of the study was pain intensity during exercise on the first postoperative day, which was measured using an 11-item verbal rating scale that was simple and easy to use, and effectively quantified pain intensity; the secondary endpoint outcome included various pain and functional recovery indicators and adverse reactions, which comprehensively assessed the effectiveness and safety of acupuncture. Sample size calculation was based on power analysis and significance levels, ensuring statistical power. The study used an intention-to-treat analysis, in which the data of all randomized patients were included in the final analysis, ensuring the principle of randomization, and reducing bias. Appropriate statistical methods were selected according to the data type, including t-tests and the Mann-Whitney U test. The study showed high scientificity and rigor in terms of research design and selection of statistical methods. The application of random allocation, multi-group control, double-blind implementation, and intention-to-treat analysis ensured the validity and reliability of the results, but there were still some limitations, including the fact that the study was conducted in a single medical center, which may have limited the external validity of the results and their wide application. Finally, the study focused on pain intensity and other short-term outcomes on the first day after surgery, and did not evaluate long-term effects.

Section 21　Introduction and Comments of *Acupuncture for the Treatment of Diarrhea-Predominant Irritable Bowel Syndrome: A Pilot Randomized Clinical Trial*

1. Introduction

IMPORTANCE　Acupuncture is a promising therapy for irritable bowel syndrome (IBS), but the use of subjective scales as an assessment is accompanied by high placebo response rates.

OBJECTIVES　To preliminarily test the feasibility of using US Food and Drug Administration (FDA)-recommended end points to evaluate the efficacy of acupuncture in the treatment of IBS.

DESIGN, SETTING, AND PARTICIPANTS　This pilot, multicenter randomized clinical trial was conducted in 4 tertiary hospitals in China from July 1, 2020, to March 31, 2021, and 14-week data collection was completed in March 2021. Individuals with a diagnosis of IBS with diarrhea (IBS-D) were randomized to 1 of 3 groups, including 2 acupuncture groups (specific acupoints [SA] and nonspecific acupoints [NSA]) and a sham acupuncture group (non-acupoints [NA]) with a 1 : 1 : 1 ratio.

INTERVENTIONS　Patients in all groups received twelve 30-minute sessions over 4 consecutive weeks at 3 sessions per week (ideally every other day).

MAIN OUTCOMES AND MEASURES　The primary outcome was the response rate at week 4, which was defined as the proportion of patients whose worst abdominal pain score (score range, 0-10, with 0 indicating no pain and 10 indicating unbearable severe pain) decreased by at least 30% and the number of type 6 or 7 stool days decreased by 50% or greater.

RESULTS　Ninety patients (54 male [60.0%]; mean [SD] age, 34.5 [11.3] years) were enrolled, with 30 patients in each group. There were substantial improvements in the primary outcomes for all groups (composite response rates of 46.7% [95% CI, 28.8%-65.4%] in the SA group, 46.7% [95% CI, 28.8%-65.4%] in the NSA group, and 26.7% [95% CI, 13.0%-46.2%] in the NA group), although the difference between them was not statistically significant (P=0.18). The response rates of adequate relief at week 4 were 64.3% (95% CI, 44.1%-80.7%) in the SA group, 62.1% (95% CI, 42.4%-78.7%) in the NSA group, and 55.2% (95% CI, 36.0%-73.0%) in the NA group (P=0.76). Adverse events were reported in 2 patients (6.7%) in the SA group and 3 patients (10%) in NSA or NA group.

CONCLUSIONS AND RELEVANCE　In this pilot randomized clinical trial, acupuncture in both the SA and NSA groups showed clinically meaningful improvement in IBS-D symptoms, although there were no significant differences among the 3 groups. These findings suggest that acupuncture is feasible and safe; a larger, sufficiently powered trial is needed to accurately assess efficacy.

2. Expert Comments

Comment 1

IBS is a functional gastrointestinal disorder with

abdominal pain, bloating, changes in defecation habits, and/or changes in stool morphology as the main clinical symptoms. IBS-D is the most common clinical subtype, and antidiarrheal and antispasmodic drugs are used as the first-line therapy. However, these drugs can only temporarily alleviate a single symptom and have frequent side effects. Long-term medication increases the incidence of adverse events such as cardiovascular disease, resulting in low patient satisfaction, which is why many patients will opt out of using such drugs. This study used a multicenter randomized controlled clinical design to objectively evaluate the effectiveness and safety of the "Xia He acupoints" and "Mu acupoints" in treating visceral diseases to provide medical evidence for the principle of acupoint compatibility for the acupuncture treatment of intestinal diseases, which can be clinically popularized and applied.

This study used the effective response rate recommended by the Food and Drug Administration (FDA) as the main outcome of acupuncture treatment for IBS-D. The multicenter randomized controlled clinical trial was performed in four tertiary hospitals in China. Ninety patients with IBS-D were randomly divided into one of three groups, including two acupuncture groups (specific acupoints and nonspecific acupoints) and a sham acupuncture group (non-acupoints) at a 1 : 1 : 1 ratio. All patients received 12 sessions over 4 consecutive weeks at a frequency of 3 sessions per week. The primary outcome was the proportion of patients with at least 30% reduction in the worst abdominal pain score and a 50% or greater reduction in the number of stool days at week 4. The results showed that both the specific acupoint group (effective response rate of 46.7%) and the non-specific acupoint group (effective response rate of 46.7%) showed clinically significant improvement, which was higher than that of the sham acupuncture group (26.7%), and the specific acupoint group showed a more stable trend in the improvement of the secondary outcomes including overall symptom relief and quality of life.

Comment 2

(1) Study design and setting

This multicenter, randomized, controlled pilot study was performed to test the feasibility of using FDA-recommended end points to evaluate the efficacy of acupuncture treatment for IBS. The study was rigorously designed and employed a randomized, patient and assessor double-blind, multi-group-controlled design to ensure the reliability of the results and reduce bias. Patients were randomly assigned to one of three groups (specific acupoints, nonspecific acupoints, and sham acupuncture) and were recruited from four tertiary hospitals, enhancing the external validity of the results. The acupuncture method and acupuncture point selection were clearly described, which contributed to the study's reproducibility.

(2) Selection and application of clinical research methodology and statistical methods

The primary outcome of the study was the composite response rate at week 4 of the treatment phase, and the secondary outcomes included the composite response rate of other time points, symptom severity, quality of life, depression, and adverse reactions, which provided multi-dimensional data to comprehensively evaluate the efficacy and safety of acupuncture. The intention-to-treat principle was applied to all efficacy analyses, and per-protocol analysis was used for the primary outcome. The results remained consistent across the two analysis methods. In addition, missing data were imputed using the last observation carried forward method. For the primary outcome, a logistic generalized linear mixed model was used to process the repeated measurement data of patients at different time points, considering individual variability and time effects. For the secondary outcome and blind quality assessment, appropriate statistical methods were selected according to the data type, including the analysis of variance and chi-square test. The research design and statistical analysis of this study were scientifically sound and rigorous; however, there were some limitations that need to be noted. First, this was a pilot trial that did not employ strict sample size estimation. Although the results can provide reference data for future large-scale studies, it may not be able to obtain reliable and accurate results. Second, although the patients were followed up for 8 weeks, the long-term efficacy and persistence of the effects of acupuncture in IBS with diarrhea treatment remain unclear. In addition, the study participants were all Chinese, which limits the generalizability of the results in other countries and races. Finally, many outcome measures relied on patient self-reports, which may be affected by subjective bias and expectation effects.

Section 22 Introduction and Comments of *Comparison of Acupuncture vs Sham Acupuncture or Waiting List Control in the Treatment of Aromatase Inhibitor-Related Joint Pain: A Randomized Clinical Trial*

1. Introduction

IMPORTANCE Aromatase inhibitors (AIs) have proven efficacy for the treatment of hormone-sensitive breast cancer; however, arthralgias (pain and stiffness) contribute to nonadherence with therapy for more than 50% of patients.

OBJECTIVE To examine the effect of acupuncture in reducing AI-related joint pain through 52 weeks.

DESIGN, SETTING, AND PARTICIPANTS A randomized clinical trial was conducted at 11 sites in the US from May 1, 2012, to February 29, 2016, with a scheduled final date of follow-up of September 5, 2017, to compare true acupuncture (TA) with sham acupuncture (SA) or waiting list control (WC). Women with early-stage breast cancer were eligible if they were taking an AI and scored 3 or higher on the Brief Pain Inventory Worst Pain (BPI-WP) item (score range, 0-10; higher scores indicate greater pain). Analysis was conducted for data received through May 3, 2021.

INTERVENTIONS Participants were randomized 2 : 1 : 1 to the TA ($n=110$), SA ($n=59$), or WC ($n=57$) group. The TA and SA protocols were composed of 6 weeks of intervention at 2 sessions per week (12 sessions overall), followed by 6 additional weeks of intervention with 1 session per week. Participants randomized to WC received no intervention. All participants were offered 10 acupuncture sessions to be used between weeks 24 and 52.

MAIN OUTCOMES AND MEASURES In this long-term evaluation, the primary end point was the 52-week BPI-WP score, compared by study group using linear regression, adjusted for baseline pain and stratification factors.

RESULTS Among 226 randomized women (mean [SD] age, 60.7 [8.6] years; 87.7% White; mean [SD] baseline BPI-WP score, 6.7 [1.5]), 191 (84.5%) completed the trial. In a linear regression, 52-week mean BPI-WP scores were 1.08 (95% CI, 0.24-1.91) points lower in the TA compared with the SA group ($P=0.01$) and were 0.99 (95% CI, 0.12-1.86) points lower in the TA compared with the WC group ($P=0.03$). In addition, 52-week BPI pain interference scores were statistically significantly lower in the TA compared with the SA group (difference, 0.58; 95% CI, 0.00-1.16; $P=0.05$). Between 24 and 52 weeks, 12 (13.2%) of TA, 6 (11.3%) of SA, and 5 (10.6%) of WC patients reported receipt of acupuncture.

CONCLUSIONS AND RELEVANCE In this randomized clinical trial, women with AI-related joint pain receiving 12 weeks of TA had reduced pain at 52 weeks compared with controls, suggesting longterm benefits of this therapy.

2. Expert Comments

Comment 1

AIs have proven efficacy for the treatment of hormone-sensitive breast cancer; however, arthralgias (pain and stiffness) contribute to nonadherence to therapy for more than 50% of patients. In this context, this paper reported the sustained benefits of acupuncture. In this trial, postmenopausal women with stage 1 to 3 breast cancer using AIs for 30 days or longer were randomly assigned to TA, SA, and WC groups. Both TA and SA consisted of 18 treatments, and 30 to 45 minutes as a session administered within the course of 12 weeks. SA was performed through shallow needle insertion using thin and short needles at non-acupuncture points. The BPI-WP score at Week 52 was measured as the primary outcome. This study showed a statistically significant reduction in the duration of joint pain at Week 52 in postmenopausal women with early breast cancer who had AI-related arthralgia compared with SA or no acupuncture (WC group). This study highlights the durability of acupuncture responses over 1 year and the importance of adequately assessing the effects of acupuncture interventions using both SA group and WC group. Given the current mixed results of pharmacological and non-pharmacological therapies for AI-associated arthralgia, and the fact that the durability of the effects of acupuncture has not been documented, the results of this study confirmed the continued benefit of acupuncture in patients with AI-associated arthralgia. This mechanism of analgesia may be related to previous reports that acupuncture at acupoints activates the vago-adrenal pathway and produces anti-inflammatory effects.

Comment 2

(1) Study design

This was a multicenter, blinded SA and WC randomized clinical trial. This study followed the consolidated standards of reporting trials (CONSORT) reporting guidelines, the standard for reporting randomized controlled trials, which met the basic conditions of the pre-publish journal.

(2) Setting

The study protocol was registered at *Clinicaltrials.gov* in advance and published prior to the study. This is an important prerequisite for the publication of high-level clinical research.

The study participants were randomly assigned to TA, SA, and WC groups, with randomization dynamically balanced by study site. For TA, stainless steel, single-use, sterile, and disposable needles were used and inserted at traditional depths and angles. The SA protocol consisted of a core standardized prescription of minimally invasive, shallow needle insertion using thin and short needles at non-acupuncture points. The WC group received no acupuncture during the initial 24 weeks of study participation. The efficacy of acupuncture treatment could be better reflected through comparisons with the two control groups.

(3) Clinical study methodology and statistical methods

The primary outcome of the study was the BPI-WP score at 52 weeks. The sample size was determined based on the primary outcome. The primary hypothesis of this study was that TA would reduce joint pain associated with AI use at 52 weeks compared to SA or WC. No adjustments for multiple comparisons were made for any secondary or post-hoc analysis, which were considered exploratory. Under intention to-treat, all evaluable 52-week assessments were used, even if the WC patients received TA after 24 weeks. The 52-week BPI-WP scores were compared by group using multivariable linear regression adjusting for the baseline score and indicator variables for study sites, with two indicator variables representing the different intervention groups. Longitudinal analyses using all assessments for each patient-reported outcome domain through Week 52 were conducted using linear mixed models, with individuals considered random effects and the assessment time (as both a linear and quadratic function) and its potential interaction with treatment considered fixed effects. Regression analyses included covariate adjustment for the baseline score, indicator variables for the study sites, and two indicator variables for the intervention group. The proportion of patients per group who discontinued use of AIs or who used any pain medications (including acetaminophen, ibuprofen, other nonsteroidal anti-inflammatory drugs, or narcotics) after the initial on-study assessment was tested. This study employed a rigorous and appropriate statistical methodology.

Section 23　Introduction and Comments of *Effect of Adjunctive Acupuncture on Pain Relief Among Emergency Department Patients With Acute Renal Colic Due to Urolithiasis: A Randomized Clinical Trial*

1. Introduction

IMPORTANCE　Renal colic is described as one of the worst types of pain, and effective analgesia in the shortest possible time is of paramount importance.

OBJECTIVES　To examine whether acupuncture, as an adjunctive therapy to analgesics, could accelerate pain relief in patients with acute renal colic.

DESIGN, SETTING, AND PARTICIPANTS　This single-center, sham-controlled, randomized clinical trial was conducted in an emergency department in China between March 2020 and September 2020. Participants with acute renal colic (Visual Analog Scale [VAS] score ≥4) due to urolithiasis were recruited. Data were analyzed from October 2020 to January 2022.

INTERVENTIONS　After diagnosis and randomization, all patients received 50 mg/2 ml of diclofenac sodium intramuscular injection immediately followed by 30-minute acupuncture or sham acupuncture.

MAIN OUTCOMES AND MEASURES　The primary outcome was the response rate at 10 minutes after needle manipulation, which was defined as the proportion of participants whose VAS score decreased by at least 50% from baseline. Secondary outcomes included response rates at 0, 5, 15, 20, 30, 45, and 60 minutes, rescue analgesia, and adverse events.

RESULTS　A total of 115 participants were screened and 80 participants (66 men [82.5%]; mean [SD] age, 45.8 [13.8] years) were enrolled, consisting of 40 per group. The response rates at 10 minutes were 77.5% (31 of 40) and 10.0% (4 of 40) in the acupuncture and sham acupuncture groups, respectively. The between-group differences were 67.5% (95% CI, 51.5% to 83.4%; $P<0.001$). The response rates of acupuncture were also significantly higher than sham acupuncture at 0, 5, 15, 20 and 30 minutes, whereas no significant difference was detected at 45 and 60 minutes. However, there was no difference between the 2 groups in rescue analgesia rate (difference 2.5%; 95% CI −8.8% to 13.2%; $P>0.99$). No adverse events occurred during the trial.

CONCLUSIONS AND RELEVANCE These findings suggest that acupuncture plus intramuscular injection of diclofenac is safe and provides fast and substantial pain relief for patients with renal colic compared with sham acupuncture in the emergency setting. However, no difference in rescue analgesia was found, possibly because of the ceiling effect caused by subsequent but robust analgesia of diclofenac. Acupuncture can be considered an optional adjunctive therapy in relieving acute renal colic.

2. Expert Comments

Comment 1

Renal colic is one of the most severe pains a patient can feel. Therefore, effective analgesia in the shortest possible time is essential for the treatment of renal colic. The mean duration of pain relief after intramuscular diclofenac sodium injection was 18.64 minutes. However, 37.5% of patients still experienced moderate or severe pain at 15 minutes. Therefore, it is very important to seek effective and feasible treatment to accelerate pain relief for patients with renal colic in the emergency department.

The study combined acupuncture with intramuscular injection of diclofenac sodium, employing an integrative approach of traditional Chinese and Western medicine to relieve renal colic. The purpose of this study was to investigate whether acupuncture as an adjunctive therapy to analgesics could accelerate pain relief in patients with acute renal colic. In this study, 80 patients with renal colic caused by urinary calculi were randomly divided into an acupuncture group or a sham acupuncture group. Patients in the acupuncture group received treatment with bilateral acupuncture at the EX-UE7 (Yaotongdian) combined with diclofenac sodium for pain relief. In contrast, patients in the sham acupuncture group were administered shallow needling at non-acupoints along with diclofenac sodium. The findings suggest that acupuncture combined with intramuscular diclofenac sodium is safe for patients with renal colic in emergency situations and provides rapid and effective pain relief compared to sham acupuncture. Acupuncture can be considered an effective adjunctive therapy for relieving acute renal colic.

The design of this study was scientifically sound and rigorous and followed a standardized and reasonable process. The conclusions are credible, and the study was labor intense, providing high-quality evidence-based support for the use of traditional Chinese acupuncture combined with Western medicine in emergency departments for the rapid relief of renal colic. This approach holds substantial value for promoting acupuncture's clinical application in treating renal colic.

Comment 2

(1) Study design

This was a single-center, sham-acupuncture-controlled, randomized clinical trial. Reporting the results according to the consolidated standards of reporting trials (CONSORT) guidelines, which is the standard for reporting randomized controlled trials, is essential for publication in high-impact journals.

(2) Process implementation

Prior to the start of the study, the study protocol was pre-registered, and both the protocol and the statistical analysis plan were published in advance, meeting the key prerequisites for the publication of high-level clinical studies.

During the protocol implementation, patients were randomly assigned to acupuncture and sham acupuncture groups, following the requirements for allocation concealment and blinding. The blinding process involved concealing group assignments using sealed envelopes, which were maintained by research assistants who were not involved in recruitment, treatment, or assessment. To ensure effective blinding, the researchers skillfully used a convenient, scientifically sound, and reasonable scheme, successfully addressing the challenge of implementing blinding in acupuncture clinical trials. Unmasked personnel included the acupuncturists and research assistants responsible for the randomization module. All other study staff members and researchers, including patients, outcome assessors, and the statistician, were masked to the grouping.

(3) Clinical research methodology and statistical methods

The calculation of the sample size was determined by the researchers based on their own previous research and clinical experience. The proportion of patients with a decrease of ≥50% from baseline in the VAS score 10 minutes after acupuncture (effective response rate) was selected as the primary outcome measure. The primary outcome measure was selected based on clinical practice, addressing the clinical goal of whether acupuncture can treat patients who experience moderate to severe pain after 10 minutes of analgesic treatment. For statistical analysis, baseline characteristics were described as follows: continuous variables were reported as mean (standard deviation) or median (interquartile range); discrete variables were described as frequencies and percentages. The analysis was based on the intention-to-treat principle and included all randomized patients. The study assessed response rates, rescue analgesia, revisit and admission rates, and adverse events. For the VAS score, a comparison between groups was assessed using a mixed-effects model with repeated measurement analysis using corresponding scale scores at all time points as dependent variables, treatment as the main factor, treatment by time as the interaction effect, the baseline value as a covariate, and a random intercept to model within-subject correlations. The difference in the VAS score at 10 minutes was estimated with analysis of covariance adjusting for the baseline VAS score for the sensitivity analysis. The clinical methodology of the study was rigorous, and the statistical method was appropriate.

Section 24 Introduction and Comments of *Effect of Acupoint Hot Compress on Postpartum Urinary Retention After Vaginal Delivery: A Randomized Clinical Trial*

1. Introduction

IMPORTANCE Acupoint hot compress during the early postpartum period may benefit patients after a vaginal delivery, but the evidence of this effect is limited.

OBJECTIVE To assess whether acupoint hot compress involving the abdominal, lumbosacral, and plantar regions could reduce the incidence of postpartum urinary retention, relieve postpartum uterine contraction pain, prevent emotional disorders, and promote lactation.

DESIGN, SETTING, AND PARTICIPANTS This multicenter randomized clinical trial was conducted at 12 hospitals in China. Pregnant patients were screened for eligibility (n=13 949) and enrolled after vaginal delivery (n=1 200) between January 17 and August 15, 2021; data collection was completed on August 18, 2021. After vaginal delivery, these participants were randomized 1∶1 to either the intervention group or control group. Statistical analysis was based on per-protocol population.

INTERVENTIONS Participants in the control group received routine postpartum care. Participants in the intervention group received routine postpartum care plus 3 sessions of a 4-hour acupoint hot compress involving the abdominal, lumbosacral, and plantar regions within 30 minutes, 24 hours, and 48 hours after delivery.

MAIN OUTCOMES AND MEASURES The primary outcome was the incidence of postpartum urinary retention, defined as the first urination occurring more than 6.5 hours after delivery and/or use of an indwelling catheter within 72 hours after delivery. The secondary outcomes were postpartum uterine contraction pain intensity (assessed with the Visual Analog Scale [VAS]), depressive symptoms (assessed with the Edinburgh Postnatal Depression Scale), and lactation conditions (including lactation initiation time, breastfeeding milk volume, feeding mood and times, and newborn weight).

RESULTS Of the 1 200 participants randomized, 1 085 completed the study (537 in the intervention group and 548 in the control group, with a median [IQR] age of 26.0 [24.0-29.0] years). Participants in the intervention group compared with the control group had significantly decreased incidence of postpartum urinary retention (relative risk [RR], 0.58; 95% CI, 0.35-0.98; P=0.03); improved postpartum uterine contraction pain when measured at 6.5 hours (median [IQR] VAS score, 1 [1-2] vs 2 [1-2]; P<0.001), 28.5 hours (median [IQR] VAS score, 1 [0-1] vs 1 [1-2]; P<0.001), 52.5 hours (median [IQR] VAS score, 1 [0-1] vs 1 [0-1]; P<0.001), and 76.5 hours (median [IQR] VAS score, 0 [0-1] vs 0 [0-1]; P=0.01) after delivery; reduced depressive symptoms (RR, 0.73; 95% CI, 0.54-0.98; P=0.01); and increased breastfeeding milk volume measured at 28.5, 52.5, and 76.5 hours after delivery. No adverse events occurred in either of the 2 groups.

CONCLUSIONS AND RELEVANCE Results of this trial showed that acupoint hot compress after vaginal delivery decreased postpartum urinary retention, uterine contraction pain, and depressive symptoms and increased breastfeeding milk volume. Acupoint hot compress may be considered as an adjunctive intervention in postnatal care that meets patient self-care needs.

2. Expert Comments

Comment 1

Postpartum urinary retention is a common complication that significantly impacts postpartum rehabilitation if not treated promptly and is an urgent problem to be solved in the obstetric clinic. In this study, 1 200 patients with urinary retention after vaginal delivery were randomly assigned to either an intervention group or a control group. In total, 1 085 patients completed the study, 537 (89.5%) in the intervention group and 548 (91.3%) in the control group. The intervention group received routine postpartum care at 30 minutes, 24 hours, and 48 hours after delivery, and acupoint hot compresses for 4 hours at a constant average temperature of (45±2)℃. The acupoints used were CV8 (Shenque), BL31-BL34 (Baliao acupoints), and KI1 (Yongquan, bilateral sides). The control group received only routine postpartum care with no acupoint hot compress treatment.

The results showed a significant effect of acupoint hot compresses. Acupoint hot compresses applied to the abdominal, lumbosacral, and plantar regions decreased the incidence of postpartum urinary retention, reduced uterine contraction pain, improved depressive symptoms, and increased breastfeeding milk volume for individuals after vaginal delivery. This traditional Chinese medicine-assisted intervention in postpartum care has shown significant therapeutic benefits for postpartum complications and meets patient self-care needs.

The conclusion of this study provides new insights and methods for the clinical treatment of postpartum urinary retention. The study's rigorous design, scientifically sound and standardized research process, and reliable conclusions provide high-quality evidence-based medical data for the clinical treatment of this condition.

Comment 2

(1) Study design and process implementation

This randomized controlled trial was conducted at 12 hospitals to evaluate the effect of acupoint hot compresses on postpartum urinary retention and other indicators of postpartum recovery. The highlights of the study design and implementation are as follows: ①The study adopted a multicenter approach, which increased the external validity and generalizability of the results. ②The study employed strict randomization and blinding procedures. Patients were randomly assigned to either an acupoint hot compress group (intervention group) or a routine postpartum care group (control group), ensuring fairness in allocation. Although the nursing staff could not be fully blinded, statisticians who were blinded to the randomization were responsible for analyzing the data. ③The intervention was well-specified, using certified medical equipment to ensure consistency and repeatability.

(2) Selection and application of clinical research methodology and statistical methods

The primary outcome of the study was the incidence of postpartum urinary retention, and the secondary outcomes included the intensity of postpartum uterine contraction pain measured with the VAS, Edinburgh Postpartum Depression Scale score, breastfeeding milk volume, weight of the newborns, and incidence of adverse events, which comprehensively assessed the impact of acupoint hot compresses on postpartum recovery. The level of significance in the calculation of the sample size of the study was set at 0.025, the power of the test was set at 80%, and the rate of loss to follow up was set at 20%, which was reasonable, and the sample size was sufficient. For the primary outcome, the incidences of postpartum urinary retention in the intervention and control groups were compared using Fisher's exact test, and the relative risk (RR) and corresponding 95% CI were calculated. For the secondary outcomes, appropriate statistical methods were selected according to the type of data, including the Wilcoxon rank-sum test and t-test. However, the study did not use an intention-to-treat analysis, which may have led to overestimation of the efficacy of the intervention. In addition, the study was conducted during postpartum hospitalization, and the long-term effect of acupoint hot compresses remains unknown.

Section 25 Introduction and Comments of *Effectiveness of Electroacupuncture or Auricular Acupuncture vs Usual Care for Chronic Musculoskeletal Pain Among Cancer Survivors: The PEACE Randomized Clinical Trial*

1. Introduction

IMPORTANCE The opioid crisis creates challenges for cancer pain management. Acupuncture confers clinical benefits for chronic nonmalignant pain, but its effectiveness in cancer survivors remains uncertain.

OBJECTIVE To determine the effectiveness of electroacupuncture or auricular acupuncture for chronic musculoskeletal pain in cancer survivors.

DESIGN, SETTING, AND PARTICIPANTS The Personalized Electroacupuncture vs Auricular Acupuncture Comparative Effectiveness (PEACE) trial is a randomized clinical trial that was conducted from March 2017 to October 2019 (follow-up completed April 2020) across an urban academic cancer center and 5 suburban sites in New York and New Jersey. Study statisticians were blinded to treatment assignments. The 360 adults included in the study had a prior cancer diagnosis but no current evidence of disease, reported musculoskeletal pain for at least 3 months, and self-reported pain intensity on the Brief Pain Inventory (BPI) ranging from 0 (no pain) to 10 (worst pain imaginable).

INTERVENTIONS Patients were randomized 2 : 2 : 1 to electroacupuncture ($n=145$), auricular acupuncture ($n=143$), or usual care ($n=72$). Intervention groups received 10 weekly sessions of electroacupuncture or auricular acupuncture. Ten acupuncture sessions were offered to the usual care group from weeks 12 through 24.

MAIN OUTCOMES AND MEASURES The primary outcome was change in average pain severity score on the BPI from baseline to week 12. Using a gatekeeping multiple-comparison procedure, electroacupuncture and auricular acupuncture were compared with usual care using a linear mixed model. Noninferiority of auricular acupuncture to electroacupuncture was tested if both interventions were superior to usual care.

RESULTS Among 360 cancer survivors (mean [SD] age, 62.1 [12.7] years; mean [SD] baseline BPI score, 5.2 [1.7] points; 251 [69.7%] women; and 88 [24.4%] non-White), 340 (94.4%) completed the primary end point. Compared with usual care, electroacupuncture reduced pain severity by 1.9 points (97.5% CI, 1.4-2.4 points; $P<0.001$) and auricular acupuncture reduced by 1.6 points (97.5% CI, 1.0-2.1 points; $P<0.001$) from baseline to week 12. Noninferiority of auricular acupuncture to electroacupuncture was not demonstrated. Adverse events were mild; 15 of 143 (10.5%) patients receiving auricular acupuncture and 1 of 145 (0.7%) patients receiving electroacupuncture discontinued treatments due to adverse events ($P<0.001$).

CONCLUSIONS AND RELEVANCE In this randomized clinical trial among cancer survivors with chronic musculoskeletal pain, electroacupuncture and auricular acupuncture produced greater pain reduction than usual care. However, auricular acupuncture did not demonstrate noninferiority to electroacupuncture, and patients receiving it had more adverse events.

2. Expert Comments

Comment 1

(1) Analysis of topic selection

The study focused on the management of chronic musculoskeletal pain, particularly in the unique group of cancer survivors. With the increasing number of cancer survivors, long-term pain has become a key factor affecting quality of life, and the limitations of conventional pharmacological treatments are especially evident in the context of the opioid crisis. By comparing the effectiveness of electroacupuncture and auricular acupuncture with conventional treatments for chronic musculoskeletal pain in cancer survivors, the study aimed to provide new evidence-based data for the management of pain with the use of non-drug therapies. This study addressed frontline clinical needs and has significant international application potential, contributing to the globalization of acupuncture and its promotion in the oncology field.

(2) Implementation of acupuncture intervention

The design of the acupuncture intervention followed rigorous scientific principles. Electroacupuncture and auricular acupuncture were used in the study. The former enhances endogenous opioid release through electrical stimulation, while the latter is easy to operate and popularize. Both intervention groups received 10 weekly sessions of either electroacupuncture or auricular acupuncture, aligning with the conventional frequency of acupuncture treatments and ensuring the rationality of the intervention. The research team consisted of experienced acupuncturists, whose professional expertise reinforced the reliability of the treatment outcomes.

The electroacupuncture intervention was delivered by licensed acupuncturists with more than 5 years of experience in oncology settings. During treatment, specific acupoint selection and acupuncture angle, the pursuit of obtaining qi sensation, and setting of electrical stimulation parameters were adopted, which reflects the professionalism and individualization of acupuncture treatment. Acupuncturists followed a standardized protocol developed by the United States military, known as battlefield acupuncture. which is simple to operate and suitable for a wide range of clinical environments, especially for non-acupuncture professionals. Both acupuncture interventions were administered once a week for 10 weeks, resulting in a coherent treatment regimen. The control group received usual care, including medication and physical therapy, which provided the necessary reference for the results, although the lack of a sham control group may have introduced bias. The professional background and skills of the therapist ensure the quality of the acupuncture intervention and also highlight the influence of the therapist's qualifications on the effectiveness of the intervention. Rigorous in design and detail-oriented in implementation, this acupuncture intervention provided a solid basis for assessing the effectiveness of acupuncture in the management of chronic pain.

Comment 2

This was a stratified, randomized, three-arm, parallel-group, multicenter clinical trial aiming to verify the efficacy of electroacupuncture and auricular acupuncture in treating chronic musculoskeletal pain in cancer survivors and to compare the therapeutic effects of auricular acupuncture relative to electroacupuncture. Participants were randomly assigned at a 2 : 2 : 1 ratio to an electroacupuncture group, auricular acupuncture group, or standard care group. The intervention groups received 10 sessions of electroacupuncture or auricular acupuncture over 10 weeks, with the primary outcome measure being the average change from baseline in the Brief Pain Inventory pain severity score at 12 weeks. The trial was conducted across six centers, with a total of 676 participants screened, and 360 enrolled. Of these, the data of 358 were included in the analysis, comprising 145 in the electroacupuncture group, 142 in the auricular acupuncture group, and 71 in the standard care group. Two participants were excluded from the final analysis due to missing data at all follow-up points.

The trial had two primary hypotheses: First, that both electroacupuncture and auricular acupuncture would be superior to conventional treatment in reducing pain severity and second, if the first hypothesis was confirmed, auricular acupuncture would be non-inferior to electroacupuncture. Dmitrienko's two-step sequential gatekeeping procedure was employed for the control of type I errors. The sample size calculation fully accounted for the direction of hypothesis testing, type I and type II errors, effect size, and threshold values. A linear mixed model was used to analyze the primary outcome measure. These statistical strategies and methods ensured the reliability of the study's conclusion that both electroacupuncture and auricular acupuncture could effectively reduce the severity of chronic musculoskeletal pain in different groups of cancer survivors. However, the noninferiority of auricular acupuncture compared to electroacupuncture could not be demonstrated.

Section 26   Introduction and Comments of *Efficacy of Acupuncture for Chronic Prostatitis/Chronic Pelvic Pain Syndrome: A Randomized Trial*

1. Introduction

BACKGROUND   Acupuncture has promising effects on chronic prostatitis/chronic pelvic pain syndrome (CP/CPPS), but high-quality evidence is scarce.

OBJECTIVE   To assess the long-term efficacy of acupuncture for CP/CPPS.

DESIGN   Multicenter, randomized, sham-controlled trial.

SETTING   Ten tertiary hospitals in China.

PARTICIPANTS   Men with moderate to severe CP/CPPS, regardless of prior exposure to acupuncture.

INTERVENTION   Twenty sessions of acupuncture or sham acupuncture over 8 weeks, with 24-week follow-up after treatment.

MEASUREMENTS   The primary outcome was the proportion of responders, defined as participants who achieved a clinically important reduction of at least 6 points from baseline on the National Institutes of Health Chronic Prostatitis Symptom Index at weeks 8 and 32. Ascertainment of sustained efficacy required the between-group difference to be statistically significant at both time points.

RESULTS   A total of 440 men (220 in each group) were recruited. At week 8, the proportions of responders were 60.6% (95% CI, 53.7% to 67.1%) in the acupuncture group and 36.8% (CI, 30.4% to 43.7%) in the sham acupuncture group (adjusted difference, 21.6 percentage points [CI, 12.8 to 30.4 percentage points]; adjusted odds ratio, 2.6 [CI, 1.8 to 4.0]; $P<0.001$). At week 32, the proportions were 61.5% (CI, 54.5% to 68.1%) in the acupuncture group and 38.3% (CI, 31.7% to 45.4%) in the sham acupuncture group (adjusted difference, 21.1 percentage points [CI, 12.2 to 30.1 percentage points]; adjusted odds ratio, 2.6 [CI, 1.7 to 3.9]; $P<0.001$). Twenty (9.1%) and 14 (6.4%) adverse events were reported in the acupuncture and sham acupuncture groups, respectively. No serious adverse events were reported.

LIMITATION   Sham acupuncture might have had certain physiologic effects.

CONCLUSION   Compared with sham therapy, 20 sessions of acupuncture over 8 weeks resulted in greater improvement in symptoms of moderate to severe CP/CPPS, with durable effects 24 weeks after treatment.

2. Expert Comments

Comment 1

(1) Analysis of topic selection

How to focus on solving the difficult and prominent

Chapter 2 Comments of Clinical Trials of Acupuncture and Moxibustion in SCI Journals

issues in clinical practice, analyze the refinement and construction of key clinical issues, and reflect their value and significance.

Solving unmet clinical needs: The ultimate goal of clinical research is to serve the clinic and solve practical problems. This study examined CP/CPPS. In clinical practice, the incidence of CP/CPPS in men is high, which seriously affects physical and mental health. Drug treatment has limitations, and the medical burden is increasing. Acupuncture and moxibustion treatment of pain is effective; therefore, it is worth exploring acupuncture and moxibustion treatment for this disease.

Drawing lessons from the previous research results: Consulting the research papers related to the disease, understanding the main problems, research hotspots, and difficulties in the historical and current research fields, discovering the problems that have not been studied in depth, and providing ideas for the topic selection of the paper. A Cochrane review of CP/CPPS showed that acupuncture may relieve symptoms and is safe. However, another study found that there was little difference in acupuncture compared to sham acupuncture, although the quality of evidence was very low. In addition, the durability of the effects of acupuncture remains unclear. Therefore, based on the results of previous studies, it is necessary to conduct high-quality clinical studies of this disease.

The results have value: The results of this study showed that 8 weeks of acupuncture improved symptoms in moderate to severe CP/CPPS and had a lasting effect for at least 24 weeks after treatment. This trial demonstrated the long-term efficacy of acupuncture and provided high-quality evidence for clinical practice and guideline recommendations. Therefore, acupuncture and moxibustion treatment has no side effects, is safe and effective, has low cost, and is worth popularizing.

(2) Implementation of acupuncture intervention

The analysis of the acupuncture intervention's implementation included considerations such as the rationality of the acupuncture treatment, details of the acupuncture points, treatment plan, auxiliary intervention measures, background of the therapist, and setting of the control group.

Clinically appropriate treatment cycle: In this case, acupuncture treatment was started on the day of randomization, and a total of 20 acupuncture sessions were performed over 8 consecutive weeks, 3 times a week for the first 4 weeks (ideally every other day) and 2 times a week for the remaining 4 weeks (ideally every 2 or 3 days). CP/CPPS is a chronic pain disease, and the frequency of treatment in this study, 2 to 3 times per week, is close to clinical practice and reduces the number of patients seeking medical treatment.

Attention paid to the details of acupuncture administration: In this study, the description of acupuncture operation is very detailed, including the selection of needles, manipulation after insertion, interval and duration of needling, manipulation of needling, and effect achieved. According to the article, a total of 23 acupuncturists performed the treatment. They could have performed both acupuncture and sham acupuncture, and, to the extent possible, the study prioritized the same acupuncturist for the treatment of a particular participant throughout the trial. The only drawback was that there was no mention of the length of practice and professional titles of the acupuncturists.

Comment 2

The objective of this randomized, single-blind, sham acupuncture controlled, multicenter clinical trial was to verify the long-term efficacy of acupuncture in treating CP/CPPS for improvement of symptoms, pain, voiding dysfunction, and quality of life. Participants were randomly assigned at a 1 : 1 ratio to receive 20 acupuncture sessions for 8 weeks in either acupuncture or sham acupuncture groups, with the primary outcome measure being the response rate to the NIH-CPSI at 8th and 32nd weeks. A total of 735 participants from 10 centers were screened, of whom 440 were enrolled, 220 in the acupuncture group and 220 in the sham acupuncture group, and 414 completed the trial, including 206 in the acupuncture group and 208 in the sham acupuncture group. The intention-to-treat analysis included 440 cases.

In this study, the sample size was estimated based on previous literature, and a generalized linear mixed model was used in the main analysis. To control for type I errors, it was stipulated that only when the evaluation results at two timepoints were positive, could long-term efficacy of acupuncture be judged. The results showed that the NIH-CPSI response rates of the acupuncture group and sham acupuncture group were 60.6%, 61.5% and 36.8%, 38.3% at the 8th and 32nd weeks, respectively, and the differences were statistically significant, indicating that acupuncture could significantly improve the symptoms of CP/CPPS and had a long-term sustained effect. Moreover, the sensitivity analysis of the main analysis results was carried out using three methods, including multiple filling of missing data, excluding the data of patients who responded that they had received sham acupuncture during the blinding evaluation, and setting the "acupuncturist" variable of as the random effect. The conclusions of the analysis were consistent, which ensured the robustness of the research results.

Section 27　Introduction and Comments of *Effect of Briefing on Acupuncture Treatment Outcome Expectations, Pain, and Adverse Side Effects Among Patients With Chronic Low Back Pain: A Randomized Clinical Trial*

1. Introduction

IMPORTANCE　In observational studies, patients' treatment outcome expectations have been associated with better outcomes (ie, a placebo response), whereas concerns about adverse side effects have been associated with an in increase in the negative effects of treatments (ie, a nocebo response). Some randomized trials have suggested that communication from clinicians could affect the treatment outcomes by changing patients' expectations.

OBJECTIVE　To investigate whether treatment outcome expectations and reported adverse side effects could be affected by different briefing contents before a minimal acupuncture treatment in patients with chronic low back pain (CLBP).

DESIGN, SETTING, AND PARTICIPANTS　This randomized single-blinded clinical trial was conducted among patients with CLBP at 1 outpatient clinic in Switzerland who had a pain intensity of at least 4 on a numeric rating scale from 0 to 10. Different recruitment channels were used to enroll patients. Data were collected from May 2016 to December 2017 and were analyzed from June to November 2018.

INTERVENTIONS　Patients were randomized to receive either a regular expectation briefing or a high expectation briefing (effectiveness) and either a regular adverse side effect briefing or an intense adverse side effect briefing (adverse side effect) in a 2×2 factorial design. The intervention (briefing sessions and written materials) was standardized and delivered before the acupuncture treatment, with additional booster informative emails provided during the 4-week, 8-session acupuncture course.

MAIN OUTCOMES AND MEASURES　The primary end point was the patients' expectations regarding the effectiveness of the acupuncture treatment (Expectation for Treatment Scale [ETS]) after the briefing and the subsequent pain intensity (Numeric Rating Scale). The primary end point for the adverse side effect briefing was the adverse side effect score at the end of the acupuncture treatment, derived from session-by-session assessments of adverse side effects.

RESULTS　A total of 152 patients with CLBP (mean [SD] age, 39.54 [12.52] years; 100 [65.8%] women) were included. The estimated group difference (regular vs high) for the ETS was −0.16 (95% CI −0.81 to 0.50, *P*=0.64), indicating no evidence for a difference between intervention groups. There was also no evidence for a difference in pain intensity at the end of the acupuncture treatment between the groups with different expectation briefings. The adverse side effects score in the group with the intense adverse side effect briefing were estimated to be 1.31 times higher (95% CI, 0.94 to 1.82; *P*=0.11) than after a regular adverse side effect briefing, but the finding was not statistically significant.

CONCLUSIONS AND RELEVANCE　In this study, suggestions regarding treatment benefits (placebo) and adverse side effects (nocebo) did not affect treatment expectations or adverse side effects. Information regarding adverse side effects might require more research to understand nocebo responses.

2. Expert Comments

Comment 1

Depending on positive and negative recommendations, different results can be elicited from the placebo or nocebo effects. Clinically, physicians recommend acupuncture and other treatments to patients during consultations and inform patients of risks and benefits. The clinician's goal in this communication is to enhance the placebo effect and minimize the nocebo effect. This study is based on the effect of different outcomes on treatment, which has certain clinical significance.

This study's design differed from previous attempts to verify the efficacy and safety of acupuncture. Acupuncture was used as a non-drug intervention model to explore the effects of varied information disclosure on the expected efficacy, pain, and adverse reactions in chronic low back pain with 150 patients with CLBP receiving acupuncture treatment with different levels of emphasis placed in the pre-treatment briefing. Based on the placebo effect, the team used a 2×2 factorial design to randomly assign patients to be informed of routine expected effectiveness information or high expected effectiveness information and routine adverse reaction information or serious adverse reaction information. The intervention information is supported by evidence on the effectiveness and adverse effects of acupuncture in the treatment of chronic low back pain. Patients received eight acupuncture sessions over a 4-week period. Oral and written information was provided before and during the acupuncture sessions, and additional email instructions were provided during the sessions. The blinding of the acupuncturists, patients, and statisticians was a highlight of the study. The results of the study showed that information on treatment effectiveness and adverse effects did not affect treatment expectations or adverse effects. This result contradicts past beliefs regarding the issue and may affect the way physicians communicate with patients in the future.

Comment 2

(1) Study design and process implementation

This study explored the impact of different briefing messages on patient expectations and clinical outcomes through a randomized, single-blind, four-arm trial design. The study used a 2×2 factorial design, incorporating two independent factors, which were divided into four groups: conventional treatment effect briefing, high expected treatment effect briefing, conventional adverse side effect briefing, and strong adverse side effect briefing. Multiple factors and their interactions could be evaluated simultaneously in the same study, and the independent and combined effects of each factor could be understood more comprehensively, which increased efficiency. Rigorous randomization and the single-blind design could help reduce bias and improve the reliability of the results. The central block randomization employed in the study and the random sequence generated by independent statisticians could improve the balance between groups. In addition, all patients received the same standardized acupuncture treatment, and the consistency of the intervention was guaranteed.

(2) Selection and application of clinical research methodologies and statistical methods

The treatment expectation scale was used to measure the treatment expectations of patients, a numeric rating scale was used to assess pain intensity, and a 13-item self-report questionnaire was used to assess the score of adverse side effects. The sample size of the study was calculated in a scientifically sound manner, and the significance level and test power were set reasonably. In addition, multiple imputations were used to handle missing data. For treatment expectations, the study used analysis of covariance to assess whether there was a difference between the conventional treatment effect briefing group and high-expectancy treatment effect briefing group, with baseline treatment expectancy scale scores and sex as covariates to control for confounders on outcomes. For pain intensity, analysis of covariance was used and adjusted for covariates such as baseline pain intensity, sex, and baseline optimism and pessimism. For the adverse side effect scores, longitudinal zero-inflated negative binomial regression was used to assess the difference in scores between the conventional adverse side effect briefing group and intense adverse side effect briefing group after each acupuncture treatment. Zero-inflated negative binomial regression could handle excessive dispersion and zero inflation.

Section 28　Introduction and Comments of *Effect of Acupuncture on Atrial Fibrillation Stratified by CHA$_2$DS$_2$-VASc Score—A Nationwide Cohort Investigation*

1. Introduction

OBJECTIVE　This research aimed to make statements regarding the reduction in atrial fibrillation (AF) risk due to acupuncture, stratified by CHA$_2$DS$_2$-VASc score.

METHODS　The Kaplan-Meier method was performed to calculate cumulative incidence of outcomes for each group, and the log-rank test were performed to compare differences between groups. Incidences and hazard ratios (HRs) were estimated by univariate Cox proportional hazards models, and adjusted HRs (aHRs) were estimated by multivariate Cox proportional hazards models including demographic covariates and comorbid status.

RESULTS　In CHA$_2$DS$_2$-VASc scores of 0-1, 2-3, 4-5 and >5, cases with acupuncture were all associated with decreased incidence of AF (aHR 0.46 with 95% CI 0.42-0.51, $P<0.001$ in the CHA$_2$DS$_2$-VASc scores of 0-1; aHR 0.53 with 95% CI 0.50-0.57, $P<0.001$ in the CHA$_2$DS$_2$-VASc scores of 2-3; aHR 0.56 with 95% CI 0.52-0.61, $P<0.001$ in the CHA$_2$DS$_2$-VASc scores of 4-5; and aHR 0.64 with 95% CI 0.55-0.74, $P<0.001$ in the CHA$_2$DS$_2$-VASc scores of >5).

CONCLUSION　Protective effect of acupuncture on AF was observed in this study, and the effect was more obvious for those with fewer comorbidities.

2. Expert Comments

Comment 1

Acupuncture and moxibustion therapy is widely used in China, but there is a lack of high-quality evidence for its benefit for most diseases. AF is a common clinical arrhythmia problem. The greatest harm of long-term onset is the formation and shedding of the thrombus in the atrium, resulting in thromboembolism of the affected organs or brain tissue, with reduction or even cessation of the blood supply. In this study, a retrospective cohort design was employed to show that acupuncture may have a protective effect on AF, and the effect was more significant in patients with low CHA_2DS_2-VASc scores (low risk of AF stroke). This finding is consistent with the basic hypothesis that acupuncture acts by activating endogenous protective mechanisms whose operation can be better stimulated when the degree of functional injury in the body is relatively low. When the degree of injury is high, the possibility that acupuncture can exert an effect is bound to be affected. Therefore, in designing confirmatory studies in the future, we can consider individuals who are likely to benefit from acupuncture and moxibustion treatment to produce confirmatory conclusions.

This was a retrospective study based on diagnosis and treatment data, and the lack of records on acupuncture programs in the diagnosis and treatment information cannot support the comparative analysis of the benefits of different acupuncture programs. Whether there are effective acupuncture timings, the dose-response relationship of acupuncture benefits, and the persistence of acupuncture effects still need to be further explored.

Comment 2

(1) Study design and implementation

A cohort study design was adopted to investigate the protective effect of acupuncture treatment on the risk of morbidity in AF stratified per the CHA_2DS_2-VASc score.

According to the PICOST (Population, Intervention, Comparison, Outcome, Study Design, and Time) principle, the participants of this study were patients enrolled in the health insurance research database of Taiwan, China, from March 1, 1995, to December 31, 2013; the exposure was acupuncture treatment, and the exposure group received acupuncture treatment for the first time at the enrollment time. The control group received non-acupuncture treatment and was matched at a 1 : 1 ratio to the exposure group (but the study did not address the key methodological issue of the matching method used) ; the outcome was AF morbidity. Acupuncture treatment and AF data were derived from the prescription and disease diagnosis information at the time of the resident's medical visit in the health insurance database. A total of 235 866 participants in the exposure group and 235 866 participants in the control group were included in the study.

(2) Selection and application of clinical research methodologies and statistical methods

In this study, survival analysis was chosen to explore the protective effect of acupuncture treatment on the risk of morbidity in AF, and the selection of methods matched the characteristics of the data. In the survival analysis, the absence of AF, withdrawal, or death as of December 31, 2013, was defined as censoring. According to the CHA_2DS_2-VASc score (0 to 1; 2 to 3; 4 to 5; >5), after stratification, the study used the Kaplan-Meier method to calculate the cumulative incidence in each group, log-rank test to compare the differences between groups, and Cox proportional hazard model to estimate the hazard ratio after adjusting for confounders. Adjustment for confounders considered demographic characteristics (specific variables not identified in the text) and concomitant underlying diseases (hyperlipidemia, chronic obstructive pulmonary disease, chronic kidney disease, hyperthyroidism, sleep disorders, and gout). In addition, the area under the receiver operating characteristic curve was used to estimate the ability of the CHA_2DS_2-VASc score to predict AF in patients who received acupuncture and those who did not; however, the predictive model used was not described.

Section 29 Introduction and Comments of *Greater Somatosensory Afference With Acupuncture Increases Primary Somatosensory Connectivity and Alleviates Fibromyalgia Pain via Insular γ-Aminobutyric: A Randomized Neuroimaging Trial*

1. Introduction

OBJECTIVE Acupuncture is a complex multi-component treatment that has shown promise for the treatment of Fibromyalgia (FM), however, clinical trials have shown mixed results, possibly due to heterogeneous

Chapter 2 Comments of Clinical Trials of Acupuncture and Moxibustion in SCI Journals

methodology and lack of understanding of the underlying mechanism of action. We sought to understand the specific contribution of somatosensory afference to improvements in clinical pain, and the specific brain circuits involved.

METHODS 76 FM patients were randomized to receive 8 weeks (2 treatments/week) of electroacupuncture (EA, with somatosensory afference) or mock laser acupuncture (ML, with no somatosensory afference). Brief Pain Inventory (BPI) Severity, resting state functional MRI (rs-fMRI), and proton magnetic resonance spectroscopy (^{1}H-MRS) in the right anterior insula (aINS) were collected at pre- and post-treatment.

RESULTS FM patients receiving EA experienced a greater reduction in pain severity compared to ML (mean difference, EA=−1.14, ML=−0.46, Group×Time interaction, P=0.036). Participants receiving EA, as compared to ML, also displayed increased resting functional connectivity between the primary somatosensory cortical representation of the leg ($S1_{leg}$; i.e. S1 subregion activated by EA) and aINS. Increase in $S1_{leg}$-aINS connectivity was associated with reductions in BPI severity (r=−0.44, P=0.01) and increases in aINS gamma-aminobutyric acid (GABA+) (r=−0.48, P=0.046) following EA. Moreover, increases in aINS GABA+ was associated with reductions in BPI severity (r=−0.59, P=0.01). Finally, post-EA changes in aINS GABA+ mediated the relationship between changes in $S1_{leg}$-aINS and BPI severity, bootstrapped CI= (−0.533, −0.037).

CONCLUSION The somatosensory component of acupuncture modulates primary somatosensory functional connectivity in association with insular neurochemistry to reduce pain severity in FM.

2. Expert Comments

Comment 1

Acupuncture has a certain clinical efficacy in the treatment of FM; however, because of methodological issues and lack of clarity regarding the potential mechanisms, its clinical efficacy and regulatory mechanisms need to be further explored. Based on previous studies, this study suggested that EA produces better analgesic efficacy through somatosensory pathways in the central nervous system than placebo acupuncture. Therefore, the purpose of this study was to explore whether acupuncture can specifically regulate brain circuits and metabolites through somatosensory afferent pathways, thereby producing analgesic effects. A randomized controlled trial design was used, with simulated laser acupuncture as a placebo control to evaluate the clinical efficacy of the EA intervention in FM. Neuroimaging techniques, ie, blood oxygenation level dependent functional magnetic resonance imaging (BOLD-fMRI) and magnetic resonance spectroscopy (MRS) were used to observe the changes in brain functional connectivity and γ-GABA levels before and after acupuncture treatment.

The authors asserted that the study had at least four strengths. ①Study design: The study combined clinical research with neuroimaging research, both clarifying the clinical efficacy of acupuncture and preliminarily exploring its potential neural regulation mechanism. ②Selection of control group: The selection of comfort acupuncture was particularly ingenious, not only avoiding the influence of acupoint palpation and tactile stimulation on the curative effect of comfort acupuncture, but also better exploring the nerve regulation pathway of EA. ③Multimodal technique: The effect of acupuncture on functional connectivity and metabolite levels in the brain was comprehensively explored through multimodal neuroimaging techniques (BOLD-fMRI and MRS). ④There is a common limitation in the study of clinical regulation mechanisms, that is, it lacks direct causal evidence to support the regulatory mechanism of acupuncture on specific neural pathways. Although this study also had this problem, it further used mediation analysis based on correlation analysis to explain the direction of the acupuncture regulatory mechanism as best as possible.

Comment 2

(1) Study design and procedure implementation

To assess the central nervous system mechanisms of action of the somatosensory afferents of acupuncture and how these mechanisms produce an analgesic response in FM. The study used a single-center, blinded, randomized, sham-controlled trial design with dynamic block randomization. No information is provided in the paper regarding the method of sample size estimation and parameter setting. According to the PICO (Participant, Intervention, Control, Outcome) principles, the participants in this study were patients with FM who met the criteria of the trial. EA was used for the intervention; the control group received ML acupuncture. The number of treatments (2 times per week with 4 weeks) and the duration of each treatment were the same for EA and ML. The primary clinical outcome was the score on the Severity subscale of the BPI, mechanistic outcomes included resting state functional magnetic resonance imaging of the primary somatosensory cortex (the variable reported in the study was $S1_{leg}$ connectivity) and ^{1}H-MRS measurements of glutamate and glutamine and GABA+ in the right anterior insula (the variable reported in the study was GABA+/Cr), and secondary clinical outcomes included the Patient-Reported Outcomes Measurement Information System anxiety and depression scale scores. All outcomes were measured before and after the trial.

(2) Selection and application of clinical research methodology and statistical methods

Seventy-nine participants were included in the study, including 40 in the test group and 39 in the control group. Data analysis was based on the per-protocol set (35 participants in the test group and 37 participants in the control group). For the clinical outcome measures, the study used a repeated-measures analysis of variance to analyze the interaction of treatment and time, main effect of the treatment factor, main effect of time, and separate effect of the treatment factor. Pearson's correlation coefficient corrected for age was used to perform association analysis on the change values of $S1_{leg}$ connectivity, GABA+, and BPI severity before and after the test. In addition, the researchers used Fisher Z-transform for one-sided testing to determine whether the relationship assessed using Pearson's correlation coefficient differed in the direction of the correlation between the test and control groups. Finally, to assess whether GABA+/Cr mediated the effect of $S1_{leg}$ connectivity on BPI severity in the test group, the investigators performed a mediation analysis to calculate 95% CI for the indirect effect after adjusting for age with the bias-corrected Bootstrap percentile method.

Section 30 Introduction and Comments of *Efficacy of Intensive Acupuncture Versus Sham Acupuncture in Knee Osteoarthritis: A Randomized Controlled Trial*

1. Introduction

OBJECTIVE To assess the efficacy of intensive acupuncture (3 times weekly for 8 weeks) versus sham acupuncture for knee osteoarthritis (KOA).

METHODS In this multicenter randomized sham-controlled trial, participants with KOA were randomly assigned to receive electro-acupuncture (EA), manual acupuncture (MA) or sham acupuncture (SA) 3 times weekly for 8 weeks. Participants, outcome assessors and statisticians were masked to treatment group assignment. The primary outcome was the response rate, which is the proportion of participants who simultaneously achieved minimal clinically important improvement in pain and function at week 8. The primary analysis was analyzed by the Z-test for proportions with the modified intention-to-treat population, which included all randomized participants who have at least one post-baseline measurement.

RESULTS Out of 480 participants recruited in the trial, 442 were evaluated for efficacy. The response rates at week 8 were 60.3% (91/151), 58.6% (85/145), and 47.3% (69/146) in the EA, MA, and SA groups, respectively. The between-group differences were 13.0% (97.5% CI, 0.2% to 25.9%; P=0.023 4) for EA vs SA and 11.3% (97.5% CI, −1.6% to 24.4%; P=0.050 7) for MA vs SA. The response rates in EA and MA groups were both significantly higher than the SA group at weeks 16 and 26.

CONCLUSION Among patients with KOA, compared with SA, intensive EA resulted in less pain and better function at week 8 and these effects persisted though week 26. Intensive MA had no benefit for KOA at week 8, although it showed benefits during follow-up.

2. Expert Comments

Comment 1

This was a multicenter randomized controlled clinical trial of acupuncture and moxibustion performed in nine hospitals in China. The study focused mainly on whether EA was effective for KOA and the long-term efficacy of EA and MA. A control study with EA and SA, and MA and SA was designed. A total of 442 patients were enrolled. The same acupoints were used for the EA and MA groups (the selection of these acupoints conformed to the clinical reality of acupuncture and can be regarded as an effective acupuncture prescription), while eight non-acupoints, away from traditional acupoints or meridians, were used for the SA group. The three groups were treated three times a week, and the needle was retained for 30 minutes each time. The treatment lasted 8 weeks, and the follow up lasted 18 weeks, for a total study duration of 26 weeks. The changes in outcome indices were observed and recorded at 4th/6th/8th weeks of treatment and 16th/26th weeks of follow up, and the results were statistically analyzed.

The results showed the following: ①Patients with

KOA had different degrees of response to EA, MA, and SA, and the response rate was the highest for EA. ②EA and MA were superior to SA for pain improvement, and this advantage persisted at 26 weeks. ③During the study period, EA significantly improved knee function and stiffness as measured with the Western Ontario and McMaster Universities Arthritis Index (WOMAC), but there was no significant difference between MA and SA. ④In the overall evaluation of the patients, EA and MA were superior to SA at 4/8/16 weeks. ⑤There were no significant changes in the scores on the 12-item Brief Health Survey in the three interventions, either in terms of physiological or of psychological effects. Only at 26 weeks, EA and MA were slightly better than SA.

The above results may suggest that: ①In this study, he choice of a dummy needle for use in the placebo group may not have been appropriate. Although there were significant differences in the effects between EA and SA, and between MA and SA, the therapeutic effects of SA could not be concealed. However, treatment efficacy declined more rapidly in the sham group during the follow-up period. According to the theory of acupuncture and moxibustion, shallow needling is also a treatment method and can have a therapeutic effect. In this study, the shallow needling points were in the muscles or joints that can affect knee joint movement and can also have a certain effect on the affected knee. Therefore, the effect of this pseudo-acupuncture design may not be obvious, but it increases the effect of pseudo-acupuncture, resulting in a reduced difference between pseudo-acupuncture and EA, and pseudo-acupuncture and MA. ②EA and MA significantly improved pain over SA. The numeric rating scale and WOMAC indicators improved, and the number of patients who required analgesic support in the three groups reflected this. However, in the improvement of stiffness and function of the affected knee, EA was superior to SA in all time periods, while the difference between MA and SA was not very large; thus, EA may be superior to MA. This phenomenon may be related to the operation design of the hand needle set. In this study, there was no additional manipulation in the MA group except for the pursuit of the feeling of deqi, which is not consistent with the purposes of MA. Generally speaking, MA should also include some manipulation in the process of needle retention to better promote the prevalence of meridian qi and achieve a better curative effect. Moreover, the addition of manual manipulation in the MA group was more compatible with the continuous sparse-dense wave electrical stimulation in the EA group (of course, this may affect the success of the blinding method). If some manipulations are appropriately added to the manipulation of the MA group, the response rate in this group may be improved.

Another interesting conclusion of this study was that "there is no meaningful impact on the efficacy of acupuncture and moxibustion experience", which may disprove "Chinese patients have more experience of acupuncture and moxibustion, and their psychological expectations of acupuncture and moxibustion will be greater".

This was an excellent clinical study of acupuncture and moxibustion published recently. Meaningful selection of clinical questions, a rigorous study design, long treatment and observation periods, high success rate of the blinding method, and attention to the qualification of acupuncturists and unified training operations across the participating centers all ensured the quality of the study.

Comment 2

Eligible participants were randomly assigned to one of three groups using a central stratified randomization system at a 1 : 1 : 1 ratio. Randomization sequences were generated by independent statisticians using SAS 9.3, and stratified by hospital, with block lengths of 6 or 9, meeting randomization grouping and allocation concealment requirements. In Table 1, the authors did not present between-group comparisons, but the baseline characteristics of the groups were similar. Except for the acupuncturist, the participants, outcome evaluator, and statistician were blinded to the grouping. With the exception of the interventions, all other procedures and measures were the same across the groups. As data were missing, baseline imputation was used for the primary analysis and last carry-forward, deletion, and multiple imputations were used for the sensitivity analysis. The analysis of the primary and secondary outcomes was based on the adjusted intentionality analysis dataset, and the outcome indicators in each group were evaluated with the same method. The results showed that the evaluation method was credible, and the data analysis method was appropriate. The design of the study was reasonable, and the study met the standards of implementation and data analysis. To sum up, the conclusion is reliable.

Section 31 Introduction and Comments of *Electroacupuncture vs Prucalopride for Severe Chronic Constipation: A Multicenter, Randomized, Controlled, Noninferiority Trial*

1. Introduction

INTRODUCTION This multicenter, randomized, noninferiority trial compared electroacupuncture with prucalopride for the treatment of severe chronic constipation (SCC).

METHODS Participants with SCC (≤2 mean weekly complete spontaneous bowel movements [CSBMs]) were randomly assigned to receive either 28-session electroacupuncture over 8 weeks with follow-up without treatment over 24 weeks or prucalopride (2 mg/d before breakfast) over 32 weeks. The primary outcome was the proportion of participants with ≥3 mean weekly CSBMs over weeks 3-8, based on the modified intention-to-treat population, with −10% as the noninferior margin.

RESULTS Five hundred sixty participants were randomized, 280 in each group. Electroacupuncture was noninferior to prucalopride for the primary outcome (36.2% vs 37.8%, with a difference of −1.6% [95% confidence interval, −8% to 4.7%], $P<0.001$ for noninferiority); almost the same results were found in the per-protocol population. The proportions of overall CSBM responders through weeks 1-8 were similar in the electroacupuncture and prucalopride groups (24.91% vs 25.54%, with a difference of −0.63% [95% confidence interval, −7.86% to 6.60%, $P=0.864$]). Except during the first 2-week treatment, no between group differences were found in outcomes of excessive straining, stool consistency, and quality of life. Adverse events occurred in 49 (17.69%) participants in the electroacupuncture group and 123 (44.24%) in the prucalopride group. One non-treatment-related serious adverse event was recorded in the electroacupuncture group.

DISCUSSION Electroacupuncture was noninferior to prucalopride in relieving SCC with a good safety profile. The effects of 8-week electroacupuncture could sustain for 24 weeks after treatment. Electroacupuncture is a promising noninferior alternative for SCC.

2. Expert Comments

Comment 1

This was the first large-scale, strictly designed, head-to-head comparative study on electroacupuncture and prucalopride in patients with SCC, based on the high-quality research published by Professor LIU Baoyan and Professor LIU Zhishun in the *Annals of Internal Medicine* to confirm the intrinsic suitability or effectiveness of acupuncture treatment for patients with chronic severe functional constipation. To clarify the external validity of acupuncture treatment of SCC. In this trial, electroacupuncture was not inferior to prucalopride in terms of the percentage of participants with mean weekly CSBMs ≥3 in weeks 3-8, with sustained efficacy and better safety. The advantage of this study was that it used the internationally recognized CSBM as the core outcome index and was based on a preliminary trial, expanding the research from the internal authenticity of acupuncture treatment of SCC to the external authenticity in a stepwise manner, with a standardized research process and strong feasibility.

This study also reported some characteristics of electroacupuncture and prucalopride. For example, electroacupuncture has a better safety profile, and the therapeutic effect accumulates with treatment time, with the curative effect exceeding that of prucalopride in 6-8 weeks, reaching a peak in 8 weeks, and maintaining a similar effect with that of prucalopride for the whole follow-up period. However, prucalopride had a faster onset of action, within 2 weeks, and was stable throughout the trial. In the EA group, the effect was stable during treatment and follow up (the proportion of patients with mean weekly CSBMs ≥3 was 36.2% and 37.6% during follow up). In addition, EA was effective in relieving incomplete emptying sensations in patients with SCC, as evidenced by a significant difference in the baseline change in mean weekly SBMs between the EA and prucalopride groups from week 3 to week 32 (difference: −0.47 to −0.74). The difference in baseline change in mean weekly CSBMs was less pronounced between the groups (difference: −0.01 to −0.14). Subjective perception is a major component of CSBM, and the participants in this study were not blinded. Therefore, the feeling of complete emptying may have been a nonspecific effect of acupuncture, for instance derived from the close interaction between physicians and patients during acupuncture treatment and the higher expectations of patients for acupuncture. However, the nonspecific and specific effects of acupuncture are inseparable.

Furthermore, there is substantial difficulty in distinguishing between patients with irritable bowel syndrome and patients with functional constipation using laxatives according to the Rome III criteria, and some patients in this study may have had irritable bowel syndrome. Second, normal transit constipation and slow transit constipation or emptying disorder constipation were not distinguished, and subgroup analysis of the relevant subtypes could better identify the dominant population of electroacupuncture treatment.

In conclusion, electroacupuncture was not inferior to prucalopride in increasing the percentage of patients with CSBMs/week ≥3 at weeks 3-8, and it had a better safety profile. The effects of EA gradually accumulated during the 8-week treatment period and lasted for 24 weeks. For patients with SCC, electroacupuncture and prucalopride had similar effects in relieving discomfort and improving quality of life. Therefore, electroacupuncture is a valuable treatment for SCC.

Comment 2

Eligible participants who completed the two-week run-in period were randomized at a 1 : 1 ratio into two groups using a centralized network or randomization system. The randomization sequence was generated by an independent third-party application of SAS 9.3. Stratification took place by location, with variable block length, and met the requirements of randomization grouping and allocation concealment. In Table 1, the authors did not did not present between-group comparisons between groups, but the baseline characteristics of the groups were similar. There was a significant difference between the two interventions, and the participants in this trial were not blinded. With the exception of the interventions, all other procedures and measures were the same across the groups. Multiple imputations based on the hypothesis of missing at random was used for missing data for the primary outcome, and the sensitivity analysis was based on the per-protocol dataset, while no imputation was used for the secondary outcome. The baseline characterization and main analysis were based on the adjusted intentionality analysis dataset. The same method was used to evaluate the outcome indicators of the participants in each group. The evaluation method was reliable, the data analysis method was appropriate, and the study design was reasonable. The study met the standards of implementation and data analysis. To sum up, the conclusion is reliable.

Section 32 Introduction and Comments of *Manual Acupuncture Versus Sham Acupuncture and Usual Care for Prophylaxis of Episodic Migraine Without Aura: Multicentre, Randomised Clinical Trial*

1. Introduction

OBJECTIVE To assess the efficacy of manual acupuncture as prophylactic treatment for acupuncture naive patients with episodic migraine without aura.

DESIGN Multicenter, randomised, controlled clinical trial with blinded participants, outcome assessment, and statistician.

SETTING Seven hospitals in China, 5 June 2016 to 15 November 2018.

PARTICIPANTS 150 acupuncture naive patients with episodic migraine without aura.

INTERVENTIONS 20 sessions of manual acupuncture at true acupuncture points plus usual care, 20 sessions of non-penetrating sham acupuncture at heterosegmental non-acupuncture points plus usual care, or usual care alone over 8 weeks.

MAIN OUTCOME MEASURES Change in migraine days and migraine attacks per four weeks during weeks 1-20 after randomisation compared with baseline (four weeks before randomisation).

RESULTS Among 150 randomised patients (mean age 36.5 [SD 11.4] years; 123 [82%] women), 147 were included in the full analysis set. Compared with sham acupuncture, manual acupuncture resulted in a significantly greater reduction in migraine days at weeks 13 to 20 and a significantly greater reduction in migraine attacks at weeks 17 to 20. The reduction in mean number of migraine days was 3.5 (SD 2.5) for manual versus 2.4 (3.4) for sham (adjusted difference −1.4, 95% confidence interval −2.4 to −0.3; P=0.005) at weeks 13 to 16 and 3.9 (3.0) for manual versus 2.2 (3.2) for sham (adjusted difference −2.1, −2.9 to −1.2; P<0.001) at weeks 17 to 20. At weeks 17 to 20, the reduction in mean number of attacks was 2.3 (1.7) for manual versus 1.6 (2.5) for sham (adjusted difference −1.0, −1.5 to −0.5; P<0.001). No severe adverse events were reported. No significant difference was seen in the proportion of patients perceiving needle penetration between manual acupuncture and sham acupuncture (79% vs 75%; P=0.891).

CONCLUSIONS Twenty sessions of manual acupuncture was superior to sham acupuncture and usual care for the prophylaxis of episodic migraine without aura. These results support the use of manual acupuncture in patients who are reluctant to use prophylactic drugs or when prophylactic drugs are ineffective, and it should be considered in future guidelines.

2. Expert Comments

Comment 1

(1) Analysis of topic selection

This was a randomized clinical trial of acupuncture intervention for migraine, a common clinical condition and one that is suitable for acupuncture treatment. Focusing on several previous randomized clinical trials that found no difference between manual acupuncture and sham acupuncture, which was associated with inappropriate placebo-controlled settings, this study utilized non-penetrating sham acupuncture controls and blinded assessments to determine the efficacy of manual acupuncture and quantify the true placebo response in preventing migraines without aura. This study better reflected the actual effects of acupuncture in treating migraines and is conducive to promoting the international application of acupuncture therapy.

(2) Implementation of acupuncture intervention

In this clinical trial, the selection of acupoints in the acupuncture group was reasonable, and the description of the acupuncture process was clear and feasible. The 14 licensed acupuncturists providing treatment had more than five years of clinical experience and participated in intensive training prior to recruitment. The overall treatment plan was reasonable and sufficient to demonstrate the clinical effects, but the study duration was not sufficiently long to observe lasting effects, which comprises a limitation. No auxiliary interventions were used in this trial. Considering the issues with sham acupuncture involving penetrating needles in previous clinical trials, non-penetrating sham acupuncture was used as a control in this trial, and compliance was excellent, which is a major strength of the study. Although to ensure successful blinding, patients who had never received acupuncture treatment were recruited, non-penetrating needles were used as controls, and the same procedure was applied, there remains some doubt as to whether the blinding was truly effective, given that the selected acupoints differed from those in real acupuncture and the needling techniques were also notably different.

Comment 2

In designing this study, the research team considered many factors that could affect the trial outcomes and rigorously followed established principles for randomized clinical trials. The study results validated the hypothesis, the statistical methods were standardized, and the graphical and textual representations were largely accurate. However, the following issues remain, which may have reduced or weakened the intergroup differences.

(1) Study design and process implementation

In the randomization design, considering a block size of five is inappropriate, as it may introduce the risk of bias. In this study, the central block randomization method was employed, and the central randomization system was used for random allocation. "The block size stratified by center was 5" which carries a risk of selection or information bias. In the three-group design with a 2 : 2 : 1 grouping ratio, where the conventional group was not needled and the other two groups were needled, it was easy to infer the group assignments within a block size of 5, which could affect the evaluation of the results. Thus, a block size of 10 is suggested as more appropriate. Furthermore, considering the stratified design, "research center" should not be used as a stratification factor, as differences among research centers relate to the quality of implementation rather than to the characteristics of the disease population or the classification of interventions.

(2) Selection and application of clinical research methodology and statistical methods

① Inclusion criteria question: The international diagnostic criteria for headache were met. However, there were two primary efficacy measures "mean change in migraine days and the number of migraine attacks per four-week cycle from week 1 to week 20 after randomization compared to baseline (four weeks before randomization)". The inclusion criteria only defined the number of headache attacks (2-8 episodes) without specifying the number of headache days, which could have introduced selection bias.

② Discussion on the selection of primary efficacy measures: Pain severity scores were not chosen as the primary efficacy measures, and the rationale for using the Visual Analog Scale (VAS) as a secondary efficacy measure should have been discussed. In future studies, the VAS could be considered as a primary efficacy indicator, with the parameters of the minimum clinically important difference being defined.

3. Author's Talk

Special attention should be given to strategies for the prevention and treatment of major diseases in research topic selection. Migraine holds the position of the second most prominent cause of disability across the globe, with over 1 billion individuals being affected. Among young and middle-aged adults in the 15-49 age bracket, it stands as the foremost disease burden for women and the second for men. A study published in *The Lancet* concerning the global burden of disease underscored the substantial impact of headache disorders, yet also pointed out their relatively scant attention within global health policies. Previous surveys have indicated a low level of adherence to preventive medications among migraine sufferers and a common occurrence of analgesic misuse. Although calcitonin gene-related peptide-targeted therapies for migraine have emerged in recent times, their prohibitively high cost has restricted their extensive application in clinical settings. For migraine patients who exhibit suboptimal responses to medications, have an intolerance to drug side effects, possess contraindications to medications, harbor concerns about potential drug interactions, or those who are reluctant to engage in pharmacological treatments, there is an immediate and pressing demand for effective and dependable non-pharmacological therapies in clinical practice.

A considerable quantity of preceding randomized controlled trials regarding acupuncture had yielded negative outcomes, prompting numerous researchers to ascribe acupuncture's effects to the placebo. Such skepticism had circumscribed the spread and recognition of the fundamental tenets of traditional acupuncture and impeded the advancement of acupuncture-related scientific investigations. Through an exhaustive review of the extant literature, we discerned crucial methodological flaws in previous studies. In a multitude of randomized controlled trials, the acupuncture group failed to accentuate the concept of deqi, which presumably attenuated the curative impacts. Concurrently, the control groups frequently employed penetrating sham needles or administered stimulation within the identical spinal segment, unwittingly augmenting their potency. These elements plausibly accounted for the negative results manifested in these studies. To surmount these obstacles, we centered on refining our study design: ①Enlisting participants bereft of prior acupuncture exposure to enhance the efficacy of the blinding protocol. ②Employing internationally acknowledged non-penetrating placebo needles for the sham acupuncture group, with interventions implemented exterior to the same spinal segment as that of the acupuncture group. ③Formulating standardized acupuncture regimens to curtail the placebo effects associated with unblinded practitioners in the treatment cohort. ④Evaluating the success of blinding subsequent to treatment to authenticate the potency of the blinding procedures.

WANG Wei
Tongji Hospital Affiliated to Tongji Medical College of Huazhong University of Science and Technology

Section 33 Introduction and Comments of *Effect of Acupuncture for Postprandial Distress Syndrome: A Randomized Clinical Trial*

1. Introduction

BACKGROUND Postprandial distress syndrome (PDS) is the most common subtype of functional dyspepsia. Acupuncture is commonly used to treat PDS, but its effect is uncertain because of the poor quality of prior studies.

OBJECTIVE To assess the efficacy of acupuncture versus sham acupuncture in patients with PDS.

DESIGN Multicenter, 2-group, randomized clinical trial.

SETTING 5 tertiary hospitals in China.

PARTICIPANTS Chinese patients aged 18 to 65 years meeting Rome IV criteria for PDS.

INTERVENTIONS 12 sessions of acupuncture or sham acupuncture over 4 weeks.

MEASURES The 2 primary outcomes were the response rate based on overall treatment effect and the elimination rate of all 3 cardinal symptoms: Postprandial fullness, upper abdominal bloating, and early satiation after 4 weeks of treatment. Participants were followed until week 16.

RESULTS Among the 278 randomly assigned participants, 228 (82%) completed outcome measurements at week 16. The estimated response rate from generalized linear mixed models at week 4 was 83.0% in the acupuncture group versus 51.6% in the sham acupuncture group (difference, 31.4 percentage points [95% CI, 20.3 to 42.5 percentage points]; $P<0.001$). The estimated elimination rate of all 3 cardinal symptoms was 27.8% in the acupuncture group versus 17.3% in the sham acupuncture group (difference, 10.5 percentage points [CI, 0.08 to 20.9 percentage points]; $P=0.034$). The efficacy of acupuncture was maintained during the 12-week posttreatment follow-up. There were no serious adverse events.

LIMITATIOM Lack of objective outcomes and daily measurement, high dropout rate, and inability to blind acupuncturists.

CONCLUSION Among patients with PDS, acupuncture resulted in increased response rate and elimination rate of all 3 cardinal symptoms compared with sham acupuncture, with sustained ef-ficacy over 12 weeks in patients who received thrice-weekly acupuncture for 4 weeks.

2. Expert Comments

Comment 1

Functional dyspepsia is a gastrointestinal disorder commonly encountered in clinical practice, which seriously impairs the physical and mental health, as well as the quality of life of patients. Currently, there is no specific treatment for this condition, and gastrointestinal motility drugs are often used in clinical practice. These drugs provide good short-term efficacy but have marked side effects with long-term use. Addressing the clinical challenges of "high incidence" "significant harm to patients" and "lack of effective interventions" the team led by Professor LIU Cunzhi from Beijing University of Chinese Medicine focused on patients with the main subtype of functional dyspepsia, PDS and conducted a study evaluating the efficacy and safety of acupuncture in treating PDS.

The design of this experiment was rigorous and could serve as a reference for future research in the areas of acupuncture program design, control group setup, and outcome indicator selection. First, a semi-standardized acupuncture intervention program was developed, balancing standardization with individualization of treatment. The study was based on the prescriptions of renowned veteran traditional Chinese medicine doctors in China, and acupoints were selected based on syndrome differentiation in traditional Chinese medicine, formulating a semi-standardized acupuncture treatment plan. This approach retained the diagnostic and therapeutic principles of traditional Chinese medicine syndrome differentiation while ensuring the standardization and reproducibility of the study. Second, the control design reflected the unique characteristics of acupuncture interventions and adhered to the principles of blinding. Shallow needling at non-meridian and non-acupoint sites was used for the control group, matching the intervention group in number, with the advantages of minimal effective stimulation, high clinical feasibility, and good blinding effect on patients. Third, the use of dual primary outcome indicators allowed for careful evaluation of acupuncture's efficacy. The study used the overall response rate and symptom elimination rate as comprehensive outcome measures, scientifically and rigorously confirming the short-term (4-week treatment) and long-term (12-week follow up) efficacy of acupuncture in treating PDS, affirming the therapeutic advantages of acupuncture for PDS intervention.

Comment 2

(1) Study design and process implementation

The study employed a multicenter, randomized, sham-controlled trial design to evaluate the efficacy of acupuncture for functional dyspepsia with PDS. The design was robust, utilizing stratified block randomization to ensure the independence and impartiality of random assignment. Participants were recruited through various channels, and the strict inclusion and exclusion criteria reduced the possible influence of confounding factors, ensuring homogeneity among patients. Blinding was implemented for patients, outcome assessors, and statistical analysts, effectively minimizing observer bias. However, the lack of blinding for the acupuncturists may have introduced implementation bias. The intervention clearly distinguished between acupuncture and sham acupuncture, facilitating a clearer understanding of the differences between specific and non-specific effects. The study employed validated tools to assess both primary and secondary outcome measures at multiple time points during the intervention and follow-up periods, ensuring systematic and continuous data collection. However, some data management details were lacking. Obtaining ethical review approval and the patients' informed consent ensured compliance with research standards. Overall, the rigorous design and standardized implementation of the study provide strong support for evaluating the efficacy of acupuncture in treating PDS.

(2) Selection and application of clinical research methodology and statistical methods

The study demonstrated high scientific rigor in its clinical methodology and statistical approaches. The multicenter, randomized, sham-controlled design and stratified block randomization further enhanced the study's internal validity. Sample size calculations were based on prior pilot data, factoring in expected response rates, elimination rates, and intraclass correlation coefficients to ensure sufficient statistical power. The primary analysis used generalized linear mixed models, which are well-suited for handling repeated measures data and accounted for group, time, and center interactions. Independent-sample *t*-tests were applied to continuous variables to ensure analytical precision. Missing data were addressed through multiple imputations, and sensitivity analyses were performed to verify the robustness of the results. Additionally, the study conducted a subgroup analysis for *Helicobacter pylori* infection, exploring differential acupuncture effects across subgroups, thereby enhancing the study's clinical relevance. However, the study did not provide detailed descriptions of multiple comparison corrections, which could have limited the interpretation of the significance of certain results. Future studies should aim to address these aspects to improve the reliability and generalizability of the findings.

Section 34 Introduction and Comments of *Electroacupuncture Trigeminal Nerve Stimulation Plus Body Acupuncture for Chemotherapy-Induced Cognitive Impairment in Breast Cancer Patients: An Assessor-Participant Blinded, Randomized Controlled Trial*

1. Introduction

Chemotherapy causes various side effects, including cognitive impairment, known as "chemobrain". In this study, we determined whether a novel acupuncture mode called electroacupuncture trigeminal nerve stimulation plus body acupuncture (EA/TNS+BA) could produce better outcomes than minimum acupuncture stimulation (MAS) as controls in treating chemobrain and other symptoms in breast cancer patients. In this assessor-and participant-blinded, randomized controlled trial, 93 breast cancer patients under or post chemotherapy were randomly assigned to EA/TNS+BA (*n*=46) and MAS (*n*=47) for 2 sessions per week over 8 weeks. The Montreal Cognitive Assessment (MoCA) served as the primary outcome. Digit span test was the secondary outcomes for attentional function and working memory. The quality of life and multiple functional assessments were also evaluated. EA/TNS+BA treated group had much better performance than MAS-treated group on reverse digit span test at Week 2 and Week 8, with medium effect sizes of 0.53 and 0.48, respectively, although no significant differences were observed in MoCA score and prevalence of chemobrain between the two groups. EA/TNS+BA also markedly reduced incidences of diarrhoea, poor appetite, headache, anxiety, and irritation, and improved social/family and emotional wellbeing compared to MAS. These results suggest that EA/TNS+BA may have particular benefits in reducing chemotherapy-induced working memory impairment and the incidence of certain digestive, neurological, and distress-related symptoms. It could serve as an effective intervention for breast cancer patients under and post chemotherapy.

2. Expert Comments

Comment 1

Trigeminal nerve stimulation as a novel, non-invasive neuromodulation technique has garnered increasing attention in the field of neuroscience. This method involves applying weak electrical currents to the head to stimulate the trigeminal nerve, thereby influencing neural circuits related to cognition and consciousness. ZHANG Zhangjin et al. demonstrated that a novel acupuncture model combining electroacupuncture trigeminal nerve stimulation with body acupuncture may be particularly effective in alleviating chemotherapy-induced working memory impairments as well as digestive, neurological, and stress-related symptoms.

In previous studies, most acupuncture points used for treating patients with cancer were located on the body and typically stimulated manually. However, this study employed combined intensive forehead and body acupoints, with additional electrical stimulation applied to the forehead acupoints. These forehead acupoints, innervated by the sensory pathways of the trigeminal nerve, play a crucial role in acupuncture's modulation of various brain functions, including the processing of pain, emotion, and cognitive information. The study found that combining electroacupuncture trigeminal nerve stimulation and body acupuncture, particularly electrical stimulation of forehead acupoints, may exert long-term additive or even synergistic effects through extensive regulation of neurochemical pathways and brain regions.

The selection of minimal acupuncture stimulation as the control in this study was well-justified, enhancing the effectiveness of blinding. This work provided robust evidence supporting the expansion of acupuncture applications in oncology, while also offering an alternative effective intervention for patients with breast cancer undergoing or recovering from chemotherapy. Additionally, it opens new avenues for acupuncture research and points to promising prospects in the field.

Comment 2

Protocol elaboration question: After the trial officially started, was the specific implementation consistent with the registered description? Were there any significant methodological changes, and why? These are not addressed in the text.

Exclusion criteria: The current study included patients who were either receiving chemotherapy or had finished chemotherapy no more than two weeks prior. The effect of acupuncture was evaluated for eight weeks after the start of the trial. It remains debatable whether patients who were undergoing chemotherapy during the entire evaluation period, or for a significant portion of it, were homogeneous with those who had completed chemotherapy prior to participation.

Sample size issue: The article mentions "A sample size of 46 each group of this study would be sufficient to detect a 30% difference in the prevalence of chemobrain between the two groups at an 80% power and a statistical level of 0.05" and no clear sample size calculation method is provided. This is very important for a clinical study.

Randomization problem: It is mentioned in the article that "based on random codes which were simple, complete, non-sequential numbers and produced in advance using a computer-generated random block". The method of generating random sequences is not clear.

The problem of statistical method: The selection basis of covariates and whether the data met the precondition of the t-test are not clarified.

Results and conclusion questions: ①The table presenting the main results is unclear. If the authors compared repeated measurement scores with the baseline score to calculate the P-value, how can the baseline score itself produce a P-value? ②Only one outcome score showed statistically significant results at weeks 2 and 8, suggesting that the current results provide very limited support for "better results in the EA/TNS+BA group". Possible reasons include that the effect of the EA/TNS+BA group is actually not superior, insufficient test power, or that the short-term effect of acupuncture is not significant. The sporadic two meaningful effect values may have occurred by chance.

The overall design and statistical methods are reasonable, but the second and sixth points mentioned above are key issues and need further verification.

Section 35 Introduction and Comments of *Effect of Acupuncture vs Sham Procedure on Chemotherapy-Induced Peripheral Neuropathy Symptoms: A Randomized Clinical Trial*

1. Introduction

INTRODUCTION Chemotherapy-induced peripheral neuropathy (CIPN) is the most common and debilitating long-term adverse effect of neurotoxic chemotherapy that significantly worsens cancer survivors' quality of life. Well-tolerated, evidence-based interventions for CIPN are needed.

METHODS This pilot randomized clinical trial compared the effect of 8 weeks of real acupuncture vs sham acupuncture or usual care to treat CIPN. The trial protocol was approved by the institutional review board of Memorial Sloan Kettering Cancer Center and follows the Consolidated Standards of Reporting Trials (CONSORT) reporting guideline. Written informed consent was obtained from all study participants. Patients with solid tumors with persistent moderate to severe CIPN (symptoms of numbness, tingling, or pain rated 4 on a Numeric Rating Scale [NRS]) who had completed 3 or more months of chemotherapy prior to study enrollment and were not taking stable neuropathic medication were eligible. Patients were allocated 1 : 1 : 1 to real acupuncture, sham acupuncture, or usual care through computer-generated randomization conducted by the Clinical Research Database in randomly permuted blocks. The real acupuncture group received ear and body acupuncture at Shen Men, point zero, and a third electrodermal active point, and bilateral body: LI4 (Hegu), PC6 (Neiguan), SI3 (Houxi), LR3 (Taichong), GB42 (Diwuhui), ST40 (Fenglong), Bafeng 2, and Bafeng 3. Electrical acupuncture was also applied bilaterally from LR-3 (negative) to GB-42 (positive) at 2 to 5 Hz for 20 minutes. The sham acupuncture group received a noninsertion procedure on nonacupoints. The usual care group did not receive any interventions throughout the study period. Investigators, study coordinators, and the statistician were blinded to the treatment assignments. The primary end point was CIPN symptom severity measured by NRS (11-point scale; 0=no symptoms and 10=worst

Chapter 2 Comments of Clinical Trials of Acupuncture and Moxibustion in SCI Journals

symptom imaginable) at week 8. In prior studies, the NRS had high reliability and validity. We targeted a sample size of 25 participants in each group. This sample size allowed us to estimate the upper bound of a 1-sided 90% confidence interval for the treatment effect on outcome (eg, sham acupuncture vs real acupuncture or usual care vs real acupuncture) to 0.35-unit SDs. Mixed-effects models with an interaction term between group and assessment time (up to 8 weeks) were fit to examine whether temporal changes in a measure differed by group. The threshold for statistical significance was set at 2-sided $P<0.05$.

RESULTS From July 2017 to June 2018, we enrolled 75 patients with solid tumors with moderate to severe CIPN (median [interquartile range] age, 59.7 [36.3-85.9] years; 60 [80%] female; 55 [73%] white; 40 [53%] with breast cancer and 12 [16%] with colorectal cancer). In all, 24 patients were randomized to real acupuncture, 23 to sham acupuncture, and 21 to usual care. Compared with usual care, NRS-measured pain, tingling, and numbness significantly decreased in real acupuncture at week 8. From baseline to week 8, mean absolute reduction in CIPN pain was greatest in real acupuncture (−1.75 [95% CI, −2.69 to −0.81]) and least in usual care (−0.19 [95% CI, −1.13 to 0.75]). At the 8-week assessment, sham acupuncture had a reduction of −0.91 (95% CI, −2.0 to 0.18). At the longer 12-week follow-up, real acupuncture had a mean absolute reduction in NRS-measured pain of −1.74 (95% CI, −2.6 to −0.83) from baseline, while sham treatment had a reduction of −0.34 (−1.3 to 0.61). Adverse events were few and mild.

DISCUSSION We found therapeutic benefit of real acupuncture for neuropathic pain that is consistent with previous pilot acupuncture CIPN trials. Distinctively, our study is the first, to our knowledge, to incorporate a sham treatment and a nontreatment control to evaluate the efficacy of acupuncture for CIPN. The addition of a sham acupuncture control in an acupuncture clinical trial is difficult owing to the challenge of incorporating a truly inert placebo. In addition, a sham control limits the ability of a small effect size to elucidate a true difference between real and sham acupuncture. Not only did our study demonstrate the feasibility of conducting a sham-controlled acupuncture trial, it generated sufficient pilot data to inform a definitive sham-controlled efficacy trial. Our trial is limited by its small sample size, single center, and short-term follow-up.

In conclusion, compared with usual care, acupuncture resulted in significant improvement in CIPN symptoms. The effect size observed between real and sham control will inform a rigorous and adequately powered trial to establish the efficacy of acupuncture for CIPN.

2. Expert Comments

Comment 1

The article published in *JAMA Network Open* in 2020, "*Effect of Acupuncture vs Sham Procedure on Chemotherapy-Induced Peripheral Neuropathy Symptoms: A Randomized Clinical Trial*" pertained to clinical study in the world at that time to evaluate the effect of acupuncture on CIPN chemotherapy-induced peripheral neuropathy with sham acupuncture and no-treatment as controls. This study not only verified the feasibility of using sham acupuncture as a control, but also showed the specific therapeutic efficacy of acupuncture intervention in CIPN.

The study addressed real clinical needs and examined meaningful research topics. According to the statistics of the World Health Organization, cancer is the second leading cause of death in the world, and chemotherapy is one of the most important clinical means to intervene in cancer. More than half of patients with cancer require chemotherapy. However, various adverse reactions, including peripheral neuropathy, cause substantial pain to patients undergoing chemotherapy and also affect the normal cycle of chemotherapy intervention, which is not conducive to the treatment and prognosis of patients. This study, aimed at major diseases, selected the right research entry point, taking a targeted approach to tackle a larger issue, and clearly put forward the clinical problem, ie, whether acupuncture is effective in the treatment of CIPN, and then precisely pinpointed the specific therapeutic efficacy of acupuncture to carry out effectiveness research. This study can qualitatively answer the critical question of whether acupuncture is effective in the intervention of the disease.

Based on previous practice, this study formulated a high-level, scientifically sound, and rigorous research program. CIPN is a complex systemic symptom, not a local or isolated one. The analgesic regimen of all patients remained unchanged during the intervention period, which also provided a basis and guarantee for researchers to observe the specific clinical efficacy of acupuncture. The acupuncture group was treated with auricular acupuncture combined with body acupuncture. The auricular points were selected as TF4 (Shen Men), point zero and a third electrodermal active point, and the body points were selected as LI4, PC6, SI3, LR3, GB42, ST40, Bafeng 2, and Bafeng 3. Traditional Chinese medicine considers that peripheral neuropathy is mostly due to the obstruction of Ying and Wei, and thus the treatment needs to harmonize Ying and Wei, and the acupoint selection should be based on promoting blood flow, unblocking the meridians, promoting blood circulation, and dredging collaterals. This study selected large meridian acupoints. Although ST40 and PC6 consider the problems of blood and collaterals, the strength of nourishing qi and blood, nourishing blood, and activating blood circulation is not enough. SP10 (Xuehai) and SP6 (Sanyinjiao) will be considered in the actual clinical treatment process. Therefore, from the perspective of clinical practice of traditional Chinese medicine acupuncture and moxibustion, the acupuncture scheme of this study was not optimal, and the acupoint selection and prescription need to be further optimized. As this was an explanatory randomized controlled trial, it is more important to highlight the intervention programs that are conducive to the efficacy of acupuncture from the perspective of design.

Comment 2

Control group setting questions: ①Although participants were randomized, what was the effect of grouping? What is critical is whether the primary outcome measure is comparable at baseline? This was not stated. ②While there are challenges with the set-up of the insertion-type sham acupuncture group, it is not impossible. Previous studies have selected acupoints unrelated to the outcome for acupuncture. Naturally, the selection of these acupoints requires researchers to have a very solid understanding of the theory of traditional Chinese medicine. The current study used a non-insertion sham acupuncture group, which failed to achieve a placebo effect.

Observation period selection questions: ①Why was 8 weeks chosen as the longest period for effect assessment? ②Why neglect the efficacy exploration of each phase within 8 weeks? This is a key point, which needs to be properly discussed in combination with the time characteristics of the onset of acupuncture and the characteristics of the disease.

Auxiliary intervention: This article does not describe whether there are other auxiliary interventions and their rationality. In other words, this study lacks discussion of confounding factors. This is very critical. It is difficult to attribute results to therapy if the groups are not comparable in terms of receiving other adjunctive interventions, among other factors.

Sample size issue: Although the article mentions "We targeted a sample size of 25 participants in each group. This sample size allowed us to estimate the upper bound of a one-sided 90% confidence interval for the treatment effect on outcome", the paper does not clarify the specific basis for the calculation of the current sample size. The sample size of the current study was small, and there are limitations such as the single-center design and short follow-up period, which all affect the promotion of the results and evaluation of the real effect.

The statistical methods were basically reasonable, but the consideration of confounding factors was insufficient. When the confounding factors are not balanced between groups, the results of inter-group comparisons are not reliable, and the results of the multi-factor analysis should be taken as the main results.

Section 36 Introduction and Comments of *Effect of Electroacupuncture vs Sham Treatment on Change in Pain Severity Among Adults With Chronic Low Back Pain: A Randomized Clinical Trial*

1. Introduction

IMPORTANCE Chronic low back pain has high societal and personal impact but remains challenging to treat. Electroacupuncture has demonstrated superior analgesia compared with placebo in animal studies but has not been extensively studied in human chronic pain conditions.

OBJECTIVE To evaluate the treatment effect of real electroacupuncture vs placebo in pain and disability among adults with chronic low back pain and to explore psychophysical, affective, and demographic factors associated with response to electroacupuncture vs placebo in treating chronic low back pain.

DESIGN, SETTING, AND PARTICIPANTS This double-blind randomized clinical trial was conducted between August 2, 2016, and December 18, 2018, at a single center in Stanford, California. Primary outcomes were collected at approximately 2 weeks before and after intervention. Participants included English-speaking adults with at least 6 months of chronic low back pain, pain intensity of at least 4 on a scale of 0 to 10, and no radiculopathy. Data analyses for this intent-to-treat study were conducted from June 2019 to June 2020.

INTERVENTIONS Twelve sessions of real or placebo (sham) electroacupuncture administered twice a week over 6 weeks.

MAIN OUTCOMES AND MEASURES The

main outcome was change in pain severity from baseline to 2 weeks after completion of treatment, measured by the National Institutes of Health Patient-Reported Outcomes Measurement Information System (PROMIS) pain intensity scale. A secondary outcome was change in the Roland Morris Disability Questionnaire (RMDQ). Baseline factors potentially associated with these outcomes included psychophysical testing (ie, thermal temporal summation, conditioned pain modulation, pressure pain threshold), participant's self-report (ie, widespread pain, coping strategies, expectations, self-efficacy, and pain catastrophizing), and demographic characteristics (eg, age, sex, and race).

RESULTS A total of 121 adults were recruited to the study, among whom 59 participants (mean [SD] age, 46.8 [11.9] years; 36 [61.0%] women) were randomized to real electroacupuncture and 62 participants (mean [SD] age, 45.6 [12.8] years; 33 [53.2%] women) were randomized to sham electroacupuncture. At baseline, the mean (SD) PROMIS T-score was 50.49 (3.36) in the real electroacupuncture group and 51.71 (4.70) in the sham acupuncture group, and the mean (SD) RMDQ score was 10.16 (4.76) in the real electroacupuncture group and 10.03 (5.45) in the sham acupuncture group. After adjusting for baseline pain scores, there was no statistically significant difference between groups in change in T-scores 2 weeks after completion of treatment (real electroacupuncture: −4.33; 95% CI, −6.36 to −2.30; sham acupuncture: −2.90; 95% CI, −4.85 to −0.95; difference: −2.09; 95% CI, −4.27 to 0.09; P=0.06). After adjusting for baseline RMDQ, there was a significantly greater reduction in RMDQ in the real electroacupuncture group (−2.77; 95% CI, −4.11 to −1.43) compared with the sham electroacupuncture group (−0.67; 95% CI, −1.88 to 0.55; difference: −2.11; 95% CI, −3.75 to −0.47; P=0.01). Within the real electroacupuncture group, effective coping at baseline was associated with greater RMDQ reduction (r=−0.32; 95% CI, −0.54 to −0.05; P=0.02), and White race was associated with worse outcomes in PROMIS score (β=3.791; 95% CI, 0.616 to 6.965; P=0.02) and RMDQ (β=2.878; 95% CI, 0.506 to 5.250; P=0.02).

CONCLUSIONS AND RELEVANCE This randomized clinical trial found no statistically significant difference in change in PROMIS pain score in real electroacupuncture vs sham electroacupuncture. There was a statistically significant treatment effect for the secondary outcome of RMDQ compared with sham electroacupuncture. Effective coping skills and non-White race were associated with response to electroacupuncture.

2. Expert Comments

Comment 1

Pain is one of the most common clinical problems worldwide, seriously affecting quality of life. Acupuncture analgesia is a hot research topic at home and abroad because of acupuncture's definite analgesic effect and because it is non-addictive and relatively safe. In particular, preclinical studies have shown that electroacupuncture may produce a stronger analgesic effect than manual acupuncture. Electroacupuncture is widely used in acupuncture analgesia. The placebo effect is controversial in acupuncture research. This single-center, parallel, randomized clinical trial compared the efficacy of real electroacupuncture and sham electroacupuncture in the treatment of chronic low back pain, and the verification of the efficacy of electroacupuncture analgesia may have an impact on the international evaluation and application of acupuncture therapy.

This study evaluated the therapeutic effects of electroacupuncture versus sham electroacupuncture in pain and disability in adults with chronic low back pain and identified factors associated with the treatment response using changes in pain and disability as clinical outcomes. In this study, 121 participants were treated with 12 sessions of electroacupuncture/sham electroacupuncture for 6 weeks. After fully considering the blinding evaluation, electroacupuncture had a significant therapeutic effect in reducing disability associated with chronic low back pain. This study introduced univariate and multivariate analysis methods to capture univariate associations between patient characteristics and clinical outcomes in the true electroacupuncture group. Racial differences were found to have an impact on the results of the study, ie, being Caucasian was associated with poorer results on pain and RMDQ scores. For the 10-week observation (2 weeks before and 2 weeks after 6 weeks of intervention) the final analysis showed that there was no significant difference in pain score change between real electroacupuncture and sham electroacupuncture. However, this was the first study to find a statistically and clinically significant effect of electroacupuncture on chronic low back pain-related disability using a randomized clinical trial design and helped elucidate the patient factors associated with the clinical response to electroacupuncture.

Comment 2

(1) Study design and process implementation

The study used a classic single-center parallel randomized controlled trial design, and the nine elements of the design can be considered as follows. ①Participants: Patients with chronic back pain. Importantly, the authors supplied a flowchart clearly presenting the context. ②Intervention: 12 applications of electroacupuncture and moxibustion within 6 weeks, each lasting 45 minutes (see the analysis of acupuncture experts for details). ③Control setting: Placebo control (sham needle) is most recommended. ④Outcomes: The change in the pain intensity score before and after treatment as the primary endpoint, which is well recognized and supported by the literature. However, it should be noted that in the attached study protocol, the investigators explicitly mentioned that the endpoint events were adjusted after the start of the study, and the reasons provided were rather far-fetched. ⑤Setting: The study being conducted in a community clinic convenient for residents increases the extrapolation of conclusions. ⑥Randomization: Block randomization (four patients per block). To increase the balance of enrollment among community clinics, the planned simple randomization was deliberately modified before the start of the study. ⑦Blinding method: Regarding the blinding of the participants, it is noteworthy that after the completion of the 12 treatment course, the participants were asked to guess their group allocation, and their judgments were included in the analysis as a binary variable. ⑧Distribution concealment: Through the standardized process as far as possible not to let the research object clear grouping, this practice is worth learning from the follow-up study. ⑨Sample size calculation: The study simultaneously answered two questions in addition to comparing the placebo group, ie, whether electroacupuncture is effective or not and what factors affect the effect of electroacupuncture in patients. The corresponding sample size calculation also included two parts. The authors first calculated the sample size for the latter problem, but the calculation was based on a correlation coefficient (0.4), and 50 patients were needed for the electroacupuncture group. Subsequently, according to 50 patients in each group of electroacupuncture and sham acupuncture, the researchers calculated that the difference between the correlation coefficients of the two groups could be explored at approximately 0.5, and the final sample was set at 60 patients in each group based on further consideration of sample loss. This choice of correlation coefficient rather than association strength is questionable. Few studies only aim to examine associations without exploring the size of the association, especially as the sample size calculation of randomized controlled trials should be carefully referred to, which is inconsistent with the primary endpoint of the study statement, especially when the authors themselves report the change in the pain intensity scores pre- and post-treatment.

(2) Selection and application of clinical research methodology and statistical methods

The effect comparison between the groups in the statistical analysis was relatively simple and direct, but the following two points should be noted. ①Missing values and outlier treatment, the valuable part of the study mentioned the exploration of the missing data mechanism and handling of missing values but unfortunately did not provide the proportion of missing values for each variable. Conversely, the authors' handling and reporting of outliers was more comprehensive and worth studying. ②It is good practice to explore the influencing factors of the treatment effect and consider multivariate analysis, but the authors' initial sample size calculation only considered the correlation coefficient between a single variable and the end event, which inevitably led to an insufficient sample size. Moreover, when choosing which variables to include in the multivariate analysis, the handing of inconsistent results between the intervention group and the control group was not clarified. Moreover, when exploring the interaction between patient grouping and other influencing factors, the selection of dependent variables and treatment of baseline variables need to be discussed, and it is more appropriate to select the primary endpoint in theory.

Section 37 Introduction and Comments of *Acupuncture as Adjunctive Therapy for Chronic Stable Angina: A Randomized Clinical Trial*

1. Introduction

IMPORTANCE The effects of acupuncture as adjunctive treatment to antianginal therapies for patients with chronic stable angina (CSA) are uncertain.

OBJECTIVE To investigate the efficacy and

safety of acupuncture as adjunctive therapy to antianginal therapies in reducing frequency of angina attacks in patients with CSA.

DESIGN, SETTING, AND PARTICIPANTS In this 20-week randomized clinical trial conducted in outpatient and inpatient settings at 5 clinical centers in China from October 10, 2012, to September 19, 2015, 404 participants were randomly assigned to receive acupuncture on the acupoints on the disease-affected meridian (DAM), receive acupuncture on the acupoints on the nonaffected meridian (NAM), receive sham acupuncture (SA), and receive no acupuncture (wait list [WL] group). Participants were 35 to 80 years of age with chronic stable angina based on the criteria of the American College of Cardiology and the American Heart Association, with angina occurring at least twice weekly. Statistical analysis was conducted from December 1, 2015, to July 30, 2016.

INTERVENTIONS All participants in the 4 groups received antianginal therapies as recommended by the guidelines. Participants in the DAM, NAM, and SA groups received acupuncture treatment 3 times weekly for 4 weeks for a total of 12 sessions. Participants in the WL group did not receive acupuncture during the 16-week study period.

MAIN OUTCOMES AND MEASURES Participants used diaries to record angina attacks. The primary outcome was the change in frequency of angina attacks every 4 weeks from baseline to week 16.

RESULTS A total of 398 participants (253 women and 145 men; mean [SD] age, 62.6 [9.7] years) were included in the intention-to-treat analyses. Baseline characteristics were comparable across the 4 groups. Mean changes in frequency of angina attacks differed significantly among the 4 groups at 16 weeks: A greater reduction of angina attacks was observed in the DAM group vs the NAM group (difference, 4.07; 95% CI, 2.43-5.71; $P<0.001$), in the DAM group vs the SA group (difference, 5.18; 95% CI, 3.54-6.81; $P<0.001$), and in the DAM group vs the WL group (difference, 5.63 attacks; 95% CI, 3.99-7.27; $P<0.001$).

CONCLUSIONS AND RELEVANCE Compared with acupuncture on the NAM, SA, or no acupuncture (WL), acupuncture on the DAM as adjunctive treatment to antianginal therapy showed superior benefits in alleviating angina.

2. Expert Comments

Comment 1

In this study, acupuncture was chosen as an auxiliary method to improve the frequency of angina pectoris in patients with CSA, and the main purpose of the study was to help patients with CSA improve their quality of life, rather than focusing on changes in index values. This is exactly the embodiment of the holistic view of traditional Chinese medicine. It is important for patients to not only to prolong their length of life but also improve their quality of life.

The research team very comprehensively considered the choice of acupuncture methods. From the perspective of clinical research methodology, the effectiveness of acupuncture can be verified according to the acupuncture treatment group and non-treatment control group. From the perspective of traditional Chinese medicine syndrome differentiation and treatment, we can further explore the efficacy of different meridian and acupoint programs for the treatment of angina pectoris by selecting acupoints along the meridians, other meridians, and false acupoints, which can well show that the therapeutic effect of the meridians and acupoints is not simply produced by stimulating skin and muscle. The setting of these three groups not only respects the international requirements for clinical research design, but also maintains the characteristics of traditional Chinese medicine.

In view of the current medical treatment mode, it is one of the greatest significances of this study to formulate an ethical and clinically meaningful research plan for acupuncture adjuvant treatment of angina pectoris. To make good use of large samples, if only 1 : 1 acupuncture and blank control are set, the sample size is wasted and the conclusion is difficult to extend to follow-up study. The acupoint selection in this study is a highlight, concise and purposeful, which provides a new idea for the clinical study of acupuncture in acupoint selection; it can both verify the safety of acupuncture and the curative effect of the heart and pericardium meridians on heart diseases in the meridian theory of traditional Chinese medicine through the selection of PC6 (Neiguan) and HT5 (Tongli) along the meridian. The previous clinical trials of acupuncture were often confined to the clinical treatment experience in the selection of acupoints, and the combination of primary and auxiliary acupoints was typically used in the research protocol, but to some extent, the more acupoints are used, the more interference information is brought to the study. For example, the same warming and tonifying acupoints may cause two different effects in individuals with body heat owing to Yang excess and cold because of Yang deficiency. This is a characteristic of traditional Chinese medicine treatment theory and a source of confounding that cannot be ignored in traditional Chinese medicine clinical research. From this study, we can see that if only the main acupoints are selected, the confounding factors between acupoints and syndromes are reduced to the greatest extent, and the results of the study are more focused on "acupuncture is really effective in improving the frequency of angina pectoris attacks".

Comment 2

(1) Study design and process implementation

This was a multicenter, randomized controlled trial conducted in five hospitals in China and included 404 patients with CSA pectoris. In this study, a variable block stratified randomization method was used, and patients were randomized into a DAM, NAM, SA and WL groups at proportions of 1∶1∶1∶1 assigned using a central randomization system to ensure balance among the groups. Patients in all groups received 16 weeks of basic antianginal therapy as recommended by the guidelines. Patients in the DAM, NAM, and SA groups were blinded to minimize the effects of expectation and subjective judgment on the results. The main outcome was the change in angina attack frequency from baseline to the 16th week, and the index was objective, measurable, and capable to evaluate the effect of acupuncture on angina symptoms, with important clinical significance. The study was rigorously designed and conducted.

(2) Selection and application of clinical research methodology and statistical methods

The study accounted for a 15% loss to follow up when estimating the sample size and ultimately recruited 404 patients aged 35 to 80 years. The study used the intention-to-treat analysis principle and Kruskal-Wallis method for statistical analysis and found that acupuncture for 16 weeks could effectively reduce the frequency of angina attacks and further explored that the benefit may be related to acupoint specificity. The study discussed some of its limitations, but other limitations remained. ① Six patients were excluded from the intention-to-treat analysis for reasons such as loss to follow up, and a prespecified sensitivity analysis was not performed to assess the impact of excluding patients on the outcome. ② A prespecified adjustment analysis was not performed for important covariates that could have affected the outcome. ③ The last observed value carried forward method was used to fill in for missing data, which is simple and easy to implement, but it might introduce bias to underestimate the treatment effect.

3. Author's Talk

The study *Acupuncture as Adjunctive Therapy for Chronic Stable Angina: A Randomized Clinical Trial*, published in *JAMA Internal Medicine*, was based on the second 973 Program project led by Professor LIANG Fanrong, titled "*Basic Research on the Meridian-Specific Regularities of Acupoint Effects and Key Influencing Factors*". Firstly, the foundation of any research question should be rooted in clinical needs. Many patients with CSA experience persistent angina symptoms despite standard western medical treatment. Frustrated by the lack of improvement, many turn to acupuncture as an adjunctive therapy. Both theoretical research and clinical practice have shown that acupuncture targeting specific acupoints can reduce the frequency and intensity of angina attacks. However, at that time, studies on acupuncture's effects on angina were characterized by an abundance of basic research but a paucity of clinical studies, often involving small sample sizes and insufficient statistical power. These limitations resulted in low-quality clinical evidence and limited application. To address these gaps, this study was designed based on the meridian-specific principles of acupoint effects. A robust study design requires meticulous preparation. Before initiating the study, our team deliberated on key questions: How willing are patients to undergo acupuncture? What type and severity of CSA cases should be included? To answer these, we conducted thorough literature reviews, extensive patient surveys, and repeated expert consultations, culminating in a well-considered study design. Rigorous clinical implementation depended on quality control. This multicenter study was conducted simultaneously across five regions in China from October 2012 to September 2015. Given the geographical dispersion of centers, maintaining consistency across sites was paramount. To achieve this, we adopted management approaches and methodologies aligned with high-quality randomized controlled trials. Standardized operating procedures were established, and a third-party company was engaged to oversee project management comprehensively.

ZHAO Ling
Chengdu University of Traditional Chinese Medicine

Chapter 2 Comments of Clinical Trials of Acupuncture and Moxibustion in SCI Journals

Section 38 Introduction and Comments of *Effect of True and Sham Acupuncture on Radiation-Induced Xerostomia Among Patients With Head and Neck Cancer: A Randomized Clinical Trial*

1. Introduction

IMPORTANCE Radiation-induced xerostomia (RIX) is a common, often debilitating, adverse effect of radiation therapy among patients with head and neck cancer. Quality of life can be severely affected, and current treatments have limited benefit.

OBJECTIVE To determine if acupuncture can prevent RIX in patients with head and neck cancer undergoing radiation therapy.

DESIGN, SETTING, AND PARTICIPANTS This 2-center, phase 3, randomized clinical trial compared a standard care control (SCC) with true acupuncture (TA) and sham acupuncture (SA) among patients with oropharyngeal or nasopharyngeal carcinoma who were undergoing radiation therapy in comprehensive cancer centers in the United States and China. Patients were enrolled between December 16, 2011, and July 7, 2015. Final follow-up was August 15, 2016. Analyses were conducted February 1 through 28, 2019.

INTERVENTION Either TA or SA using a validated acupuncture placebo device was performed 3 times per week during a 6- to 7-week course of radiation therapy.

MAIN OUTCOMES AND MEASURES The primary end point was RIX, as determined by the Xerostomia Questionnaire in which a higher score indicates worse RIX, for combined institutions 1 year after radiation therapy ended. Secondary outcomes included incidence of clinically significant xerostomia (score >30), salivary flow, quality of life, salivary constituents, and role of baseline expectancy related to acupuncture on outcomes.

RESULTS Of 399 patients randomized, 339 were included in the final analysis (mean [SD] age, 51.3 [11.7] years; age range, 21-79 years; 258 [77.6%] men), including 112 patients in the TA group, 115 patients in the SA group, and 112 patients in the SCC group. For the primary aim, the adjusted least square mean (SD) xerostomia score in the TA group (26.6 [17.7]) was significantly lower than in the SCC group (34.8 [18.7]) ($P=0.001$; effect size=−0.44) and marginally lower but not statistically significant different from the SA group (31.3 [18.6]) ($P=0.06$; effect size=−0.26). Incidence of clinically significant xerostomia 1 year after radiation therapy ended followed a similar pattern, with 38 patients in the TA group (34.6%), 54 patients in the SA group (47.8%), and 60 patients in the SCC group (55.1%) experiencing clinically significant xerostomia ($P=0.009$). Post hoc comparisons revealed a significant difference between the TA and SCC groups at both institutions, but TA was significantly different from SA only at Fudan University Cancer Center, Shanghai, China (estimated difference [SE]: TA vs SCC, −9.9 [2.5]; $P<0.001$; SA vs SCC, −1.7 [2.5]; $P=0.50$; TA vs SA, −8.2 [2.5]; $P=0.001$), and SA was significantly different from SCC only at the University of Texas MD Anderson Cancer Center, Houston, Texas (estimated difference [SE]: TA vs SCC, −8.1 [3.4]; $P=0.016$; SA vs SCC, −10.5 [3.3]; $P=0.002$; TA vs SA, 2.4 [3.2]; $P=0.45$).

CONCLUSIONS AND RELEVANCE This randomized clinical trial found that TA resulted in significantly fewer and less severe RIX symptoms 1 year after treatment vs SCC. However, further studies are needed to confirm clinical relevance and generalizability of this finding and to evaluate inconsistencies in response to sham acupuncture between patients in the United States and China.

2. Expert Comments

Comment 1

This study focused on solving a difficult and prominent issue in clinical practice, that is, RIX, a common side effect of radiotherapy in patients with head and neck cancer. RIX severely affects the quality of life of patients, and the effect of existing treatment methods is limited. In this study, the effects of TA, SA, and SCC for the prevention of RIX were systematically compared through a randomized controlled trial design, and a safe and effective non-drug treatment was explored, which has high clinical application value.

Acupuncture intervention was carried out in a scientifically sound and rational manner. Standardized and validated acupuncture protocols and acupoints were used in the study to ensure the consistency and repeatability of the treatment. Each treatment was conducted by an experienced acupuncturist to ensure the suitability and safety of the operation. Although the study design was reasonable, there remain some limitations. First, there are differences in the treatment environment between China and the United States, which may have affected the consistency of the results. Second, the setting of the control group is reasonable, but there was lack of in-depth analysis of the differences in efficacy between different control groups, especially a comparison between the sham acupuncture group and standard nursing group, which may have affected the accurate evaluation of the real effect of acupuncture. In addition, although the depth of acupuncture and the feeling of deqi are described, the possible influence of individual differences on the effect of acupuncture, such as the patient's constitution and sensitivity to acupuncture, are not mentioned. Finally, the study did not adequately consider the possible impact of adjunctive therapeutic measures (eg, oral moisturizers, saliva substitutes) on the efficacy of acupuncture and did not explore the use of these measures in combination with acupuncture therapy.

Comment 2

(1) Study design and process implementation

The study adopted a two-center, multi-arm, double-blind randomized controlled trial design, and the nine elements related to the design could be considered as follows. ①Participants: Patients with head and neck cancer who received radiotherapy but note that the Chinese patients were inpatients and the American patients were outpatients, and they had not received acupuncture treatment before. ②Intervention: Acupuncture 3 days a week for 6-7 weeks (see the analysis of acupuncture experts for details). ③Controls: Sham needles were used for the placebo control, and standard treatments (such as brushing, fluoride toothpaste, dental floss, and other types of oral care) were used for the standard control. ④Outcomes: Self-reported xerostomia was selected as the primary endpoint. ⑤Setting: Cancer hospitals in China and the United States. ⑥Randomization method: Central randomization was used, and two covariate adaptive randomization strategies were integrated, ie, minimization method and stratified randomization (according to disease stage, age, sex, average planned parotid dose, with or without induction therapy, and with or without chemotherapy). Covariate-adaptive randomization strategies are widely used in clinical trials to balance covariates and maintain randomization, especially when there are many important prognostic factors to be managed, as in this case. ⑦Blinding: Patients and reviewers were blinded; although the patients may not have been strictly blinded, the investigators did not investigate patient awareness. ⑧Concealment of distribution: Not clearly reported. ⑨Sample size calculation: Although there was no preliminary trial or literature data to support the sample size calculation, the researchers gave full play to the advantages of the clinical background and defined the size of clinically meaningful effect values. According to 0.5 standard deviation (supported by literature here), 100 patients in each group would have sufficed. Further accounting for 25% loss to follow up, 399 patients were randomized.

(2) Selection and application of clinical research methodology and statistical methods

The effect comparison among the three groups in the statistical analysis was relatively simple and direct, but the following two points should be noted. ①Analysis of covariance (ANCOVA): In the analysis of the primary endpoint (xerostomia score 1 year after radiotherapy), the investigator used ANCOVA to better control the baseline xerostomia score and center effect, which is also common in randomized controlled trials, especially when the sample size is relatively small. The main purpose was to solve the problem that even if adaptive randomization of covariates is adopted, there may remain risk of unbalanced baseline covariates, and covariance analysis can better handle this problem. ②Mixed model analysis: Because for each subject, the xerostomia score was measured at 5 time points (including baseline, the end of radiotherapy in the 7th week, 3 months, 6 months, and 12 months), the researchers used mixed model analysis to handle the correlation between multiple time points within individuals.

Section 39 Introduction and Comments of *Acupuncture Versus Cognitive Behavioral Therapy for Insomnia in Cancer Survivors: A Randomized Clinical Trial*

1. Introduction

BACKGROUND Insomnia is a common and debilitating disorder experienced by cancer survivors. While cancer survivors expressed interest in using non-pharmacological treatment to manage insomnia, the comparative effectiveness between acupuncture and Cognitive Behavioral Therapy for Insomnia (CBT-I) for this disorder is unknown.

METHODS This randomized trial compared 8 weeks of acupuncture ($n=80$) and CBT-I ($n=80$) in cancer survivors. Acupuncture involved stimulating specific points on the body with needles. CBT-I included sleep restriction, stimulus control, cognitive restructuring, relaxation training, and education. We measured insomnia severity (primary outcome), pain, fatigue, mood, and quality of life post-treatment (8 weeks) with follow-up until 20 weeks. We used linear mixed-effects models for analyses. All statistical tests were two-sided.

RESULTS The mean age was 61.5 years, 56.9% were women. CBT-I was more effective than acupuncture post-treatment ($P<0.001$); however, both acupuncture and CBT-I produced clinically meaningful reductions in insomnia severity (acupuncture: −8.31 points, 95% CI: −9.36 to −7.26; CBT-I: −10.91 points, 95% CI: −11.97 to −9.85) and maintained improvements up to 20 weeks. Acupuncture was more effective for pain at end of treatment; both groups had similar improvements in fatigue, mood, and quality of life and reduced prescription hypnotic medication use. CBT-I was more effective for those who were male ($P<0.001$), white ($P=0.003$), highly educated ($P<0.001$), and had no pain at baseline ($P<0.001$).

CONCLUSIONS While both treatments produced meaningful and durable improvements, CBT-I was more effective and should be the first line of therapy. The relative differences in the comparative effectiveness between the two interventions for specific groups should be confirmed in future adequately powered trials to guide more tailored interventions for insomnia.

2. Expert Comments

Comment 1

The incidence of insomnia among patients with cancer reaches an astonishing 60%, as they face the numerous challenges associated with the disease, highlighting the severe issues in mental health and sleep quality within this patient group. If effective intervention is not implemented in time, insomnia is likely to turn into a persistent and incurable chronic morbid state, which will lead to a series of chain reactions, such as the aggravation of psychological anxiety, depression, and decline of physiological function, which will pose a double threat to the overall health of patients.

In this context, acupuncture therapy and CBT-I, as two high-profile non-drug treatments, have attracted increasing attention for their potential in alleviating insomnia symptoms. However, it is regrettable that although these two therapies have shown positive therapeutic prospects, clinicians still lack awareness of them, and they have not been given full attention and utilization in practice. This not only reflects the limitations of insomnia treatment strategies in the current clinical field, but also reveals the urgency of improving clinician awareness and acceptance of new therapies.

This study was concerned with this clinical difficulty and prominent issue. Through in-depth analysis of the current clinical situation, the authors accurately extracted the key challenges and potential development opportunities that hinder the progress of insomnia treatment, aiming to show the far-reaching value and significance of these non-drug treatments in improving the sleep quality of patients and improving their overall health through systematic research and discussion.

The study paid special attention to the balance between innovation and feasibility, striving to build a solid bridge between theoretical exploration and practical application. Through in-depth theoretical research and practical verification, the authors expected to promote the wide application and continuous optimization of acupuncture and moxibustion therapy and CBT-I in clinical practice and provide solid theoretical support and practical guidance for the continuous improvement of clinical practice. The topic also focuses on the rationality and scientificity of acupuncture intervention in the treatment process, as well as the standard control of acupuncture details. The effect and safety of acupuncture treatment can be improved by further refining the acupuncture treatment plan and standardizing the treatment operation. In addition, the planning of treatment programs and qualifications of therapists are also important factors affecting the effectiveness of treatment. Therefore, the authors suggest that priority should be given to professionals with rich experience in insomnia treatment to ensure that patients can profit from the best treatment results.

This topic has important theoretical value and practical significance and will play an active role in promoting the further deepening and expansion of clinical research and promotion of overall improvement in medical perspective. It is expected that the research and discussion of this topic will bring new ideas and breakthroughs in the field of clinical treatment of insomnia after cancer.

Comment 2

(1) Study design

This was a randomized controlled trial designed to compare the effects of acupuncture and CBT-I on insomnia in cancer survivors. The two-center, parallel-group, randomized controlled efficacy trial design avoided selection bias and increased the intrinsic validity of the results by randomizing participants to acupuncture and CBT-I. Studies were stratified by study site through replacement block randomization and assigned using the sealed envelope method, which ensured the concealment of the randomization process and helped reduce selection bias.

The main researchers, such as principal investigator, co-investigators, and statisticians, were blinded to prevent bias from affecting the results of the study and ensure that the data analysis would be more objective.

The study described in detail the inclusion and exclusion criteria for participants, ensuring the homogeneity of the study population. The inclusion criteria included a clear definition of insomnia severity and treatment completion time, while the exclusion criteria considered the impact of other sleep and psychiatric disorders, ensuring the reliability and interpretability of the results.

The outcome variables defined in advance were divided into primary and secondary outcome variables. The primary outcome variable was the insomnia severity index (the primary time point was 8 weeks after the end of treatment, and the secondary time point was 20 weeks after the end of treatment). The secondary outcome variable was the Pittsburgh Sleep Quality Index, which ensured the rigor of the study design and improved the quality of the study results.

(2) Process implementation

The implementation of both interventions was carried out by trained professionals, which further improved the internal validity of the study. Adverse events were recorded in detail during the intervention, providing comprehensive safety data. The assessment of treatment expectations and tracking of sleep medication use added to the comprehensiveness and credibility of the findings.

(3) Selection and application of clinical research methodology and statistical methods

In the early stage of the trial, the sample size was estimated based on the results of a preliminary trial, which is time efficient and cost effective.

Regarding the statistical analysis, the study used a linear mixed-effects model to analyze the primary and secondary outcomes, considering the correlation of repeated measurement data. This method can effectively handle missing data and further verify the robustness of the results by adjusting for the baseline expected values. The interpretation of effect sizes using Cohen's d augmented the clinical significance of the results.

In addition to the main analysis, the study also conducted subgroup analysis based on sex, race, education level, and baseline pain status, which helped elucidate differences across subgroups and provided a basis for individualized treatment. However, the researchers also clearly indicated that because of the small sample size, the results of these subgroup analyses are only of exploratory significance and need to be verified by larger studies in the future.

To sum up, this paper is highly scientifically sound and rigorous in terms of study design, process implementation, methodology selection, and statistical analysis, and the results are reliable and have clinical application value. However, the paper also noted that the selected population was not completely random and selection bias could have been involved; specifically, all participants were highly educated. The study could be expanded to include a more diverse sample in the future.

Section 40 Introduction and Comments of *Effect of Acupuncture vs Sham Acupuncture or Waitlist Control on Joint Pain Related to Aromatase Inhibitors Among Women With Early-Stage Breast Cancer: A Randomized Clinical Trial*

1. Introduction

IMPORTANCE Musculoskeletal symptoms are the most common adverse effects of aromatase inhibitors and often result in therapy discontinuation. Small studies suggest that acupuncture may decrease aromatase inhibitor-related joint symptoms.

OBJECTIVE To determine the effect of acupuncture in reducing aromatase inhibitor-related joint pain.

DESIGN, SETTING, AND PATIENTS Randomized clinical trial conducted at 11 academic centers and clinical sites in the United States from March 2012 to February 2017 (final date of follow-up, September 5, 2017). Eligible patients were postmenopausal women with early-stage breast cancer who were taking an aromatase inhibitor and scored at least 3 on the Brief Pain Inventory Worst Pain (BPI-WP) item (score range, 0-10; higher scores indicate greater pain).

INTERVENTIONS Patients were randomized 2 : 1 : 1 to the true acupuncture (n=110), sham acupuncture (n=59), or waitlist control (n=57) group. True acupuncture and sham acupuncture protocols consisted of 12 acupuncture sessions over 6 weeks (2 sessions per week), followed by 1 session per week for 6 weeks. The waitlist control group did not receive any intervention. All participants were offered 10 acupuncture sessions to be used between weeks 24 and 52.

MAIN OUTCOMES AND MEASURES The primary end point was the 6-week BPI-WP score. Mean 6-week BPI-WP scores were compared by study group using linear regression, adjusted for baseline pain and stratification factors (clinically meaningful difference specified as 2 points).

RESULTS Among 226 randomized patients (mean [SD] age, 60.7 [8.6] years; 88% white; mean [SD] baseline BPI-WP score, 6.6 [1.5]), 206 (91.1%) completed the trial. From baseline to 6 weeks, the mean observed BPI-WP score decreased by 2.05 points (reduced pain) in the true acupuncture group, by 1.07 points in the sham acupuncture group, and by 0.99 points in the waitlist control group. The adjusted difference for true acupuncture vs sham acupuncture was 0.92 points (95% CI, 0.20-1.65; $P=0.01$) and for true acupuncture vs waitlist control was 0.96 points (95% CI, 0.24-1.67; $P=0.01$). Patients in the true acupuncture group experienced more grade 1 bruising compared with patients in the sham acupuncture group (47% vs 25%; $P=0.01$).

CONCLUSIONS AND RELEVANCE Among postmenopausal women with early-stage breast cancer and aromatase inhibitor-related arthralgias, true acupuncture compared with sham acupuncture or with waitlist control resulted in a statistically significant reduction in joint pain at 6 weeks, although the observed improvement was of uncertain clinical importance.

2. Expert Comments

Comment 1

(1) Background and significance

This study focused on arthralgia in patients with cancer treated with aromatase inhibitors, a relatively common problem in patients with breast cancer affecting quality of life. Through the study of this specific population, we can propose new notions and methods for cancer pain management.

(2) Study design

This study proposed a clear research hypothesis that real acupuncture would reduce aromatase inhibitor-related joint pain at 6 weeks (according to BPI-WP) compared with sham acupuncture or no acupuncture (waiting treatment control group), and based on previous studies. A 2-point decrease in the BPI-WP score was identified as the clinically meaningful change. This laid a solid foundation for the selection of clinical outcome indicators, the sample size calculation, and the analysis and interpretation of the results.

A waiting treatment control group design was used to address concerns regarding the placebo effect in previous studies. This design can better evaluate the effect difference between real acupuncture and sham acupuncture and provides a more reliable basis for the interpretation of the results. In this study, special attention was paid to the training of acupuncture operators and the evaluation of their mastery, which ensured the effect of acupuncture.

(3) Limitations analysis

The article clearly listed several limitations, such as the inability to achieve blinding when patients are randomly assigned to the waiting treatment control group, and that the beliefs of patients in the real acupuncture group regarding the treatment could have affected the results. The main outcome was based on relatively short-term measures and lacked long-term follow-up data over 12 months, suggesting that further studies are needed to assess the persistence of treatment effects.

(4) Community participation and accessibility

The slow recruitment of participants and cost of intervention mentioned in the study reflect the challenges of promoting acupuncture treatment in the actual clinical environment, which need to be considered and addressed in future studies.

(5) Future research directions

As this study failed to assess the maintenance and durability of efficacy, future studies should focus on this aspect and explore the differences in response to acupuncture in different patient groups.

(6) Statistical analysis

① Poisson regression was used to estimate risk differences and relative risks, and Poisson regression models were used in the study along with robust standard errors. This method is suitable for the analysis of count data and can better handle the frequency of events. ② Mixed model analysis: A linear mixed model (SAS proc mixed) was used in the statistical analysis, which showed that the researchers considered the variability among individuals and the structure of repeated measures, thus improving the accuracy of the model. ③ Correction for multiple comparisons: In the comparison of the primary endpoint, the investigators used Bonferroni adjustment to control for the error rate of multiple comparisons, setting a significance level of $α=0.025$. This measure helped reduce the likelihood of false-positive results. ④ Data completeness: In the analysis, the investigators focused on the availability of follow-up data from different groups, and the results showed that the data reporting rate was similar across groups ($P=0.93$), which reduced concerns regarding bias stemming from differences between groups. ⑤ Assessment of clinical significance: Although statistical results showed a significant difference in joint pain reduction between the real and sham acupuncture groups and the waiting control group, the investigators noted that the clinical significance of the observed improvement remained uncertain, reflecting a distinction between statistical and clinical significance.

Overall, this study has important clinical significance in topic selection and a rigorous design, but there are also some limitations, which can be further explored in future studies. In this paper, the statistical analysis method was rigorous, and the characteristics of the data and needs of the research design were fully considered.

Comment 2

(1) Research design and process implementation

The study adopted a multicenter, randomized, controlled design with the following characteristics. ① The study adopted a three-group design, namely, a real acupuncture group, sham acupuncture group, and waiting treatment group, which is a classic design in clinical acupuncture research. Moreover, the study clarified in advance that the real acupuncture and sham acupuncture groups and the real acupuncture and waiting treatment groups would be compared twice, which could not only evaluate the specific effect of acupuncture, but also evaluate the overall effect of real acupuncture by comparing real acupuncture with awaiting treatment. Studies have shown that acupuncture has a strong placebo effect, and because of the characteristics of acupuncture and moxibustion therapy, the commonly used sham acupuncture is usually not a blank control without therapeutic effect; thus, sham acupuncture usually has a certain effect, which has a certain impact on the study. In this study, a waiting treatment group was added, which can better compensate for this problem. ② The study adopted a 2∶1∶1 ratio across groups, which allowed more participants to enter the real acupuncture treatment group and was more in line with ethical requirements. ③ Shallow needling of non-acupoints was used in the sham acupuncture group, and sham auricular point therapy was also provided in the sham acupuncture group. The superposition of the two sham interventions may increase the effect in the sham acupuncture group. ④ The minimum clinically significant difference was defined in advance as a 2-point decrease in the BPI-short form score, and based on this difference, the sample size was estimated and the final conclusion was determined.

(2) Selection and application of clinical research methodology and statistical methods

Overall, the statistical methods of this study were standardized. ① Sample size calculation: The sample size calculation process adjusted the test level α based on two comparisons determined in advance and considered the proportion of non-compliance, dropout rate, and proportion of possible contamination, but the number of cases finally determined based on the above considerations was not provided. ② Statistical analysis: The statistical analysis was mainly based on the multi-factor analysis method, and the possible influencing factors in the research process were fully considered. Furthermore, the detailed report of the complex mixed effects model is more comprehensive, giving a specific covariance matrix, random effects, and fixed effects factors, which is helpful for readers to fully understand the details of the analysis. The key contents such as the processing of missing data and adjustment of inspection level were also clearly reported. For the blinding evaluation, although there was a statistical difference in the proportion of correct guesses between the real and sham acupuncture groups, the interaction analysis showed that the results of guesses had no effect on the results of the study. For acupuncture research, it is difficult to achieve true blindness owing to the particularity of acupuncture therapy, and it is necessary to evaluate the success of blinding even if sham acupuncture is implemented.

Section 41 Introduction and Comments of *Effect of Acupuncture vs Sham Acupuncture on Live Births Among Women Undergoing in Vitro Fertilization: A Randomized Clinical Trial*

1. Introduction

IMPORTANCE Acupuncture is widely used by women undergoing in vitro fertilization (IVF), although the evidence for efficacy is conflicting.

OBJECTIVE To determine the efficacy of acupuncture compared with a sham acupuncture control performed during IVF on live births.

DESIGN, SETTING, AND PARTICIPANTS A single-blind, parallel-group randomized clinical trial including 848 women undergoing a fresh IVF cycle was conducted at 16 IVF centers in Australia and New Zealand between June 29, 2011, and October 23, 2015, with 10 months of pregnancy follow-up until August 2016.

INTERVENTIONS Women received either acupuncture ($n=424$) or a sham acupuncture control ($n=424$). The first treatment was administered between days 6 to 8 of follicle stimulation, and 2 treatments were administered prior to and following embryo transfer. The sham control used a noninvasive needle placed away from the true acupuncture points.

MAIN OUTCOMES AND MEASURES The primary outcome was live birth, defined as the delivery of 1 or more living infants at greater than 20 weeks' gestation or birth weight of at least 400 g.

RESULTS Among 848 randomized women, 24 withdrew consent, 824 were included in the study (mean [SD] age, 35.4 [4.3] years); 371 (45.0%) had undergone more than 2 previous IVF cycles, 607 proceeded to an embryo transfer, and 809 (98.2%) had data available on live birth outcomes. Live births occurred among 74 of 405 women (18.3%) receiving acupuncture compared with 72 of 404 women (17.8%) receiving sham control (risk difference, 0.5% [95% CI, −4.9% to 5.8%]; relative risk, 1.02 [95% CI, 0.76 to 1.38]).

CONCLUSIONS AND RELEVANCE Among women undergoing IVF, administration of acupuncture vs sham acupuncture at the time of ovarian stimulation and embryo transfer resulted in no significant difference in live birth rates. These findings do not support the use of acupuncture to improve the rate of live births among women undergoing IVF.

2. Expert Comments

Comment 1

This was a multiple-center, randomized-assignment, parallel-controlled, single-blind, sham-acupuncture controlled trial. The study design covered three acupuncture sessions of 25 minutes on days 6 to 8 of induction, before and after embryo transfer. The results showed that there was no statistically significant difference between acupuncture and sham acupuncture in the live birth rate of women undergoing IVF, and therefore did not support the use of acupuncture as an auxiliary means to improve the live birth rate of women undergoing IVF. As the first multicenter, large-sample, randomized controlled trial, the study demonstrated a high level of rigor in its design. However, the selection of a suitable population, design, and operation of the acupuncture program need to be further studied.

First, the effect of acupuncture depends on the acupuncture scheme (such as acupoint collection, stimulation amount, and intervention timing) and on the patient's physical condition. Therefore, it is necessary to set reasonable inclusion and exclusion criteria in clinical studies to explore the IVF population suitable for acupuncture treatment and to further clarify the efficacy and action mechanism of acupuncture in IVF.

Second, the acupuncture program of IVF mainly includes the selection of acupoints, amount of stimulation, and timing of the intervention. Stimulating quantity is a main factor affecting the curative effect of acupuncture and moxibustion. Correctly grasping the dose-effect relationship and conducting in-depth exploration have always been key considerations in clinical research. Since only three acupuncture treatments were performed in this trial, the amount of stimulation may have been insufficient, and thus the negative conclusion may be related to the failure to reach the required amount of acupuncture treatments.

Finally, the acupuncture protocol of the trial was determined based on the Delphi consensus, which has a certain gap with clinical practice; the acupoint compatibility is inconsistent with the previous study protocol, and its rationality remains to be discussed. Therefore, the key to improving the quality of clinical research and credibility of conclusions is to implement a strict research design that meets the requirements of evidence-based medicine.

Future clinical studies of acupuncture-assisted IVF should follow the strict evidence-based medical research model. First, we should choose an effective research scheme after preliminary clinical observation to carry out a case sequence study or small sample independent randomized controlled trial and constantly optimize and improve the research scheme according to the results of the trial. Multicenter and large sample randomized controlled trials should be carried out after accumulating a large reliable dataset and implementing mature research protocols.

Comment 2

(1) Study design and process implementation

This was a single-blind, parallel-group, randomized controlled trial designed to assess the effect of acupuncture on live birth rates in women undergoing IVF. The study was conducted at 16 IVF centers in Australia and New Zealand, with a final sample size of 848 women. The advantage of the study design was the large sample size, which can provide more statistically significant results, while the multicenter setting enhanced the external validity of the results. In addition, the study effectively reduced potential confounders by stratified randomization based on the number of embryo transfer cycles, age, and study site. However, the study also had some limitations. For example, there was imbalance in the stage of embryo transfer between the control and treatment groups, which may have affected the reliability of the results. In addition, the sample size did not meet the expected target because some patients refused to participate because of the widespread use of community acupuncture, which may have affected the generalizability and representativeness of the results.

(2) Selection and application of clinical research methodology and statistical methods

In terms of clinical research methodology, the study strictly followed the design specifications of randomized controlled trials, including randomization, stratification, and single-blind methods, which played an important role in controlling bias and improving the credibility of the results. The main analysis adopted the intention-to-treat principle, and further verified the robustness of the results through sensitivity analysis, showing the scientific rigor of the study in terms of data analysis. However, there is still room for improvement regarding the statistical methods. First, while the study primarily relied on risk differences and relative risks for group comparisons, it did not adjust for multiple comparisons, which may have increased the risk of false positives. Second, when facing the problem of an insufficient sample size, although the study carried out sensitivity analysis, it failed to strictly follow the original intention of sample size estimation, which may have led to some uncertainty in the interpretation of the results. In addition, the impact of imbalances in the study, such as differences in the stage of embryo transfer in the control group was not fully explained, which to some extent undermined the rigor of the conclusions.

To sum up, the design and implementation of this study were advantageous in several respects, including a large sample size, multicenter design, and rigorous randomization process, but there remain some issues that need to be further explored, such as the insufficient sample size, insufficient adjustment for multiple comparisons, and potential impact of uneven embryo transfer stages. Nevertheless, the results provided important clinical evidence for the use of acupuncture in IVF, but caution should be exercised in interpreting and generalizing the conclusions.

Section 42　Introduction and Comments of *Effect of Electroacupuncture on Urinary Leakage Among Women With Stress Urinary Incontinence: A Randomized Clinical Trial*

1. Introduction

IMPORTANCE Electroacupuncture involving the lumbosacral region may be effective for women with stress urinary incontinence (SUI), but evidence is limited.

OBJECTIVE To assess the effect of electroacupuncture vs sham electroacupuncture for women with SUI.

DESIGN, SETTING, AND PARTICIPANTS Multicenter, randomized clinical trial conducted at 12 hospitals in China and enrolling 504 women with SUI between October 2013 and May 2015, with data collection completed in December 2015.

INTERVENTIONS Participants were randomly assigned (1 : 1) to receive 18 sessions (over 6 weeks) of electroacupuncture involving the lumbosacral region (n=252) or sham electroacupuncture (n=252) with no skin penetration on sham acupoints.

MAIN OUTCOMES AND MEASURES The primary outcome was change from baseline to week 6 in the amount of urine leakage, measured by the 1-hour pad test. Secondary outcomes included mean 72-hour urinary incontinence episodes measured by a 72-hour bladder diary (72-hour incontinence episodes).

RESULTS Among the 504 randomized participants (mean [SD] age, 55.3 [8.4] years), 482 completed the study. Mean urine leakage at baseline was 18.4 g for the electroacupuncture group and 19.1 g for the sham electroacupuncture group. Mean 72-hour incontinence episodes were 7.9 for the electroacupuncture group and 7.7 for the sham electroacupuncture group. At week 6, the electroacupuncture group had greater decrease in mean urine leakage (−9.9 g) than the sham electroacupuncture group (−2.6 g) with a mean difference of 7.4 g (95% CI, 4.8 to 10.0; P<0.001). During some time periods, the change in the mean 72-hour incontinence episodes from baseline was greater with electroacupuncture than sham electroacupuncture with between-group differences of 1.0 episode in weeks 1 to 6 (95% CI, 0.2-1.7; P=0.01), 2.0 episodes in weeks 15 to 18 (95% CI, 1.3-2.7; P<0.001), and 2.1 episodes in weeks 27 to 30 (95% CI, 1.3-2.8; P<0.001). The incidence of treatment-related adverse events was 1.6% in the electroacupuncture group and 2.0% in the sham electroacupuncture group, and all events were classified as mild.

CONCLUSIONS AND RELEVANCE Among women with stress urinary incontinence, treatment with electroacupuncture involving the lumbosacral region, compared with sham electroacupuncture, resulted in less urine leakage after 6 weeks. Further research is needed to understand long-term efficacy and the mechanism of action of this intervention.

Chapter 2 Comments of Clinical Trials of Acupuncture and Moxibustion in SCI Journals

2. Expert Comments

Comment 1

Female SUI is a common clinical disease, with a prevalence rate as high as 49%. Currently, there is no effective way to cure SUI with the means available to contemporary medicine. The treatment effect of pelvic floor muscle training is usually limited, while some patients with severe disease face high cost and recurrence risk even if surgery is used. Traditional acupuncture and moxibustion therapy has certain advantages in the treatment of SUI, but previous studies generally had limitations such as small sample sizes, design defects, and high risk of bias, which severely limit the treatment's clinical application. Based on this practical clinical problem, LIU Baoyan and LIU Zhishun's research team in China included 504 patients in a multicenter randomized controlled study and divided the patients into an electroacupuncture group and a sham electroacupuncture group, which received bilateral electroacupuncture at BL33 (Zhongliao) and BL35 (Huiyang) points and sham electroacupuncture at sham points three times a week for 6 weeks. The results showed that electroacupuncture was significantly better than sham electroacupuncture in reducing the amount of urine leakage and frequency of urinary incontinence, and the difference was clinically significant. The curative effect could be maintained for 24 weeks after stopping the treatment, and adverse events rarely occurred during the treatment. The clinical value of the selected topic is high, the details of acupuncture intervention measures were completely disclosed, and the selection and location of acupoints, angle of acupuncture, manipulation of acupuncture, specific parameters of electroacupuncture, and treatment cycle and other specific details were introduced in detail. The study's scientifically sound and strict methodological design (including a large sample and multicenter recruitment) helped overcome the limitations of previous studies. The study provided high-quality evidence-based data for the effectiveness and safety of acupuncture and moxibustion in the treatment of female SUI. However, as no skin penetration and current output were used in the sham acupuncture control group, how could the effects of the blinding method be ensured? More details are needed for evaluation, and blinding may be more secure in future studies if placebo control is used with penetrating acupuncture combined with no current output.

Comment 2

(1) Study design and process implementation

This was a 30-week multicenter, randomized, sham electroacupuncture-controlled trial conducted in 12 hospitals in China and included 504 female patients with SUI. The study used a fixed-block stratified randomization method, and the patients were allocated to receive electroacupuncture or sham electroacupuncture treatment according to a ratio of 1 : 1 through a centralized randomization system, which ensured balance between the groups. Patients were blinded using a placebo and sham electroacupuncture design, and the blinding effect was tested to minimize the effects of expectation and subjective judgment on the results. The main outcome was the change in urine leakage from baseline to the 6th week, which was objectively measurable with a 1-hour urine pad test and could effectively evaluate the effect of acupuncture treatment of SUI, which had important clinical significance. The study was rigorously designed and conducted.

(2) Selection and application of clinical research methodology and statistical methods

The sample size of the study was estimated, considering 20% loss to follow up and pre-set subgroup analysis, and finally 504 female patients aged 40-75 years were included. The study used intention-to-treat analysis principles to fit a mixed-effects model, using baseline leak as the covariate, treatment as the fixed effect, and center and the interaction between center and treatment as the random effects considering across center differences. The analysis method fully considered repeated measurement data and adjusted for important covariates, which could effectively handle the variability among patients. The use of multiple imputations to impute the primary outcome under the missing at random hypothesis reduces bias compared with a single imputation method. Four sensitivity analyses (one prespecified and three post-hoc analyses) were conducted to assess the impact of missing data on the results and verify their robustness; a post-hoc subgroup analysis was conducted to explore the impact of electroacupuncture on SUI of varying severity. The paper fully discussed the limitations of the trial, and the selection and application of the methodology and statistical methods of the clinical study were reasonable and appropriate.

Section 43 Introduction and Comments of *Effect of Acupuncture and Clomiphene in Chinese Women With Polycystic Ovary Syndrome: A Randomized Clinical Trial*

1. Introduction

IMPORTANCE Acupuncture is used to induce ovulation in some women with polycystic ovary syndrome (PCOS), without supporting clinical evidence.

OBJECTIVE To assess whether active acupuncture, either alone or combined with clomiphene, increases the likelihood of live births among women with polycystic ovary syndrome.

DESIGN, SETTING, AND PARTICIPANTS A double-blind (clomiphene vs placebo), single-blind (active vs control acupuncture) factorial trial was conducted at 21 sites (27 hospitals) in mainland China between July 6, 2012, and November 18, 2014, with 10 months of pregnancy follow-up until October 7, 2015. Chinese women with polycystic ovary syndrome were randomized in a 1 : 1 : 1 : 1 ratio to 4 groups.

INTERVENTIONS Active or control acupuncture administered twice a week for 30 minutes per treatment and clomiphene or placebo administered for 5 days per cycle, for up to 4 cycles. The active acupuncture group received deep needle insertion with combined manual and low-frequency electrical stimulation; the control acupuncture group received superficial needle insertion, no manual stimulation, and mock electricity.

MAIN OUTCOMES AND MEASURES The primary outcome was live birth. Secondary outcomes included adverse events.

RESULTS Among the 1 000 randomized women (mean [SD] age, 27.9 [3.3] years; mean [SD] body mass index, 24.2 [4.3]), 250 were randomized to each group; a total of 926 women (92.6%) completed the trial. Live births occurred in 69 of 235 women (29.4%) in the active acupuncture plus clomiphene group, 66 of 236 (28.0%) in the control acupuncture plus clomiphene group, 31 of 223 (13.9%) in the active acupuncture plus placebo group, and 39 of 232 (16.8%) in the control acupuncture plus placebo group. There was no significant interaction between active acupuncture and clomiphene ($P=0.39$), so main effects were evaluated. The live birth rate was significantly higher in the women treated with clomiphene than with placebo (135 of 471 [28.7%] vs 70 of 455 [15.4%], respectively; difference, 13.3%; 95% CI, 8.0% to 18.5%) and not significantly different between women treated with active vs control acupuncture (100 of 458 [21.8%] vs 105 of 468 [22.4%], respectively; difference, −0.6%; 95% CI, −5.9% to 4.7%). Diarrhea and bruising were more common in patients receiving active acupuncture than control acupuncture (diarrhea: 25 of 500 [5.0%] vs 8 of 500 [1.6%], respectively; difference, 3.4%; 95% CI, 1.2% to 5.6%; bruising: 37 of 500 [7.4%] vs 9 of 500 [1.8%], respectively; difference, 5.6%; 95% CI, 3.0% to 8.2%).

CONCLUSIONS AND RELEVANCE Among Chinese women with PCOS, the use of acupuncture with or without clomiphene, compared with control acupuncture and placebo, did not increase live births. This finding does not support acupuncture as an infertility treatment in such women.

2. Expert Comments

Comment 1

PCOS is a common cause of infertility in women. Clinically, the failure rate (anovulation) of clomiphene citrate alone in the treatment of PCOS is as high as 23.4%. This was a randomized controlled trial designed to evaluate the effect of acupuncture combined with clomiphene citrate on improving the live birth rate of patients with PCOS, which is of high clinical value. In addition, this study innovatively used a 2×2 factorial design to analyze the overall and independent component effects of clomiphene and acupuncture, which can help clinicians more accurately determine the respective and combined effects of acupuncture and clomiphene. However, in the design of acupuncture interventions, there are several aspects worthy of in-depth consideration to carry out further research. First, the acupoint selection and intervention program of acupuncture more greatly considered the stimulation of acupuncture to the nervous system. PCOS is a complex disease; if infertility is treated according to the diagnosis of traditional Chinese medicine, selection of acupoints on the Conception Vessel and the Kidney Meridian of Foot-Shaoyin should be considered. It is worth considering whether future research can achieve a better curative effect if it is based on traditional dialectical acupoint selection along the meridians. Second, the real acupuncture program mainly used points on the abdomen and lower extremities, while the placebo acupuncture program mainly used points on the upper extremities. Whether this design would lead to a poor blinding effect is also worth serious consideration. Future studies may consider real acupuncture points adjacent to the sham acupuncture sites to achieve better blinded results. Third, as a disease that affects both the reproductive and endocrine systems, it is necessary to record the concomitant medication of patients to improve the symptoms of endocrine disorders. Future research can design a table to collect the information of concomitant medication and perform relevant statistical analysis. Overall, the study has high value in terms of clinical topic selection and a novel clinical design method, providing high-quality evidence for adjuvant acupuncture treatment of PCOS.

Comment 2

This study was widely influential and has attracted wide attention in China. The study, conducted in 21 centers in mainland China, used a two-by-two factorial design with four groups, and included a total of 1 000 women with PCOS to assess the effects of acupuncture and clomiphene and their interactions. The study design included four groups of acupuncture combined with clomiphene, control acupuncture (shallow acupuncture at non-shoulder points) combined with clomiphene, acupuncture combined with clomiphene placebo, and control acupuncture combined with clomiphene placebo. Acupuncture was administered twice a week. The study provided evidence of the beneficial effects of clomiphene in the Chinese population and found that neither acupuncture combined with clomiphene nor placebo increased the live birth rates, pregnancy rates, twin rates, and ovulation rates.

The large sample size and factorial design are significant characteristics of this study, enhancing its scientific and clinical value. The dropout rate was low, the report was rigorous and standardized, and the statistical analysis was thorough, providing a clear guide for the rational treatment of PCOS infertility in the clinic. The factorial design and statistical analysis scheme of the study were greatly changed compared with the initial study protocol, which is an important limitation of the self-report of the study in this paper. The basis of the study emphasized the preliminary research evidence and clinical status of acupuncture treatment of PCOS and related infertility and provided nine international clinical studies and a series of small sample randomized controlled trials as support, but it will be more convincing if there are preliminary clinical studies or large sample-size (more than 1 000 participants) clinical studies in China as support. In addition, the inclusion criteria for the study did not specify whether the enrolled participants had a desire to become pregnant or whether they were women of gestational age, and the primary outcome of the study was the live birth rate. The clinical plan, including the acupoint selection, acupoint setting for sham acupuncture, course of treatment, frequency of acupuncture, and design of follow-up course of treatment, would be more convincing if it was based on powerful evidence and a theoretical basis from early clinical and basic research. The study mentioned that the acupuncturists were graduate students in traditional Chinese medicine and emphasized that they were specifically trained according to the study protocol. A more detailed description of their qualifications and clinical experience would have been better according to the requirement of international reporting guidelines.

Section 44   Introduction and Comments of *The Long-Term Effect of Acupuncture for Migraine Prophylaxis: A Randomized Clinical Trial*

1. Introduction

IMPORTANCE   The long-term prophylactic effects of acupuncture for migraine are uncertain.

OBJECTIVE   To investigate the long-term effects of true acupuncture compared with sham acupuncture and being placed in a waiting-list control group for migraine prophylaxis.

DESIGN, SETTING, AND PARTICIPANTS   This was a 24-week randomized clinical trial (4 weeks of treatment followed by 20 weeks of follow-up). Participants were randomly assigned to true acupuncture, sham acupuncture, or a waiting-list control group. The trial was conducted from October 2012 to September 2014 in outpatient settings at 3 clinical sites in China. A total of 249 participants 18 to 65 years old with migraine without aura based on the criteria of the International Headache Society, with migraine occurring 2 to 8 times per month.

INTERVENTIONS   Participants in the true acupuncture and sham acupuncture groups received treatment 5 days per week for 4 weeks for a total of 20 sessions. Participants in the waiting-list group did not receive acupuncture but were informed that 20 sessions of acupuncture would be provided free of charge at the end of the trial.

MAIN OUTCOMES AND MEASURES   Participants

used diaries to record migraine attacks. The primary outcome was the change in the frequency of migraine attacks from baseline to week 16. Secondary outcome measures included the migraine days, average headache severity, and medication intake every 4 weeks within 24 weeks.

RESULTS A total of 249 participants 18 to 65 years old were enrolled, and 245 were included in the intention-to-treat analyses. One hundred eighty-nine (77.1%) were women. Baseline characteristics were comparable across the 3 groups. The mean (SD) change in frequency of migraine attacks differed significantly among the 3 groups at 16 weeks after randomization ($P<0.001$); the mean (SD) frequency of attacks decreased in the true acupuncture group by 3.2 (2.1), in the sham acupuncture group by 2.1 (2.5), and the waiting-list group by 1.4 (2.5); a greater reduction was observed in the true acupuncture than in the sham acupuncture group (difference of 1.1 attacks; 95% CI, 0.4-1.9; $P=0.002$) and in the true acupuncture vs waiting-list group (difference of 1.8 attacks; 95% CI, 1.1-2.5; $P<0.001$). Sham acupuncture was not statistically different from the waiting-list group (difference of 0.7 attacks; 95% CI, −0.1 to 1.4; $P=0.07$).

CONCLUSIONS AND RELEVANCE Among patients with migraine without aura, true acupuncture may be associated with long-term reduction in migraine recurrence compared with sham acupuncture or assigned to a waiting list.

2. Expert Comments

Comment 1

(1) Topic analysis

Approximately 25% to 38% of patients with migraine need preventive and drug treatment, but such treatment is often accompanied by adverse reactions, and overuse of analgesics or specific anti-migraine treatment may lead to drug overuse headache. Acupuncture and moxibustion are widely used in the treatment of migraine at home and abroad, especially for patients who are refractory to medication. Acupuncture has been shown to be effective in reducing migraine pain intensity, attack frequency, and duration, but previous studies have some limitations attributable to their small sample size. While expanding the sample size, this clinical trial also focused on the long-term effects of acupuncture, which is crucial for the successful prevention and reduction of migraine attacks.

(2) Implementation of acupuncture intervention

Acupuncture intervention is meaningful because acupuncture can relieve pain during a migraine attack (acute effect) and prevent migraine attacks (long-term effect); in the acupuncture intervention, GB20 (Fengchi) and GB8 (Shuaigu) were selected according to the meridian syndrome differentiation of the headache area, and the left and right points were used alternately for unilateral treatment. In the actual operation of acupuncture and description in the paper, the specification of the needle, operation of the needle, parameters of obtaining the qi sensation, and electroacupuncture stimulation (as well as the electroacupuncture stimulator) were clearly explained. The treatment was administered 20 times (once a day, 30 minutes each time, 5 consecutive days, 2 days off) for 4 weeks, and the overall intervention time was neither long nor short. No other auxiliary interventions were used in this trial. All therapists had received at least 5 years of training and had at least 4 years of clinical experience; the control group received sham acupuncture; that is, four non-acupoints were selected, without obtaining the qi sensation, and the electric stimulation and treatment time were the same as those for the electroacupuncture group. The above sham acupuncture method was simple and practical.

Comment 2

The design and implementation of this clinical study were scientifically sound and rigorous. The study was conducted in China with a multicenter, randomized, controlled trial design, which enhanced the scientificity and generalizability of the results. The study protocol was registered in advance and well implemented. During the implementation of the study, detailed operational standards and quality control measures were established for each stage, including participant screening, grouping, treatment, and follow up. In addition, the acupuncture protocol used in the study had a good clinical and theoretical basis and clear guidance and requirements for the addition and subtraction of acupoints, acupuncture parameters, deqi, and other factors. The study also clearly discussed the qualifications and experience requirements for acupuncturists. A series of measures taken ensured the standardization, individualization, and quality control of the acupuncture treatment.

The study used both a sham acupuncture control and a waiting treatment group (blank group). Such a control format facilitates the observation of the effects of sham acupuncture and provides a basis for the analysis of the components of acupuncture efficacy; however, it precludes blinding of patients in the waiting treatment group and of acupuncturists and other research workers who have contact with patients. Furthermore, the primary outcome of this study was the difference in the cumulative frequency of migraine attacks from baseline (cumulative frequency of migraine attacks during the 4 weeks prior to enrollment) during weeks 13-16 (4 weeks total). Outcome and secondary outcome data were collected through patient diaries. This is a typical patient self-reported outcome. Such outcomes, especially symptomatic outcomes, are greatly influenced by subjective factors, and the need to use blinding methods to overcome information bias is obvious. In addition, the English description of the primary outcome in the article is easy for readers to misunderstand; specifically, that the study spanned 4 weeks. The study was well discussed, especially regarding the reduction of disease in the waiting treatment group during the observation period and reliability of baseline disease data. If we can increase the comparison of the significance and results between the placebo acupuncture group and waiting treatment group, the significance and value of the study will be enhanced.

Section 45 Introduction and Comments of *Rewiring the Primary Somatosensory Cortex in Carpal Tunnel Syndrome With Acupuncture*

1. Introduction

Carpal tunnel syndrome (CTS) is the most common entrapment neuropathy, affecting the median nerve at the wrist. Acupuncture is a minimally-invasive and conservative therapeutic option, and while rooted in a complex practice ritual, acupuncture overlaps significantly with many conventional peripherally-focused neuromodulatory therapies. However, the neurophysiological mechanisms by which acupuncture impacts accepted subjective/psychological and objective/physiological outcomes are not well understood. Eligible patients ($n=80$, 65 female, age: 49.3±8.6 years) were enrolled and randomized into three intervention arms: (i) Verum electro-acupuncture "local" to the more affected hand; (ii) verum electro-acupuncture at "distal" body sites, near the ankle contralesional to the more affected hand; and (iii) local sham electro-acupuncture using non-penetrating placebo needles. Acupuncture therapy was provided for 16 sessions over 8 weeks. Boston Carpal Tunnel Syndrome Questionnaire (BCTQ) assessed pain and paraesthesia symptoms at baseline, following therapy and at 3-month follow-up. Nerve conduction studies assessing median nerve sensory latency and brain imaging data were acquired at baseline and following therapy. Functional magnetic resonance imaging assessed somatotopy in the primary somatosensory cortex using vibrotactile stimulation over three digits (2, 3 and 5). While all three acupuncture interventions reduced symptom severity, verum (local and distal) acupuncture was superior to sham in producing improvements in neurophysiological outcomes, both local to the wrist (ie. median sensory nerve conduction latency) and in the brain (ie. digit 2/3 cortical separation distance). Moreover, greater improvement in second/third interdigit cortical separation distance following verum acupuncture predicted sustained improvements in symptom severity at 3-month follow-up. We further explored potential differential mechanisms of local versus distal acupuncture using diffusion tensor imaging of white matter microstructure adjacent to the primary somatosensory cortex. Compared to healthy adults ($n=34$, 28 female, 49.7±9.9 years old), patients with carpal tunnel syndrome demonstrated increased fractional anisotropy in several regions and, for these regions we found that improvement in median nerve latency was associated with reduction of fractional anisotropy near (i) contralesional hand area following verum, but not sham, acupuncture; (ii) ipsilesional hand area following local, but not distal or sham, acupuncture; and (iii) ipsilesional leg area following distal, but not local or sham, acupuncture. As these primary somatosensory cortex subregions are distinctly targeted by local versus distal acupuncture electrostimulation, acupuncture at local versus distal sites may improve median nerve function at the wrist by somatotopically distinct neuroplasticity in the primary somatosensory cortex following therapy. Our study further suggests that improvements in primary somatosensory cortex somatotopy can predict long-term clinical outcomes for carpal tunnel syndrome.

2. Expert Comments

Comment 1

CTS involves a group of symptoms and signs of median nerve compression in the carpal tunnel and is one of the most common peripheral nerve compression syndromes. The prevalence of CTS in adults is approximately 2.7% to 5.8%, and its lifetime incidence is as high as 10% to 15%. This was a placebo-controlled, randomized parallel group longitudinal neuroimaging study designed to evaluate the efficacy of acupuncture in the treatment of CTS and has high clinical value. However, there are several aspects worthy of further consideration regarding the design of the acupuncture interventions, which would facilitate carrying out more in-depth research. First, the susceptibility and severity of CTS vary significantly among individuals of different ages, sexes, and occupations. CTS usually occurs between the ages of 36 and 60 years; the ratio of women to men is as high as 2 : 1 to 5 : 1; and individuals who engage in repetitive wrist movements for a long time, such as computer programmers, maintenance workers, painters and others, are more likely to be affected. This study could have performed further analyses based on the results obtained and observe whether there are different treatment effects across different age stages, sexes, and occupations. Second, the evaluation of acupuncture efficacy in this study only considered three time points, namely, before treatment, at the end of treatment, and at the end of follow up. Setting up evaluation time points during treatment can better reflect the changes in acupuncture efficacy, considering acupuncture time and dosage, to better guide the clinician in selecting the best course of treatment. Third, the points used in the two groups of real acupuncture treatment groups were located in the upper or lower limbs, while both upper and lower limbs were targeted in the sham acupuncture group, and the position of the points was obviously different. Whether this design would lead to a poor blinding effect is worth considering. A double simulation design can be considered in future studies; for example, the acupoint selection scheme can include upper limb real acupuncture combined with lower limb sham acupuncture and upper limb sham acupuncture combined with lower limb real acupuncture, so that patients cannot distinguish the treatment received according to the location of acupoint selection to achieve a better blinding effect. Overall, the study examined a valuable clinical topic and had a novel clinical design, providing high-quality evidence of the effectiveness of acupuncture in the treatment of CTS.

Comment 2

(1) Study design

This study investigated the effect of acupuncture treatment for CTS on remodeling of the primary somatosensory cortex (S1). A randomized (replacement block randomization), controlled (placebo or sham acupuncture control), and single-blind (patient-blind and physician-informed) parallel-group longitudinal neuroimaging design was used. The potential confounding factors were effectively controlled, and the reliability and scientificity of the results were ensured by comparing the efficacy of real acupuncture with that of sham acupuncture. Outcome variables were also defined in advance, and the measure of symptom severity was the BCTQ, which was measured at the start of treatment, after treatment, and at the 3-month follow up. For nerve conduction studies, the median sensory nerve conduction latency was measured before and after treatment. For the finger separation distance, the measurement index was D2/D3 separation, measured before and after treatment.

(2) Process implementation

In the implementation process, three intervention methods were used, ie, local acupuncture, distal acupuncture, and sham acupuncture; the balance among the groups was ensured by computer-generated random block assignment. Acupuncture treatment was performed by an experienced, licensed acupuncturist, reducing manipulation variability. In addition, multiple assessment tools were used, including the BCTQ to assess symptoms, nerve conduction studies to assess wrist nerve function, and functional magnetic resonance imaging to assess cortical neuroplasticity, with comprehensive coverage of subjective and objective indicators to ensure a multidimensional study.

(3) Selection and application of clinical research methodology and statistical methods

In the statistical analysis stage, repeated measures analysis of variance was used to evaluate the changes in the BCTQ score, nerve conduction study, and finger separation distance, and post-hoc testing was conducted to handle longitudinal data and multi-group comparisons. However, there were some problems. For the BCTQ score, the interaction between group (true acupuncture, sham acupuncture) and time (baseline, post-treatment, 3-month follow up) obtained with repeated measures analysis of variance in the paper is trend-significant ($P=0.098$), with no statistical significance according to the results. In addition, for post-hoc testing, the study analyzed the change in indicators (such as the BCTQ score), which essentially means applying new statistical methods (such as the two independent samples t-test), and the term post-hoc testing may not be applicable here.

Overall, the study combined traditional clinical evaluation methods and advanced neuroimaging techniques for an in-depth exploration of the mechanism of acupuncture treatment for CTS, and strictly followed the standards of clinical research methodology in the design and implementation process to ensure the scientificity and reliability of the results. Through multi-level and multi-dimensional evaluation methods, as well as rigorous statistical analyses, the neurophysiological mechanism of acupuncture treatment of CTS was effectively revealed. However, the study also had some limitations, such as no prior sample size estimation, a relatively small sample size, and limited data for long-term follow up. Future studies can consider increasing the sample size and extending the follow-up period to further verify and expand the existing findings. Second, the paper did not test whether the assumption of homogeneity of variance had been met when using repeated measures analysis of variance.

Section 46   Introduction and Comments of *A Randomised Controlled Trial Examining the Effect of Acupuncture at the EX-HN3 (Yintang) Point on Pre-operative Anxiety Levels in Neurosurgical Patients*

1. Introduction

Pre-operative anxiety is an unpleasant state of psychological distress that occurs in up to 87% of patients awaiting neurosurgical procedures. Sedative medication is undesirable in this population due to the need for early postoperative neurological assessment. Acupuncture has previously been shown to reduce pre-operative anxiety, but studies involving neurosurgical patients are lacking. This single-center, prospective, randomised controlled trial was designed to determine the effect of acupuncture at the EX-HN3 (Yintang) on pre-operative anxiety levels in neurosurgical patients. The study was prospectively registered before participant recruitment. After measuring baseline anxiety levels, 128 patients were randomly allocated in a 1∶1 ratio by a web-based computer program to receive either acupuncture at the EX-HN3 point (acupuncture group) or no intervention (control group). Participants were not blinded, but all analyses were performed by a member of the research team who was unaware of the group allocation. The primary outcome measure was anxiety level after 30 min, as measured by the six-item short form of the State-Trait Anxiety Inventory (STAI-S6) (possible score range 20-80). Sixty-two patients in each group were subsequently analysed. Median (IQR [range]) STAI-S6 score reduced significantly in the acupuncture group (46.7 [36.7-53.3] {23.3-70.0} to 40.0 [30.0-46.7] {20.0-53.3}, $P<0.001$), with no change seen in the control group (41.7 [33.3-53.3] {20.0-76.7} to 43.3 [36.7-50.0] {20.0-76.7}, $P=0.829$). There were no adverse events in either group. Acupuncture at the EX-HN3 point reduces pre-operative anxiety levels in patients awaiting neurosurgery.

2. Expert Comments

Comment 1

(1) Analysis of topic selection

The topic selection focused on how to solve a difficult and prominent issue in clinical practice, analyze the refinement and construction of the key clinical issue, and reflect its value and significance.

This single-center, prospective, randomized, controlled trial addressed the clinical reality of "preoperative anxiety" in neurosurgery, using needle stimulation and pressing of the EX-HN3 acupoint, and performed comparisons with a waiting list group. The main outcome measure was the anxiety level (STAI-S6 score) after 30 minutes. Secondary outcome measures included changes in anxiety levels (Amsterdam Preoperative Anxiety and Information Scale), postoperative pain scores in the post anesthesia care unit, opioid requirements, and incidence of postoperative nausea and vomiting. The results showed that the STAI-S6 score in the acupuncture group was significantly lower than that in the control group. There were no adverse events in either group. It was confirmed that acupuncture treatment of the EX-HN3 acupoint could reduce the preoperative anxiety level of neurosurgical patients.

In recent years, the concept of enhanced recovery after surgery (ERAS) has attracted much attention. Its purpose is to effectively reduce surgical trauma and stress by taking a series of measures following evidence-based medical data in the perioperative period to promote the rapid recovery of patients. Acupuncture and moxibustion are expected to play an important role in perioperative management. This study examined a clinical problem faced by patients in neurosurgery, integrated external treatment of traditional Chinese medicine, had clear research objectives and clear research ideas, simple and feasible operation, and good clinical guiding significance.

(2) The implementation of acupuncture intervention

The implementation of the acupuncture intervention was analyzed, with issues including the rationality of acupuncture treatment, details of acupuncture, treatment plan, auxiliary intervention measures, background of the therapist, and setting of the control group.

In this study, the acupuncture intervention scheme was applied to the EX-HN3 acupoint by pressing the needle and applying rotary pressing manipulation every 10 minutes, which was easy to operate and easy to learn and use, without other auxiliary measures, being convenient for clinical promotion. However, whether the scheme was suitable for the clinical practice of acupuncture and moxibustion and can obtain the best curative effect can be further studied. First, regarding the acupoint selection, is EX-HN3 the most effective acupoint? Are there better synergistic acupoint combinations? The second concerns the amount of stimulation; the amount of stimulation in the skin is smaller when the needle (0.2 mm × 1.5 mm) is pressed every 10 minutes. What is the curative effect compared with acupuncture? Is there any basis for stimulation every 10 minutes? The frequency of pressing (tid, bid, qd, etc.), the design of matching acupoints, and the strength of pressing manipulation can be further refined. The third pertains to the selection of the control group. Enrolling a group of patients waiting for surgery does not help control for the placebo effect, so we can design a scientific acupuncture group.

Comment 2

This was a randomized controlled trial designed to evaluate the effect of acupuncture at EX-HN3 on relieving preoperative anxiety in neurosurgical patients. The study used a rigorous randomization method, ie, the randomized permutation block method, to divide patients into a test group and a control group, but did not describe the process of patient recruitment, and it is not clear whether the random sequence was destroyed after patient assignment. Blinding researchers and participants in acupuncture therapy clinical studies is challenging, but the use of allocation concealment during patient recruitment can effectively reduce bias. At the same time, using sham acupuncture as a control can effectively eliminate the subjective influence of not receiving acupuncture treatment. On the population side, the exclusion of patients with psychiatric disorders, prior acupuncture treatment experience, and acupuncture for the prevention of nausea and vomiting was effective in avoiding problems with the patient's understanding of the anxiety scale, as well as psychological resistance or comfort because of previous acupuncture treatment. In the statistical analysis, the study should also consider variations in efficacy among different subgroups, for example, approximately 50% of the patients had severe anxiety, and the influence of effect modifiers (such as anxiety severity) on the effect of acupuncture should be explored. In the methodological part of the study, the extent of clinically meaningful improvement in anxiety levels (30% score reduction) was identified, but in the outcome part, the proportion of patients who achieved clinically meaningful improvement was not analyzed. In general, the study design could be further improved, especially in the aspects of concealed grouping, sham acupuncture control, subgroup analysis, and result reporting, to further explore the dominant population of acupuncture and provide higher quality evidence-based medical data for acupuncture to alleviate the preoperative anxiety of neurosurgical patients.

Section 47   Introduction and Comments of *Acupuncture As an Integrative Approach for the Treatment of Hot Flashes in Women With Breast Cancer: A Prospective Multicenter Randomized Controlled Trial (AcCliMaT)*

1. Introduction

PURPOSE   To determine the effectiveness of acupuncture for the management of hot flashes in women with breast cancer.

PATIENTS AND METHODS   We conducted a pragmatic, randomized controlled trial comparing acupuncture plus enhanced selfcare versus enhanced self-care alone. A total of 190 women with breast cancer were randomly assigned. Random assignment was performed with stratification for hormonal therapy; the allocation ratio was 1 : 1. Both groups received a booklet with information about climacteric syndrome and its management to be followed for at least 12 weeks. In addition, the acupuncture group received 10 traditional acupuncture treatment sessions involving needling of predefined acupoints. The primary outcome was hot flash score at the end of treatment (week 12), calculated as the frequency multiplied by the average severity of hot flashes. The secondary outcomes were climacteric symptoms and quality of life, measured by the Greene Climacteric and Menopause Quality of Life scales. Health outcomes were measured for up to 6 months after treatment. Expectation and satisfaction of treatment effect and safety were also evaluated. We used intention-to-treat analyses.

RESULTS   Of the participants, 105 were randomly assigned to enhanced self-care and 85 to acupuncture plus enhanced self-care. Acupuncture plus enhanced self-care was associated with a significantly lower hot flash score than enhanced self-care at the end of treatment ($P<0.001$

and at 3-and 6-month post-treatment follow-up visits (P=0.002 8 and 0.001, respectively). Acupuncture was also associated with fewer climacteric symptoms and higher quality of life in the vasomotor, physical, and psychosocial dimensions ($P<0.05$).

CONCLUSION Acupuncture in association with enhanced self-care is an effective integrative intervention for managing hot flashes and improving quality of life in women with breast cancer.

2. Expert Comments

Comment 1

(1) Topic analysis

Breast cancer is one of the most common malignant tumors in women, and its treatment is often accompanied by varied side effects, of which hot flashes are one of the most common symptoms experienced by patients with breast cancer receiving chemotherapy or corticosteroid therapy. This study focused on the comprehensive efficacy of acupuncture combined with self-care in the treatment of hot flashes and improvement of quality of life in women with breast cancer. The study design fully considered the individual differences and disease characteristics of patients and used a multicenter, randomized controlled trial design to ensure the reliability and reproducibility of the results. Acupuncture combined with enhanced self-care provides a non-drug, low-cost, and effective treatment option for patients with breast cancer who experience hot flashes, helping alleviate the symptom, improve quality of life, and reduce the physical and mental burden of patients.

(2) The implementation of acupuncture intervention

The study implemented acupoint selection based on syndrome differentiation. What are the criteria for different syndromes? Is subjectivity possible? In terms of acupoint selection, no more than 11 acupoints are used for each treatment, and the number of acupoints varies greatly among different syndromes. During the evaluation, different syndrome types and different acupoint selection can also be used for subgroup analysis, and the results may thus become more rigorous. Generally, the frequency of acupuncture in clinical trials is three times a week or once every other day. In this study, 10 acupuncture treatments were provided and one should consider whether the low acupuncture frequency was not in line with clinical practice.

Comment 2

(1) Study design and process implementation

This practical multicenter, randomized, controlled trial compared the effectiveness of acupuncture and intensive self-care combined therapy versus intensive self-care alone in the treatment of hot flashes in women with breast cancer, rather than using a placebo control to assess the specific effect. The experimental group was treated with acupuncture combined with moxibustion, and the patient's syndrome type was considered to select acupuncture points and moxibustion treatment, closely aligned with clinical practice.

The study was rigorously conducted; given the lack of guidelines for the management of menopausal syndrome in women with a history of breast cancer, the intensive self-care program was based on the consensus of team experts. Moreover, at periodic visits, the researchers also assessed patients' adherence to the intensive self-care recommendations.

Conversations between the acupuncturist and patient were kept to a minimum to limit nonspecific therapeutic effects.

(2) Selection and application of clinical research methodology and statistical methods

Overall, the statistical method of this study was standardized. ①Randomization: Stratification was conducted based on the presence or absence of corticosteroid therapy (gonadotropin-releasing hormone agonist), with good control for hormonal effects on the study outcome. ②Sample size calculation: Sample size estimation conducted based on the pre-test results can improve accuracy; although the study was terminated early because not all patients were enrolled as designed, this had a limited impact on the outcome of the study. ③Statistical analysis: Overall, the analysis was standardized, but there are several points that could have been better managed, such as the use of corticosteroid therapy as a stratification factor for randomization, but in fact, almost all patients received breast cancer corticosteroid therapy, and nearly half of the participants received gonadotropin-releasing hormone analogue combination therapy, which may have affected the implementation of stratified randomization. It even led to the adjustment of the randomization method, but the article did not provide relevant details. Moreover, t-test was used for statistical analysis of the primary efficacy index, without considering the influence of baseline and other possible factors on the results.

Section 48 Introduction and Comments of *Acupuncture for Chronic Severe Functional Constipation: A Randomized Trial*

1. Introduction

BACKGROUND Acupuncture has been used for chronic constipation, but evidence for its effectiveness remains scarce.

OBJECTIVE To determine the efficacy of electroacupuncture (EA) for chronic severe functional constipation (CSFC).

DESIGN Randomized, parallel, sham-controlled trial.

SETTING 15 hospitals in China.

PARTICIPANTS Patients with CSFC and no serious underlying pathologic cause for constipation. Intervention: 28 sessions of EA at traditional acupoints or sham EA (SA) at nonacupoints over 8 weeks.

MEASUREMENTS The primary outcome was the change from baseline in mean weekly complete spontaneous bowel movements (CSBMs) during weeks 1 to 8. Participants were followed until week 20.

RESULTS 1 075 patients (536 and 539 in the EA and SA groups, respectively) were enrolled. The increase from baseline in mean weekly CSBMs during weeks 1 to 8 was 1.76 (95% CI, 1.61 to 1.89) in the EA group and 0.87 (CI, 0.73 to 0.97) in the SA group (between-group difference, 0.90 [CI, 0.74 to 1.10]; $P<0.001$). The change from baseline in mean weekly CSBMs during weeks 9 to 20 was 1.96 (CI, 1.78 to 2.11) in the EA group and 0.89 (CI, 0.69 to 0.95) in the SA group (between-group difference, 1.09 [CI, 0.94 to 1.31]; $P<0.001$). The proportion of patients having 3 or more mean weekly CSBMs in the EA group was 31.3% and 37.7% over the treatment and follow-up periods, respectively, compared with 12.1% and 14.1% in the SA group ($P<0.001$). Acupuncture-related adverse events during treatment were infrequent in both groups, and all were mild or transient.

LIMITATIONS Longer-term follow-up was not assessed. Acupuncturists could not be blinded.

CONCLUSION Eight weeks of EA increases CSBMs and is safe for the treatment of CSFC. Additional study is warranted to evaluate a longer-term treatment and follow-up.

2. Expert Comments

Comment 1

(1) The topic selection is suitable for clinical practice

This study focuses on CSFC, a condition with a global incidence of up to 16% that significantly reduces patients' quality of life. Patients with constipation usually experience persistent symptoms. Traditional drugs, such as laxatives and prokinetics, are widely used, but their efficacy is limited, accompanied by strong recurrence, poor compliance, and other issues. Therefore, finding an effective and safe alternative therapy is crucial. By introducing EA into the treatment of CSFC, this study fills a gap in non-pharmacological constipation and provides robust clinical evidence that supports the use of acupuncture treatment for the disease, underscoring the clinical relevance and social impact of the chosen topic.

In this study, EA served as the core intervention of the selected topic, supported by both traditional Chinese medicine theory and modern medical research. Acupoint selection was based on the traditional Chinese medicine concept that "spleen and stomach are the foundation of acquired constitution" emphasizing the improvement of large intestine conduction and defecation by regulating functions of the spleen and stomach. This theoretical basis is further strengthened by modern research showing that EA can promote gastrointestinal motility and improve gut dynamics, which reinforces the scientific rationale of this study.

(2) The design of the experiment is rigorous, and the results convincing

EA has attracted increasing attention due to its minimal adverse and strong regulation effects on the body; however, its clinical efficacy still requires confirmation through rigorous trials. While existing literature includes clinical trial results on acupuncture for constipation, most studies are limited to small sample sizes, single-center studies, and a lack of large-scale, multi-center randomized controlled trials. The current study collected data from 1 075 patients across 15 hospitals, providing a robust sample size and strengthening the credibility of its conclusions. This large-scale investigation not only contributes to raising the profile of EA within the international medical community but also broadens the potential for applying acupuncture in the treatment of functional disorders.

(3) Analysis of the implementation of acupuncture intervention

This study demonstrates scientific rigor and precision in the implementation of acupuncture intervention. The selection of acupoints and formulation of the acupuncture

Chapter 2 Comments of Clinical Trials of Acupuncture and Moxibustion in SCI Journals

protocol were carefully and scientifically designed by the researchers. ST25 (Tianshu), SP14 (Fujie), and ST37 (Shangjuxu) were selected as the primary acupoints for electroacupuncture intervention. These acupoints are traditionally associated with the regulation of gastrointestinal function in traditional Chinese medicine, and modern research also supports their effectiveness in promoting intestinal peristalsis. This integration of Chinese and Western medical insights in acupoint selection strengthens the credibility of the study findings.

Additionally, the acupuncture procedures used in this study paid careful attention to stringent standardization measures, such as the control of acupuncture depth and stimulation frequency and intensity, to ensure repeatability and consistency of the treatment process.

(4) Design of the sham acupuncture control group

The design of the control group is a key feature of this study. To minimize the impact of psychological expectations on the study outcomes, a SA control was used, which was relatively effective in controlling the placebo effect. The SA group was punctured at the superficial layer of non-acupoints without electrical stimulation, which simulated the operation of EA to the maximum extent. Subjects without prior acupuncture experience were included to distinguish between the two groups based on appearance. Shallow puncture at non-acupoints reduced the physiological and psychological effects of acupuncture as much as possible. This design enhances the study results, making them more reliable, and could provide a methodological reference for similar research designs.

(5) Optimizable aspect

Although the study design is rigorous, areas for potential optimization still exist. For example, although the study addressed the qualifications and training of therapists, it did not elaborate on how the consistency of treatment in each center was guaranteed. Variations in operating habits and skill levels among therapists may have subtle impacts on treatment outcomes, and future studies could thus further enhance operational consistency through more detailed operating specifications and regular supervision, potentially using *Kappa* consistency analysis to evaluate the consistency of interventions or assessment results among multiple investigators.

In addition, although the study adopted a multicenter design, it was not completely blinded, and the therapist was aware of the grouping, which may have introduced observer bias. In this paper, shallow needling of non-acupoints without electrical stimulation was used to achieve the blind method, which may pose several issues. First, numerous acupoints exist in the human body, and "Ashi points" without fixed positions can be found; therefore, shallow needling at non-acupoints could potentially trigger therapeutic effects that weaken specific therapeutic effects of the experimental group, as would be observed in the comparative statistics of the two groups. Second, positional differences can occur between acupoints and non-acupoints, and if both groups are treated in the same space at the same time, subjects may notice differences in acupoint selection. Perhaps placing the two groups in relatively independent rooms could help ensure better blinding. Third, with no electrical stimulation, the needle used for acupuncture does not oscillate with the current, which creates a sensory difference between the two methods. This may make it easier for subjects who have undergone EA treatment in the past to break the blindness. However, the implementation of blinding in acupuncture clinical trials is challenging. Therefore, future studies should consider enhanced blinding techniques or minimizing potential bias through multipoint monitoring.

Comment 2

(1) Study design and process implementation

This was a large-sample, multicenter, randomized, controlled, superiority and confirmatory study with the following main characteristics. ①The study clearly put forward the clinical hypothesis of superiority and was designed accordingly. ②The study recruited 1 075 participants from 15 centers in China, resulting in a large sample size and good representativeness. ③A sham acupuncture control was used to control the placebo effect of acupuncture, and the specific therapeutic effect of acupuncture was evaluated. ④A defecation diary was used to record the patient's defecation, which ensured the accuracy of the data. ⑤An independent data safety monitoring committee was set up to monitor the research process and safety.

(2) Selection and application of clinical research methodology and statistical methods

Overall, the statistical methods were standardized. ①Test hypothesis: A clear superiority test hypothesis was proposed, and the results of the study also reached the threshold set by the superiority assumption. ②Sample size calculation: The sample size was estimated based on preliminary test results, and the sample size estimation was accurate. ③Statistical analysis: Multivariate analysis was the main method of statistical analysis, and covariates that may have affected the results were included. The multiple imputation method was used to handle missing data, which is more rigorous and reliable than the last observation carried forward method. Additionally, a pattern-mixture model was used to analyze the sensitivity of multiple imputations to evaluate the robustness of the multiple imputation results, which is worth studying. ④Evaluation of blinding: Although sham acupuncture control can achieve better blinding of patients, whether the blinding is really successful remains a concern. Therefore, it is necessary to carry out blind evaluation of clinical trials with sham acupuncture control. It is recommended to use a special blinding evaluation index for blinding evaluation and report the results in detail.

Section 49　Introduction and Comments of *Acupuncture for Menopausal Hot Flashes: A Randomized Trial*

1. Introduction

BACKGROUND　Hot flashes (HFs) affect up to 75% of menopausal women and pose a considerable health and financial burden. Evidence of acupuncture efficacy as an HF treatment is conflicting.

OBJECTIVE　To assess the efficacy of Chinese medicine acupuncture against sham acupuncture for menopausal HFs.

DESIGN　Stratified, blind (participants, outcome assessors, and investigators, but not treating acupuncturists), parallel, randomized, sham-controlled trial with equal allocation.

SETTING　Community in Australia.

PARTICIPANTS　Women older than 40 years in the late menopausal transition or postmenopause with at least 7 moderate HFs daily, meeting criteria for Chinese medicine diagnosis of kidney yin deficiency.

INTERVENTIONS　10 treatments over 8 weeks of either standardized Chinese medicine needle acupuncture designed to treat kidney yin deficiency or noninsertive sham acupuncture.

MEASUREMENTS　The primary outcome was HF score at the end of treatment. Secondary outcomes included quality of life, anxiety, depression, and adverse events. Participants were assessed at 4 weeks, the end of treatment, and then 3 and 6 months after the end of treatment. Intention-to-treat analysis was conducted with linear mixed-effects models.

RESULTS　327 women were randomly assigned to acupuncture (n=163) or sham acupuncture (n=164). At the end of treatment, 16% of participants in the acupuncture group and 13% in the sham group were lost to follow-up. Mean HF scores at the end of treatment were 15.36 in the acupuncture group and 15.04 in the sham group (mean difference, 0.33 [95% CI, −1.87 to 2.52]; P=0.77). No serious adverse events were reported.

LIMITATION　Participants were predominantly Caucasian and did not have breast cancer or surgical menopause.

CONCLUSION　Chinese medicine acupuncture was not superior to noninsertive sham acupuncture for women with moderately severe menopausal HFs.

2. Expert Comments

Comment 1

Topic analysis: The incidence of perimenopausal vasomotor symptoms (VMS) is high, and the quality of life of patients with severe VMS is compromised. Although hormone replacement therapy (menopausal hormone therapy) is a recognized treatment measure, the acceptance of patients is not high. Acupuncture is a commonly used method for the treatment of VMS, but there are different opinions on its therapeutic effect, and high-quality clinical evidence is lacking. This study enrolled patients with the kidney yin deficiency syndrome of VMS, and a randomized controlled trial was conducted in 15 acupuncture clinics to evaluate the efficacy of acupuncture in the treatment of perimenopausal hot flashes, which has important clinical significance.

Implementation of acupuncture intervention: In terms of setting and implementation of intervention measures, this study has certain reference significance, such as including an acupuncture group and a placebo acupuncture group with the non-acupoint and non-puncture method, acupuncture performed by acupuncture therapists with more than 5 years of experience, and a management plan of hormone replacement therapy for participants. However, the study concluded that for patients with VMS kidney yin deficiency syndrome, 8-week standardized acupuncture treatment did not reduce menopausal HF more effectively than non-invasive sham acupuncture. This merits in depth discussion. Acupoint selection, acupuncture operation, and course of treatment are the core elements of acupuncture prescription per the consensus of the acupuncture industry. Is the acupoint selection and course of treatment in this study a better choice for the treatment of VMS with kidney yin deficiency syndrome? Are the six acupoints of KI6 (Zhaohai), KI7 (Fuliu), SP6 (Sanyinjiao), LR3 (Taichong), CV4 (Guanyuan), and HT6 (Yinxi) consistent with the etiology and pathogenesis of this disease? Given that only 10 treatments over 8 weeks (twice a week for the first 2 weeks and once a week thereafter) were administered, does the frequency of treatment meet the demand for the amount of treatment? Do the results of the study reflect the true clinical value of acupuncture in the treatment of this condition? In fact, the authors also expressed thoughts on personalized treatment and acupuncture "dosage" in the article.

Comment 2

(1) Study design and process implementation

This study was rigorously designed to evaluate the effect of acupuncture on VMS in menopausal women and to ensure the scientificity and reliability of the results through a multicenter, stratified, and randomized trial method. Stratified randomization was performed by an acupuncturist using a password-protected electronic system to ensure secrecy and fairness of distribution. Participants were recruited through multiple channels with strict inclusion criteria to ensure homogeneity; the sample size was reasonably calculated, considering the expected effects and attrition rates. Although acupuncturists were not blinded, other participants and assessors were, reducing bias. Interventions were standardized for the acupuncture and sham acupuncture groups, using noninsertive blunt needles to simulate the acupuncture process. The primary outcome measure was the hot flash score, assessed using a validation tool, and the systematic data collection covered the baseline, treatment, and follow up. Although the details of data management and protection measures were insufficiently described, the study did obtain ethical approval and followed the relevant standards, and the overall design was scientifically sound and reasonable. However, there is still room for improvement regarding quality control and control of confounding factors.

(2) Selection and application of clinical research methodology and statistical methods

The clinical research methodology and statistical methods of this study were rigorously selected, and a multicenter, randomized, sham-controlled trial design was adopted to effectively evaluate the efficacy of acupuncture and moxibustion on VMS in menopausal women. The risk of bias was controlled using computer-generated random sequence and spreadsheet hidden assignment for the allocation of participants to the control group and the blinding method. The primary outcome measures were assessed using standardized instruments, and statistical analyses were performed using linear mixed-effects models for repeated measures and intention-to-treat analysis to enhance the robustness of the results. Multiple imputations and sensitivity analysis were used to examine the robustness of the missing data. However, the study did not specify the correction measures for multiple comparisons and the subgroup analysis strategy, which may have an impact on the interpretation of the results. Although significance levels were set, and effect sizes were reported, there was insufficient discussion on clinical significance. Overall, the study provided credible evidence for the efficacy of acupuncture in menopausal women, but, in the future, further optimization should be made in terms of multiple comparison correction, subgroup analysis, and interpretation of clinical significance to enhance the broad applicability and clinical value of the study.

Section 50 Introduction and Comments of *Transcutaneous Acupoint Electrical Stimulation Pain Management After Surgical Abortion: A Cohort Study*

1. Introduction

INTRODUCTION Transcutaneous acupoint electrical stimulation (TEAS) is a standard therapy for painful conditions. This study evaluated pain-relieving effects of treatment with TEAS before and after surgical abortion.

METHODS In this cohort study 140 nulliparae requesting pregnancy termination with intravenous anesthesia from August to December 2013 at the outpatient clinic of Wenzhou Medical University First Affiliated Hospital were recruited and divided into three cohorts who received TEAS pre-, post-, and both pre- and post-operation, alongside a control group. The cohorts underwent TEAS treatment for 30 min before and/or after the procedure while the control group received no TEAS treatment. Pain levels were evaluated upon recovery at 10, 30, and 45 min, respectively, after abortion.

RESULTS Mean Visual Analog Scale (VAS) scores in pre-operation cohorts, but not the post-operation cohort, were significantly lower than those obtained for the control group at 10 min ($P<0.01$). VAS scores at 30 min and 45 min postoperatively were similar in each cohort but lower than control values ($P<0.001$). More cohort patients reported mild or no pain than control patients ($P<0.05$); the preoperation cohorts had more women with no pain compared with the post-operation group ($P<0.05$). There were no differences among groups in medical treatment required after 45 min. There were fewer complications of nausea and vomiting in the cohorts compared with the control group ($P<0.05$).

CONCLUSIONS Performing TEAS before and after surgical abortion provides postoperative pain relief. However, receiving TEAS before surgery allowed more women to experience mild or no pain.

IMPLICATIONS Transcutaneous acupoint electrical stimulation shows potential as an adjunct to conventional pain treatment following surgical abortion in nulliparae.

2. Expert Comments

Comment 1

This study focused on pain management during surgical abortion, a topic of significant clinical interest. Surgical abortion is a common gynecological operation, and pain management during the procedure is directly linked to the patient's surgical experience and postoperative recovery. Although general anesthesia can effectively control intraoperative pain, postoperative pain remains a common issue, and it is particularly important to explore more effective postoperative analgesia methods. This study provided a potential, non-pharmacological analgesic option for clinical use by evaluating the analgesic effect of TEAS before and after surgical abortion.

The study divided the patients into four groups: Preoperative, postoperative, combination of preoperative and postoperative, and control groups to comprehensively evaluate the analgesic effect of TEAS at different time points. The reliability of the findings was ensured by standardized TEAS treatment parameters and a clinically recognized pain assessment method (VAS score). Moreover, the study also had a certain scientific basis for the selection of analgesic acupoints according to contemporary anatomical findings that there are medial crural cutaneous branches of the saphenous nerve in the superficial layer of the SP8 (Diji) acupoint and tibial nerve in the deep layer. The saphenous nerve and sympathetic nerve innervating the smooth muscle of the uterus derive from the same nerve segment, and the tibial nerve and sensory and parasympathetic nerve fibers of the uterus derive from the same nerve segment. The nerve fibers of the SP6 (Sanyinjiao) point mainly derive from the L4-S2 nerve segments, and the nerve fibers of the uterus mainly derive from the T11-L2, S2-S4 nerve segments, which share the same or adjacent nerve segment distributions. This may be the anatomical basis for the analgesic effect of SP8 and SP6 before and after surgical abortion.

The results of this study showed that patients treated with preoperative TEAS had significantly lower pain scores than those in the control group in the early postoperative period (10 minutes), indicating that preoperative TEAS demonstrated a significant preemptive analgesic effect. Although pain scores in the postoperative groups converged at 30 and 45 minutes, patients preoperatively treated with TEAS showed a lower incidence of pain in the early postoperative period, suggesting the effectiveness of the preemptive analgesia strategy. In addition, the study also found that TEAS treatment significantly reduced the incidence of postoperative nausea and vomiting, further supporting its clinical value.

In conclusion, this study provided strong evidence for the application of TEAS for analgesia during surgical abortion. Preoperative TEAS treatment significantly reduced the early postoperative pain score and incidence of pain and reduced the incidence of postoperative side effects such as nausea and vomiting. Therefore, TEAS was suggested as a safe and effective non-pharmacological analgesic option for use in clinical practice, helping improve patient surgical experience and postoperative recovery quality. Future studies should further explore the optimal treatment parameters and acupoint selection of TEAS to enhance its analgesic effect and promote its wide clinical application.

Comment 2

This study used a cohort study design to assess the effect of TEAS on pain before and after surgical abortion, with visual analog scale measures of pain scores and pain incidence as primary outcomes. The final 140 patients included in the study were all from the same time period in the region, and the population origins of the TEAS-exposed group and non-exposed group were considered relatively similar. The study provided a detailed report on the operational procedures and technical parameters of TEAS, which can be used as a reference for evidence users. However, the study was limited in the following respects: ①The study did not calculate the sample size, and the final sample size was small, resulting in insufficient statistical power. ②The report of the pain score was insufficient in the Results section, and the pain score value of the non-exposure group was not reported. ③The study did not account for confounding factors. As this study had an observational design, it was extremely crucial to adjust for confounding factors when assessing the differences in outcome efficacy between groups and to clearly report the effect indicators before and after adjustment and their 95% confidence intervals. ④As described by the authors, the study did not identify the best acupoints at different stages (preoperative, intraoperative, and postoperative), mainly because of the small sample size, and could not conduct subgroup or exploratory analysis on the effect modifiers that may have affected the treatment effect, such as acupoints, pain level, and sub-population, to provide personalized guidance.

Section 51   Introduction and Comments of *Electroacupuncture Versus Gabapentin for Hot Flashes Among Breast Cancer Survivors: A Randomized Placebo-Controlled Trial*

1. Introduction

PURPOSE Hot flashes are a common and debilitating symptom among survivors of breast cancer. This study aimed at evaluating the effects of electroacupuncture (EA) versus gabapentin (GP) for hot flashes among survivors of breast cancer, with a specific focus on the placebo and nocebo effects.

PATIENTS AND METHODS We conducted a randomized controlled trial involving 120 survivors of breast cancer experiencing bothersome hot flashes twice per day or greater. Participants were randomly assigned to receive 8 weeks of EA or GP once per day with validated placebo controls (sham acupuncture [SA] or placebo pill [PP]). The primary end point was change in the hot flash composite score (HFCS) between SA and PP at week 8, with secondary end points including group comparisons and additional evaluation at week 24 for durability of treatment effects.

RESULTS By week 8, SA produced significantly greater reduction in HFCS than did PP (−2.39; 95% CI, −4.60 to −0.17). Among all treatment groups, the mean reduction in HFCS was greatest in the EA group, followed by SA, GP, and PP (−7.4 vs −5.9 vs −5.2 vs −3.4; $P \leqslant 0.001$). The pill groups had more treatment-related adverse events than did the acupuncture groups: GP (39.3%), PP (20.0%), EA (16.7%), and SA (3.1%), with $P=0.005$. By week 24, HFCS reduction was greatest in the EA group, followed by SA, PP, and GP (−8.5 vs −6.1 vs −4.6 vs −2.8; $P=0.002$).

CONCLUSION Acupuncture produced larger placebo and smaller nocebo effects than did pills for the treatment of hot flashes. EA may be more effective than GP, with fewer adverse effects for managing hot flashes among breast cancer survivors; however, these preliminary findings need to be confirmed in larger randomized controlled trials with long-term follow-up.

2. Expert Comments

Comment 1

(1) Topic analysis

How the chosen topic focuses on solving a difficult and prominent issue in clinical practice, analyze the refinement and development of the key clinical issue, and reflect its value and significance.

Focus on a hot issue: Breast cancer is one of the most common malignant tumors among women in China, and its incidence ranks first among female malignant tumors, increasing by year and trending toward younger patients. However, this study specifically focused on the symptom of hot flashes after breast cancer surgery. The topic is narrow yet precise, and it aligns well with the strengths of acupuncture.

Basic research support: It is stated in the research background that acupuncture is a non-pharmacological therapy that may be helpful in the treatment of hot flashes. EA in particular has been shown to affect endorphins and other central neuropeptides, providing biological plausibility support for the treatment of hot flashes using this modality. Previous basic research served as support for this clinical study.

Placebo effect of acupuncture: The placebo effect of acupuncture and moxibustion is a multidimensional and complex phenomenon, involving many aspects of patients' psychological and physiological reactions as well as research methodology. The placebo effect of acupuncture is complex and worthy of further discussion. This study did not avoid addressing its associated placebo and nocebo effects.

(2) The implementation of acupuncture intervention

The analysis of acupuncture intervention implementation was discussed, including the rationale for acupuncture treatment, details of acupuncture, treatment plan, adjunctive interventions, background of the therapist, and setting of the control group.

Treatment frequency: In this study, the intervention was conducted twice a week in the first 2 weeks, then once a week in the next 6 weeks, with 10 treatments conducted in 8 weeks. The treatment frequency was relatively low, and the duration too long. Better results may have been achieved with an increased frequency.

Background of the therapists: This was a single-center trial with two participating acupuncturists of 8 and 20 years of experience, respectively. The difference in the experience of the two acupuncturists is substantial and raises the question of whether this may have led to result variations.

Comment 2

The study, published in the *Journal of Clinical Oncology*, employed a four-arm randomized controlled trial design with the participants randomized to EA, SA, GP, and PP groups. The primary objective of the study was to compare the efficacy of SA and PP in reducing hot flashes in breast cancer survivors to assess the placebo and nocebo effects of non-pharmacological therapy. The sample size calculation based on this explicit assumption ensured the validity of the statistical design and sufficient statistical power, while effectively controlling for type I errors in multiple comparisons. The study assigned the participants to four groups to more comprehensively explore the effects of different treatments. The differences between real treatment and placebo could be further explored through the inclusion of the EA and GP groups. Although the sample size of these two groups was insufficient to support the evaluation of their efficacy, the study provided important preliminary data for future large-scale studies.

Randomization and blinding in the study design effectively improved the quality of the study and reduced the risk of bias. Participants were assigned with the use of computer-generated random numbers and stratified according to hormone therapy status to ensure equilibrium across the groups. The use of opaque envelopes and the unblocked randomization design increased the unpredictability of the randomization process, thereby reducing the risk of selection bias. Patients, lead investigators, and statisticians were blinded to reduce information bias. In terms of statistical analysis, the study used a mixed linear model to analyze repeated measures data, which makes full use of data at different time points, improves statistical efficiency, and can evaluate the impact of individual differences.

Overall, the study validated the main hypothesis through a sound design and randomization method and provided insights into the differences in the effects of different treatments. The study provided important clinical evidence for the application of non-pharmacological treatments for managing hot flashes among breast cancer survivors.

Section 52 Introduction and Comments of *Alexander Technique Lessons or Acupuncture Sessions for Persons With Chronic Neck Pain*

1. Introduction

BACKGROUND Management of chronic neck pain may benefit from additional active self-care-oriented approaches.

OBJECTIVE To evaluate clinical effectiveness of Alexander Technique Lessons or Acupuncture Sessions (ATLAS) usual care for persons with chronic, nonspecific neck pain.

DESIGN Three-group randomized, controlled trial.

SETTING U. K. primary care.

PARTICIPANTS Persons with neck pain lasting at least 3 months, a score of at least 28% on the Northwick Park Questionnaire (NPQ) for neck pain and associated disability, and no serious underlying pathology.

INTERVENTION 12 acupuncture sessions or 20 one-to-one Alexander lessons (both 600 minutes total) plus usual care versus usual care alone.

MEASUREMENTS NPQ score (primary outcome) at 0, 3, 6, and 12 months (primary end point) and Chronic Pain Self-Efficacy Scale score, quality of life, and adverse events (secondary outcomes).

RESULTS 517 patients were recruited, and the median duration of neck pain was 6 years. Mean attendance was 10 acupuncture sessions and 14 Alexander lessons. Between-group reductions in NPQ score at 12 months versus usual care were 3.92 percentage points for acupuncture (95% CI, 0.97 to 6.87 percentage points) ($P=0.009$) and 3.79 percentage points for Alexander lessons (CI, 0.91 to 6.66 percentage points) ($P=0.010$). The 12-month reductions in NPQ score from baseline were 32% for acupuncture and 31% for Alexander lessons. Participant self-efficacy improved for both interventions versus usual care at 6 months ($P<0.001$) and was significantly associated ($P<0.001$) with 12-month NPQ score reductions (acupuncture, 3.34 percentage points [CI, 2.31 to 4.38 percentage points]; Alexander lessons, 3.33 percentage points [CI, 2.22 to 4.44 percentage points]). No reported serious adverse events were considered probably or definitely related to either intervention.

LIMITATION Practitioners belonged to the 2 main U.K.-based professional associations, which may limit generalizability of the findings.

CONCLUSION Acupuncture sessions and Alexander Technique lessons both led to significant reductions in neck pain and associated disability compared with usual care at 12 months. Enhanced self-efficacy may partially explain why longer-term benefits were sustained.

2. Expert Comments

Comment 1

This study systematically evaluated the clinical efficacy of ATLAS in patients with chronic nonspecific neck pain using a randomized controlled clinical trial design and was conducted in a primary health care center in the United Kingdom. The study both provided strong evidence for ATLAS treatment of chronic neck pain and emphasized the importance of psychological factors in clinical outcomes, which has significant implications for guiding clinical practice, optimizing treatment options, and improving the quality of life of patients.

In total, 517 patients with chronic nonspecific neck pain were randomly divided into three groups: acupuncture plus usual care, Alexander Technique training plus usual care, and usual care alone. The former two groups received 12 sessions of 50-minute acupuncture therapy and 20 one-on-one Alexander Technique training sessions, respectively, in addition to usual care. The primary outcome measure was the NPQ score, and the secondary outcome measures included current pain intensity, the Short Form 12, version 2 (SF-12v2), and patients' self-efficacy. The study's strength lies in its use of a large sample, parallel randomized controlled trial design, scientifically reasonable outcome measures, and a follow-up period of up to 12 months, providing strong support for evaluating long-term efficacy. The results showed that ATLAS can effectively relieve symptoms in patients with chronic neck pain, improve quality of life, and significantly enhance self-efficacy, revealing the important role of positive psychological changes in the sustained relief of chronic neck pain. The study also indicated that acupuncture, as a non-invasive and low-risk intervention, shows promise as an important complementary alternative for the treatment of chronic pain.

Comment 2

This pragmatic randomized controlled trial was designed to evaluate the long-term clinical efficacy of acupuncture and Alexander Technique lessons compared to usual care in patients with chronic neck pain. Broader inclusion criteria were used to enhance the generalizability of the results. The participants were randomly assigned to receive acupuncture or Alexander Technique lessons in addition to usual care or usual care alone. This design aimed to assess whether additional interventions augmenting existing usual care could lead to significant clinical improvements.

Dynamic block randomization was implemented through a secure randomization system, ensuring the rigor and unpredictability of group assignments. Both the acupuncturists and course instructors were members of professional associations, which to some extent guaranteed the standardization and consistency of the interventions. Statistical analysis followed an intention-to-treat approach, ensuring that all randomly assigned participants were included in the analysis to reduce selection bias. To address missing data, the study used a repeated-measures mixed-effects model to analyze the NPQ score at 12 months as the main outcome measure, and multiple sensitivity analyses were conducted to ensure the robustness of the results. Although the study performed two primary hypothesis tests to compare the effects of the two interventions, a correction for multiple testing was not mentioned, which may comprise a limitation. However, as both hypothesis tests reached statistical significance, the interpretation of the findings may not have been materially affected.

Although blinding was difficult to achieve owing to the nature of the intervention, several measures were taken during the design, implementation, and statistical analysis phases, effectively reducing potential bias and improving the reliability and validity of the results.

Chapter 3

Content and Interpretation of the *Tianjin Consensus on Clinical Research of Traditional Chinese Medicine Initiated by Researchers*

Section 1 Tianjin Consensus on Clinical Research of Traditional Chinese Medicine Initiated by Researchers

The *Tianjin Consensus on Clinical Research of Traditional Chinese Medicine Initiated by Researchers* was specifically formulated to further standardize the project selection, design evaluation, process management, and quality control of traditional Chinese medicine clinical researches, improve the quality of traditional Chinese medicine clinical researches, promote the healthy development, and enhance the ability of traditional Chinese medicine medical and health institutions to diagnose, treat, prevent, and control diseases.

1. Clinical researches initiated by researchers comprises an activity carried out by medical and health institutions to study the diagnosis, treatment, rehabilitation, prognosis, etiology, prevention, and health maintenance of diseases, with individuals or groups (including medical and health information) as the research object, not for the purpose of registration of products such as drugs and medical devices (including *in vitro* diagnostic reagents).

2. The Clinical Research Center of Traditional Chinese Medicine was established relying on the First Teaching Hospital of Tianjin University of Traditional Chinese Medicine and giving full play to the guiding role of the World Federation of Acupuncture-Moxibustion Societies (WFAS), World Federation of Chinese Medicine Societies, China Association of Acupuncture and Moxibustion, and China Association of Chinese Medicine. The aims include adopting innovative and open management mechanisms and operation modes, establishing a multidisciplinary professional clinical research methodology team, building a clinical research evaluation technology platform, organizing and conducting clinical research of traditional Chinese medicine initiated by researchers, accumulating high-quality clinical evidence, and enhancing and highlighting the clinical value of traditional Chinese medicine.

3. Aims also include improving and revising the *Management Standards for Clinical Research of Acupuncture and Moxibustion*, and the *Management Standards for Clinical Research of Traditional Chinese Medicine*, standardizing behavior in the process of clinical research of traditional Chinese medicine to protect the rights and interests of the participants, validating the research results, establishing the reliability of the research conclusions, and providing a basis for the safe and effective use of traditional Chinese medicine.

4. Relying on the Clinical Research Center of Traditional Chinese Medicine, the aim is to organize research efforts at home and abroad; focus on the difficulties of major and common diseases such as stroke, dementia, hypertension, pain, and depression; fully utilize the advantages of acupuncture and moxibustion; clarify the scope of treatment; and compensate for the shortcomings of drug therapy and for the deficiencies of pharmacotherapy. Acupuncture and moxibustion clinical diagnosis and treatment programs and high-quality clinical evidence, complementing the advantages of traditional Chinese medicine and western medicine, and reflecting the ability and level of diagnosis and treatment in China, have been popularized and applied at home and abroad through clinical guidelines. Concurrently, we should utilize the means of contemporary science and technology to clarify and explain the principles of acupuncture and moxibustion treatment, innovate and develop acupuncture and moxibustion theory, develop intelligent acupuncture and moxibustion diagnosis and treatment equipment, and strive to produce original results to lead the global academic development of acupuncture and moxibustion adhering to international standards, enhance the clinical value of acupuncture and moxibustion in preventing and treating diseases, and promote acupuncture and moxibustion worldwide.

Chapter 3 Content and Interpretation of the *Tianjin Consensus on Clinical Research of Traditional Chinese Medicine Initiated by Researchers*

5. The First Teaching Hospital of Tianjin University of Traditional Chinese Medicine will provide special funds and strive for support from all sides at home and abroad to establish a multi-funding mechanism to ensure the continuous development of clinical research initiated by researchers.

6. We should actively strive for the guidance, assistance, and support of national and local competent departments, and contribute more greatly to the modernization and internationalization of traditional Chinese medicine.

Authors: LIU Baoyan, ZHANG Yanjun, WANG Jingui

Expert group for consensus formulation (in *Pinyin* of order): DU Yuzheng (First Teaching Hospital of Tianjin University of Traditional Chinese Medicine), DU yuanhao (First Teaching Hospital of Tianjin University of Traditional Chinese Medicine), FAN Guanwei (First Teaching Hospital of Tianjin University of Traditional Chinese Medicine), FEI Yutong (Beijing University of Chinese Medicine), FU Wenbin (Guangdong Provincial Hospital of Traditional Chinese Medicine), GANG Weijuan (China Academy of Chinese Medical Sciences), GUO Yi (Tianjin University of Traditional Chinese Medicine), HAO Chongyao (Shanxi University of Traditional Chinese Medicine), HU Siyuan (First Teaching Hospital of Tianjin University of Traditional Chinese Medicine), HUANG Yuhong (Second Teaching Hospital of Tianjin University of Traditional Chinese Medicine), KONG Fanming (First Teaching Hospital of Tianjin University of Traditional Chinese Medicine), LI Huanan (First Teaching Hospital of Tianjin University of Traditional Chinese Medicine), LIU Baoyan (China Academy of Chinese Medical Sciences), LIU Cunzhi (Beijing University of Chinese Medicine), LIU Guozheng (*Journal of Traditional Chinese Medicine*), LU Liming (Guangzhou University of Traditional Chinese Medicine), MAO Jun (Memorial Sloan-Kettering Cancer Center, USA), NI Guangxia (Nanjing University of Traditional Chinese Medicine), RONG Peijing (China Academy of Chinese Medical Sciences), SUN Xin (West China Hospital), WANG Baohe (First Teaching Hospital of Tianjin University of Traditional Chinese Medicine), WANG Bin (First Teaching Hospital of Tianjin University of Traditional Chinese Medicine), WANG Jingui (First Teaching Hospital of Tianjin University of Traditional Chinese Medicine), WANG Shu (Affiliated Hospital of Tianjin Academy of Traditional Chinese Medicine), WANG Xianliang (First Teaching Hospital of Tianjin University of Traditional Chinese Medicine), WU Xiaodong (China Academy of Chinese Medical Sciences), ZHANG Hong (Chengdu University of Traditional Chinese Medicine), ZHANG Yanjun (First Teaching Hospital of Tianjin University of Traditional Chinese Medicine), ZHAO Ling (Chengdu University of Traditional Chinese Medicine), ZHUANG Pengwei (First Teaching Hospital of Tianjin University of Traditional Chinese Medicine)

Section 2 Interpretation of the *Tianjin Consensus on Clinical Research of Traditional Chinese Medicine Initiated by Researchers*

On November 11, 2023, the 16th International Symposium on Acupuncture and Moxibustion was held in Tianjin, China, sponsored by the First Teaching Hospital of Tianjin University of Traditional Chinese Medicine and the World Federation of Acupuncture-Moxibustion Societies (WFAS), and hosted by the National Acupuncture and Moxibustion Clinical Medical Research Center of Traditional Chinese Medicine. During the meeting, 30 experts in traditional Chinese medicine and methodology were invited to hold a closed-door meeting on the topic of the construction of a clinical research system of traditional Chinese medicine initiated by researchers and conducted in-depth discussions on the organizational structure, safeguard mechanisms, and research focus of clinical research of traditional Chinese medicine initiated by researchers. Finally, the *Tianjin Consensus on Clinical Research of Traditional Chinese Medicine Initiated by Researchers* (hereinafter referred to as the *Tianjin Consensus*) was formed.

1. Background of the Formation of the *Tianjin Consensus*

Traditional Chinese medicine has unique characteristics and advantages. As traditional Chinese medicine is increasingly widely used worldwide, the importance of clinical research has become increasingly prominent, and the evidence-based sources of decision-making transformation in clinical practice also require high-quality clinical data. In recent years, significant progress has been made in the clinical and mechanism research of traditional Chinese medicine in the treatment of several major and common diseases, such as cardiovascular and cerebrovascular diseases, cancer, metabolic diseases, pain syndromes, and gastrointestinal dysfunction. Clinical research results have been published in the *JAMA*, *The Lancet*, *New England Journal of Medicine*, *Annals of Internal Medicine*, *The BMJ*, and other authoritative international journals, showcasing the clinical effectiveness of traditional Chinese medicine and promoting the incorporation of Chinese programs into international clinical practice guidelines. With the increasing influence of traditional Chinese medicine in the world, the support of the development of modern science and technology, and the deepening integration of multiple disciplines, its modernization process is also accelerating. With the global pursuit of a healthy lifestyle, the unique concepts and treatment methods contained in traditional Chinese medicine will be more popularized, and it is expected that in the future, traditional Chinese medicine will play a more important role in the field of global health.

Clinical research initiated by researchers refers to the activities carried out by medical and health institutions to study the diagnosis, treatment, rehabilitation, prognosis, etiology, prevention, and health maintenance of individuals with varied diseases, with individuals or groups (including medical and health information) as the participant, not for the purpose of registration of drugs and medical devices. For the innovation and development of traditional Chinese medicine, the role of clinical research of traditional Chinese medicine initiated by researchers has become increasingly prominent, and its importance has been widely recognized.

There remain many problems in the clinical research of traditional Chinese medicine initiated by researchers: ① The phenomenon of "scattered studies" is increasingly prevalent, the degree of organization is obviously insufficient, with each unit often carrying out research independently, lacking unified planning and coordination, resulting in a large number of low-level clinical research repetition, affecting the progress of scientific research, leading to waste of resources, and increasing the possibility of misleading clinical practice. ② Lack of a clinical research evaluation system in line with the characteristics of traditional Chinese medicine. The existing evaluation system cannot accurately measure the value and efficacy of clinical research in traditional Chinese medicine, which limits further development in clinical research in this field. ③ Scientific research activities cannot progress smoothly because clinical research is limited by insufficient funding; sufficient and sustained research funds are also an important bottleneck affecting clinical research.

Therefore, solving these problems, improving the organization of traditional Chinese medicine clinical researches, establishing a scientific evaluation system, and ensuring sufficient research funds have become important issues to be urgently solved in the current *Tianjin Consensus*.

2. Interpretation of the *Tianjin Consensus*

(1) Strive for policy support

National and local authorities play a vital role in the clinical researches of traditional Chinese medicine initiated by researchers. Traditional Chinese medicine clinical research urgently needs to win multi-directional policy support, promote the implementation of action plans through industry forces, and strive for a more favorable environment and conditions for the development of clinical research of traditional Chinese medicine.

(2) Build a research platform and a talent team

Adhering to the concept of resource integration and collaborative innovation, this effort provides strong support for clinical research of traditional Chinese medicine by building a professional team and technology platform of multi-disciplinary integration. We should pool the strength of multi-disciplinary scientific research; set up professional teams for clinical research; attract the active participation of well-known universities, medical institutions, scientific research institutes and research and development enterprises at home and abroad; jointly build an innovative system of deep collaboration across medicine, science, research, production, and government; establish a professional clinical research methodology team with multi-disciplinary integration; form a community of clinical research of traditional Chinese medicine through a scientific and effective organizational structure; concentrate superior resources; and carry out large sample, multi-center, and high-quality clinical research.

(3) Form an operation mechanism for the clinical research community

To build an efficient three-level network structure of the national traditional Chinese medicine clinical research community, the first-level units are the head medical unit or scientific research institution, which should have strong scientific research strength and whose main responsibilities include top-level design, overall coordination, supervision of operation implementation and quality control, data collection and analysis, and result release. The secondary-level units are composed of medical institutions or universities with strong scientific research capabilities in various regions, mainly responsible for assisting the first-level units in communicating with each other, participating in research programs and planning, and be held responsible for ethical review, implementation plans, and sample and data collection. The third-level units comprise municipal hospitals, primary medical institutions, or small research institutions, whose main task is to participate in data collection and result promotion. Optimal allocation and efficient utilization of resources can be realized, and a complete scientific research chain from top-level design to grass-roots practice can be formed, through this three-level network architecture.

(4) Standardize the research process and behavior, focus on critical issues and challenges, and promote innovation and development

Perfecting and revising the relevant management norms is a key step to ensuring the quality of clinical research in traditional Chinese medicine. These norms attach importance to the authenticity and reliability of research results and emphasize protecting the rights and interests of the participants. By standardizing all aspects of the research process, we can prevent the occurrence of research deviations and misconduct, ensure the standardization and scientific of clinical research of traditional Chinese medicine, provide a basis for the safe and effective use of traditional Chinese medicine, and help enhance public trust and acceptance of traditional Chinese medicine.

The *Tianjin Consensus* clearly indicates the major and common diseases that should be focused on in clinical research of traditional Chinese medicine, emphasizes the advantages of acupuncture and moxibustion and other characteristic therapies of traditional Chinese medicine, and concentrates incorporating key technological advances and overcoming clinical problems in the field of traditional Chinese medicine. Through the combination of traditional Chinese and western medicine and complementary advantages, a more targeted and effective Chinese diagnosis and treatment program could be formed to enhance the clinical value and international influence of traditional Chinese medicine. Contemporary science and technology are used to reveal the therapeutic principles of acupuncture and other therapies, promote theoretical innovation and technological progress, enhance the scientific and credibility of traditional Chinese medicine, and lay the foundation for the internationalization of traditional Chinese medicine.

(5) Construct a diversified financing system

Funding is an important condition for ensuring the continuous development of clinical research in traditional Chinese medicine. The *Tianjin Consensus* proposes striving for the support of various resource sources at home and abroad, building a diversified financing system, strengthening the supervision and evaluation of the use of funds to ensure the sustainability and stability of clinical research initiated by researchers, and strengthening the transformation and application of clinical research results to ensure that the research results serve the clinic and bring substantial benefits to patients. This mechanism could help alleviate the shortage of research funds and provide material guarantees for the further development of the clinical research of traditional Chinese medicine.

In summary, it is of great consequence to vigorously develop "Clinical Research of Traditional Chinese Medicine Initiated by Researchers" to enhance the international status of Traditional Chinese Medicine and promote the modernization and internationalization of traditional Chinese medicine. By concentrating resources, establishing a characteristic evaluation system, increasing research funds, and setting up a multi-disciplinary talent team, we can lay the foundation for the long-term development of traditional Chinese medicine, promote its wider application and value in the world, and more substantially contribute to the cause of safeguarding human health.

Authors: SHI Jiangwei, SHEN Yan, ZHUANG Pengwei, YANG Changquan (First Teaching Hospital of Tianjin University of Traditional Chinese Medicine, National Clinical Research Center for Chinese Medicine Acupuncture and Moxibustion)

Principal reviewers: ZHANG Yanjun, WANG Jingui, FAN Guanwei (First Teaching Hospital of Tianjin University of Traditional Chinese Medicine, National Clinical Research Center for Chinese Medicine Acupuncture and Moxibustion; LIU Baoyan, LIU Zhishun, HE Liyun (China Academy of Chinese Medical Sciences)

Appendix: Disease Index (ICD-11)

Table 1 The International Classification of Diseases Covered in This Book (ICD-11)

Disease Types	Section (Chapter 2)
02 Neoplasms	
Malignant neoplasms of rectosigmoid junction, unspecified (2B91.Z)	11
Carcinoma of breast, specialised type (2C60)	22; 34; 40; 47; 51
Malignant neoplasms, stated or presumed to be primary, of specified sites, except of lymphoid, haematopoietic, central nervous system or related tissues, unspecified (2D3Z)	3; 38
Unspecified carcinoma of unspecified site (2D41)	39
05 Endocrine, nutritional or metabolic diseases	
Polycystic ovary syndrome (5A80.1)	43
Depressive disorders, unspecified (6A7Z)	15; 18
Other specified neurocognitive disorders (6B0Y)	46
Post traumatic stress disorder (6B40)	1
Disorders due to use of opioids (6C43)	13
Opioid dependence, current use (6C43.20)	5
08 Diseases of the nervous system	
Parkinson disease (8A00.0)	2; 12; 19
Migraine without aura (8A80.0)	32
Migraine, unspecified (8A80.Z)	44
Carpal tunnel syndrome (8C10.0)	45
11 Diseases of the circulatory system	
Stable angina (BA40.1)	37
Atrial fibrillation, unspecified (BC81.3Z)	28
13 Diseases of the digestive system	
Temporomandibular joint disorders (DA0E.8)	7
Adhesions of large intestine with obstruction (DB30.2)	16
Crohn disease, unspecified site (DD70.Z)	17
Functional dyspepsia (DD90.3)	33
Irritable bowel syndrome, diarrhoea predominant (DD91.01)	21
Functional constipation (DD91.1)	31; 48
14 Diseases of the skin	
Chronic urticaria (EB00.1)	9
15 Diseases of the musculoskeletal system or connective tissue	
Inflammatory arthropathies, unspecified & Knee joint (FA2Z&XA8RL1)	8; 30

Appendix: Disease Index (ICD-11)

(Continued)

Disease Types	Section (Chapter 2)
Degenerative condition of spine, unspecified (FA8Z)	52
16 Diseases of the genitourinary system	
Menopausal hot flush (GA30.4)	49
Calculus of upper urinary tract, unspecified (GB70.Z)	23
Stress incontinence associated with pelvic organ prolapse (GC40.50)	42
18 Pregnancy, childbirth or the puerperium	
Induced abortion, complete or unspecified, with other complication (JA60.Z)	10
Other specified complications of the puerperium (JB44.Y)	24
21 Symptoms, signs or clinical findings, not elsewhere classified	
Intervertebral disc stenosis of neural canal, lumbar region (ME93.43)	6
Chronic primary visceral pain (MG30.00)	26
Chronic widespread pain (MG30.01)	29
Chronic primary musculoskeletal pain (MG30.02)	27; 36
Chronic cancer pain (MG30.10)	14; 25
Chronic peripheral neuropathic pain (MG30.51)	35
Acute postoperative pain, not elsewhere classified (MG31.2)	20; 50
Dysphasia(MA80.1)	4
24 Factors influencing health status or contact with health services	
Contact with health services for assisted reproductive technology (QA30.1)	41

功能来改善大肠传导，促进排便。这一理论基础结合现代研究发现的电针在促进胃肠蠕动、改善肠道动力方面的潜力，进一步强化了本研究的科学依据。

（2）试验设计严谨，结果具有说服力

电针以不良反应少、整体调节性强的特点，逐渐受到关注，但其临床有效性仍需通过严谨的试验证实。现有文献虽然有关于针刺治疗便秘的临床试验结果，但多集中于小样本、单中心研究，缺乏大规模、多中心的随机对照试验。本研究收集了15家医院的1075例患者，样本量充足，结论说服力强。不仅有助于提升电针在国际医学界的认可度，也为针刺在功能性疾病中的应用提供了更广阔的前景。

（3）针刺干预的实施分析

本研究在针刺干预的具体实施中展现了严格的科学性和精确性。首先，穴位的选择和针刺方案的制定经过研究者的深思熟虑的科学设计，选择了天枢、腹结和上巨虚作为电针干预的主要穴位，这些穴位在传统中医中被认为与调理胃肠功能密切相关，且现代研究也支持它们在促进肠蠕动方面的有效性。这种基于中西医结合的穴位选择增强了研究结果的可信度。

此外，本研究的针刺操作注重细节，研究采取了严格的标准化措施，如针刺深度、刺激频率和强度的控制等，确保了治疗过程的可重复性和一致性。

（4）假针对照组的设计

对照组的设计是本研究的一大亮点。为了避免心理预期对研究结果的影响，研究采用了假电针对照，这种对照方法相对有效地控制了安慰剂效应。假电针组在非穴位浅层刺入且不进行电刺激，最大限度地模拟了电针的操作，没有针刺经验的受试者可能在外观上很难察觉两组的差别，非穴位点的浅刺尽量减少了针刺的生理效应和心理效应。这一设计使得研究结果更为可靠，可以为类似的研究设计提供方法借鉴。

（5）可优化方面

尽管研究设计严谨，本研究仍有可以进一步优化的方面。例如，虽然研究考虑到了治疗师的资质和培训，但并未详细阐述每家中心的治疗一致性如何得到保障。不同治疗师的操作习惯和技术水平可能会对治疗效果产生微妙的影响，未来研究可以通过更详细的操作规范和定期监督来进一步提高操作一致性，如可以使用Kappa一致性分析检测多个研究者干预或评估结果的一致性。

另外，研究虽然采用了多中心设计，但未能实现完全盲法操作，治疗师知晓分组情况，这可能引入一定的观察者偏倚。文中采用了非穴位浅刺且不加电的方法来实现盲法，可能存在以下问题：一是人体的穴位众多，更是存在没有固定位置的"阿是穴"，采用非穴位的浅刺可能也会带来相关的针刺疗效，在两组的对比统计之下使得试验组的特异性治疗效果减弱；二是穴位与非穴位点存在位置差异，两组受试者同时在同一空间下治疗可能会发现取穴差异，或许两组在相对独立的诊室中治疗更能保证蒙蔽效果；三是不加电的设计下，针身可能并不会如真正通电般随着电流的通过而抖动，两者存在感觉上的差异,这一设计可能会使以往做过电针治疗的受试者更容易破盲。不过盲法的实施在针刺的临床研究中本身就困难较大,故在未来研究中可考虑更新盲法的实施方式及更全面的盲法程序设置,或通过多点监控减少潜在的偏倚。

2. 述评二

(1)研究设计和过程实施

该项研究是一项大样本、多中心、随机、对照、优效性设计,属于验证性研究。主要有以下几方面特点:①研究明确提出了优效性的临床假设,并进行对应的研究设计;②研究基于中国15家中心的1075例受试者,样本量大,具有较好的代表性;③采用了假针刺对照,控制了针刺的安慰剂效应,对针刺的特异性疗效进行了评价;④采用了排便日记记录患者排便情况,保证了数据的准确性;⑤设立了独立的数据安全监测委员会,对研究过程及安全性进行监测。

(2)临床研究方法学及统计学方法的选择及应用

整体上看,本项研究的统计学方法较为规范。①检验假说:提出了明确的优效性检验假设,且研究结果也达到了优效性设定的界值。②样本量计算:基于前期预试验结果进行样本量估计,样本量估计较为准确。③统计分析:以多因素分析方法为主,纳入了可能影响结果的协变量。缺失数据处理采用了多重填补法,相对于末次观测值结转的方法来说更为严谨可靠;同时,采用混合模式模型进行多重填补的敏感性分析,以评估多重填补结果的稳健性,值得借鉴。④盲法评价:假针刺对照虽然可以较好地实现患者的盲法,但盲法是否真正成功仍然备受关注。因此,对假针刺对照的临床试验开展盲法评价是有必要的。推荐采用专门的盲法评价指数进行盲法评价,并详细报告结果。

第四十九节 "Acupuncture for Menopausal Hot Flashes: A Randomized Trial" 相关介绍和述评

一 论文介绍

1. 中文题目:针刺治疗更年期潮热症:一项随机试验

2. 作者:Carolyn Ee, Charlie Xue, Patty Chondros, Stephen P. Myers, Simon D. French, Helena Teede, Marie Pirotta

3. 主要单位:Department of General Practice, University of Melbourne; Royal Melbourne Institute of Technology (RMIT) University; NatMed Research Unit, Southern Cross University

4. 发表期刊：*Annals of Internal Medicine*

5. 发布日期：2016年1月19日

6. SCI源文献：EE C, XUE C, CHONDROS P, et al. Acupuncture for Menopausal Hot Flashes: A Randomized Trial [J]. Ann Intern Med, 2016, 164 (3): 146-154.

7. 内容简介：本研究为分层、盲法、平行、随机、假针刺对照试验。为了探索对于更年期潮热（hot flashes，HF）患者，针刺在HF评分方面是否比假针刺的治疗效果更好，将327例受试者随机分配至针刺组和假针刺组，并分别进行干预，观察两组受试者治疗前后HF评分的情况。得出结论：对于中重度更年期HF患者，针刺治疗并不优于非刺入式假针刺治疗。

针刺组和假针刺组均进行为期8周、共10次治疗，前2周为每周治疗2次，之后6周为每周1次。

针刺组采用治疗肾阴虚证的标准化中医针刺，使用0.32 mm×40 mm无菌一次性不锈钢针灸针，针刺6个穴位直至得气，留针20 min，在留针10 min时手动行针1次。采用穴位包括双侧照海（KI6）、双侧复溜（KI7）、双侧三阴交（SP6）、双侧太冲（LR3）、关元（CV4）、双侧阴郄（HT6）。

对照组采用非刺入式假针刺疗法，使用经过验证的Park假针刺装置，即一根0.35 mm×40 mm钝针，由塑料垫圈和塑料导管（基座）支撑，通过双面胶固定在皮肤上，而针体随操作缩回自身内部，造成刺入皮肤的视觉和触觉印象。基座用于所有患者的治疗，包括针刺组。穴位包括双侧3个远离针刺组所选穴位的非穴位置，针灸师询问感受并在10 min时假装行针，不产生得气。余治疗方案与针刺组一致。

二 专家述评（针灸学专家，临床研究方法学及卫生统计学专家）

1. 述评一

选题分析：围绝经期血管舒缩症状（vasomotor symptoms，VMS）的发病率较高，严重影响患者的生活质量。激素替代治疗（menopausal hormone therapy，MHT）虽是公认的治疗措施，但患者的接受度并不高。针刺是治疗VMS的常用手段，但对于其治疗效果的优劣存在不同意见，且缺少高质量的临床证据。该研究以VMS肾阴虚证患者为研究对象，在15家针灸诊所进行随机对照试验，以评价针刺治疗围绝经期HF的疗效，选题具有较重要的临床意义。

针刺干预的实施：在干预措施的设置、实施方面，该研究有一定的借鉴意义，如设置针刺组与采用非穴非刺入方式的安慰针刺组，要求针灸师有5年以上经验，以及受试者MHT的管理方案等。但该研究认为：对于VMS肾阴虚证患者，为期8周的标准化针刺治疗并没有比非刺入性假针刺更有效地减少更年期HF症状。对此，值得深入讨论。取穴、针刺操作、疗程等是针刺处方的核心要素，此为针灸业界共识。本研究的取穴、疗程是否是治疗VMS肾阴虚证的较佳选择？照海、复溜、三阴交、太冲、关元、阴郄6个穴位是否高度符合本病证的病因病机？8周内仅给予10次治疗（前2周为每周2次，之后6周为每周1次），是否达到应有的治疗量的需求？研究结果是否反映了针刺治疗本病的真实临床价值？实际上，作者在文章中也对个性化治疗、针刺频次有所思考。

2. 述评二

（1）研究设计和过程实施

本研究设计严谨，旨在评估针刺对更年期女性VMS的效果，通过多中心、分层随机化试验，确保研究结果的科学性和可靠性。分层随机化按针灸师进行分层，使用受密码保护的电子系统确保分配的隐蔽性和公正性。受试者通过多种渠道招募，纳入标准严格，确保同质性；样本量计算合理，考虑了预期效应和流失率。虽然针灸师未盲化，但其他参与者和评估员实现了盲法，减少了偏倚。针刺组和假针刺组的干预措施标准化，使用非刺入性钝针模拟针刺过程。主要结局为潮热评分，通过验证工具评估，系统地收集覆盖基线、治疗期间和随访阶段的数据。本研究对数据管理和保护措施的细节描述较少，尽管研究获得伦理批准并遵循规范，整体设计科学合理，但在质量控制和对混杂因素的控制上仍有改进空间。

（2）临床研究方法学及统计学方法的选择及应用

本研究的临床研究方法学和统计学方法选择严谨，采用多中心、随机、假对照试验设计，有效评估针刺对更年期女性VMS的疗效。研究通过计算机生成随机序列和电子表格隐藏分配，实现了对照和盲法，控制了偏倚风险。主要结局使用标准化工具进行评估，统计分析采用线性混合效应模型处理重复测量数据，并进行意向性治疗分析以增强结果的稳健性。研究对缺失数据采用多重插补和敏感性分析，验证了数据的稳健性。然而，研究未详细说明多重比较的校正措施和亚组分析策略，这可能对结果的解读产生一定影响。尽管设定了显著性水平并报告了效应量，但对临床显著性的讨论仍不足。整体而言，研究为针刺治疗更年期HF女性提供了可信的证据，但未来应在多重比较校正、亚组分析和临床意义的解读方面进一步优化，以提升研究的广泛适用性和临床价值。

第五十节 "Transcutaneous Acupoint Electrical Stimulation Pain Management After Surgical Abortion: A Cohort Study"相关介绍和述评

一 论文介绍

1. 中文题目：经皮穴位电刺激治疗手术流产后疼痛：一项队列研究
2. 作者：Xiaozhen Feng, Tianshen Ye, Zedong Wang, Xiufang Chen, Wenjie Cong,

Yong Chen, Pinjie Chen, Chong Chen, Beibei Shi, Wenxia Xie

3．主要单位：温州医科大学附属第一医院针推理疗科，温州医科大学附属第一医院老年医学科，温州医科大学附属第一医院妇产科

4．发表期刊：*International Journal of Surgery*

5．发布日期：2016年4月26日

6．SCI源文献：FENG X Z, YE T S, WANG Z D, et al. Transcutaneous acupoint electrical stimulation pain management after surgical abortion: A cohort study [J]. Int J Surg, 2016, 30: 104-108.

7．内容简介：本研究为队列研究。为了探索经皮穴位电刺激（transcutaneous acupoint electrical stimulation，TEAS）对于接受手术流产患者的镇痛作用，将140例受试者随机分为术前组（术前接受TEAS）、术后组（术后接受TEAS）、术前和术后结合组（术前和术后均接受TEAS）及对照组，并分别进行干预，对4组受试者手术流产前和术后复苏10、30、45 min时的疼痛情况进行评估[使用平均视觉模拟量表（visual analog scale，VAS）评分]。得出结论：在手术流产前、后进行TEAS均可减轻术后疼痛，而在流产手术前进行TEAS可以让更多患者体验到轻度疼痛或无痛。

TEAS治疗使用便携式电池电针仪（HANS-100A），电流1~30 mA，2/100 Hz疏密波，脉冲持续0.5 ms。将电极置于双侧地机（SP8）、三阴交（SP6），刺激强度逐渐增加，直至受试者感觉到神经支配区域有麻电感。

术前组、术前和术后结合组受试者在术前接受30 min的TEAS治疗。术后组、术前和术后结合组受试者在术后接受30 min的TEAS治疗。

对照组无相应治疗。

二　专家述评（针灸学专家，临床研究方法学及卫生统计学专家）

1．述评一

这篇研究聚焦手术流产过程中的疼痛管理，这是一个具有显著临床意义的课题。手术流产作为常见的妇科手术之一，其过程中的疼痛管理直接关系到患者的手术体验和术后恢复。鉴于全身麻醉虽然能在手术期间有效控制疼痛，但术后疼痛仍是一个普遍存在的问题，因此，探索更为有效的术后镇痛方法显得尤为重要。这项研究通过评估在手术流产前后进行TEAS对患者的镇痛效果，为临床提供了一种潜在的、非药物的镇痛选择。

该研究将受试者分为术前接受TEAS组、术后接受TEAS组、术前和术后均接受TEAS组及对照组4个组别，以全面评估在不同时间点进行TEAS对手术流产患者的镇痛效果。通过标准化的TEAS治疗参数和临床上公认的疼痛评估方法（VAS评分），确保了研究结果的可靠性。同时，该研究在镇痛穴位的选择上也有一定的科学依据。现代解剖学发现，地机穴浅层有隐神经小腿内侧皮支，深层有胫神经分布，而隐神经与

支配子宫平滑肌运动的交感神经来自同一神经节段，胫神经与子宫的感觉神经和副交感神经纤维来自同一神经节段。三阴交穴处的神经纤维主要来自L4～S2神经节段，子宫处的神经纤维主要来自T11～L2、S2～S4等神经节段，两者具有相同或邻近的神经节段分布特点。这可能是地机、三阴交用于手术流产前后镇痛的解剖学基础。

该研究结果显示，术前接受TEAS治疗的受试者在术后早期（10 min）的疼痛评分显著低于对照组，表明术前TEAS具有显著的预先镇痛效果。尽管术后各组的疼痛评分在30 min和45 min时趋于一致，但术前接受TEAS治疗的受试者在术后早期表现出更低的疼痛发生率，这提示预先镇痛策略的有效性。此外，研究还发现TEAS治疗能够显著降低受试者术后恶心、呕吐的发生率，进一步证明了其临床价值。

综上所述，本研究为TEAS在手术流产镇痛中的应用提供了有力证据。术前给予TEAS治疗能够显著降低受试者术后早期的疼痛评分和疼痛发生率，同时减少术后恶心、呕吐等不良反应的发生。这一发现为临床提供了一种安全、有效的非药物镇痛选择，有助于改善患者的手术体验和术后恢复质量。未来研究应进一步探索TEAS的最佳治疗参数和穴位选择，以优化其镇痛效果并推动其在临床中的广泛应用。

2. 述评二

该研究采用队列研究设计评估手术流产前后使用TEAS止痛的效果，以VAS评分和疼痛发生率作为主要结局。研究最终纳入的140例受试者均来自区域内同一时间段内，TEAS暴露组与非暴露组人群来源可认为具有一定相似性。研究详细报告了TEAS操作流程和技术参数，可以为证据使用者提供参考。然而，该研究在设计方面尚存在一定的局限性：①研究未计算样本量，且最终纳入样本量较小，统计学效能不足；②结果部分对疼痛评分的报告不够充分，未报告非暴露组疼痛评分数值；③未考虑混杂因素对结果的影响，由于本研究为观察性研究设计，在评估组间疗效差异时需要对混杂因素进行调整，并明确报告调整前后效应指标及其95%可信区间；④正如作者所描述，研究未探索在术前、术中和术后不同阶段的最佳穴位，主要原因在于样本量较小，不能对穴位、疼痛程度、亚人群等可能影响治疗效果的效应修饰因子进行亚组或探索性分析，从而提供个性化指导。

第五十一节 "Electroacupuncture Versus Gabapentin for Hot Flashes Among Breast Cancer Survivors: A Randomized Placebo-Controlled Trial" 相关介绍和述评

一 论文介绍

1. 中文题目：电针对比加巴喷丁治疗乳腺癌幸存者潮热：一项随机安慰剂对照

试验

2. 作者：Jun J. Mao, Marjorie A. Bowman, Sharon X. Xie, Deborah Bruner, Angela DeMichele, John T. Farrar

3. 主要单位：Perelman School of Medicine at the University of Pennsylvania, Wright State University Boonshoft School of Medicine, Emory University Nell Hodgson Woodruff School of Nursing

4. 发表期刊：*Journal of Clinical Oncology*

5. 发布日期：2015年8月24日

6. SCI源文献：MAO J J, BOWMAN M A, XIE S X, et al. Electroacupuncture Versus Gabapentin for Hot Flashes Among Breast Cancer Survivors: A Randomized Placebo-Controlled Trial [J]. J Clin Oncol, 2015, 33 (31): 3615-3620.

7. 内容简介：本研究为四臂、随机对照临床试验，旨在探讨电针（electroacupuncture，EA）与加巴喷丁（gabapentin，GP）对乳腺癌幸存者潮热症状的干预效果。将120例乳腺癌患者随机分配到EA组、假针刺（sham acupuncture，SA）组、加巴喷丁（GP）组和安慰剂（placebo pill，PP）组，比较EA与药物治疗在缓解潮热症状方面的效果，并关注安慰剂和反安慰剂效应。得出结论：8周治疗后，EA组在缓解潮热症状方面优于GP组和PP组，且EA组的不良反应较少；24周随访显示，EA组的效果持续时间最长。

EA组和SA组在前2周每周接受2次治疗，后6周每周接受1次治疗，共治疗10次，疗程8周。

EA组采用直径0.25 mm、长30 mm或40 mm的一次性针具，针刺部位根据患者的症状选择，标准取穴包括四肢、背部和头部共11个穴位，如足三里（ST36）、三阴交（SP6）等，并结合经络辨证选择其他4个穴位进行加减。针刺达到得气（即患者感到酸、胀、麻等）后，连接电针仪，使用2 Hz频率治疗，留针30 min，在治疗开始、中间和结束时对针具进行轻微提插捻转。

SA组采用不能刺入皮肤的假针具，类似舞台匕首的设计，针柄能够回缩，营造出针刺的视觉效果，但实际未进行针刺，仅为轻微表面接触。针刺部位选择在与标准经络无关的非穴位置，整个过程中避免达到得气。针刺过程中不通电流，而是将电针仪的旋钮调至另一个通道，使受试者能够看到指示灯闪烁，但实际上并未接收到电流。其他操作和EA组相同。

GP组服用GP，前3天于睡前服用1次（300 mg），接下来3天每天服用2次（600 mg），后50天每天服用3次（900 mg），共8周；从第9周开始减少药量，前3天每天服用2次（600 mg），然后再连续3天每天服用1次（300 mg），之后停药。将剂量为300 mg的GP药片封装于较大的不透明明胶空心胶囊中以遮蔽药物。PP组安慰剂胶囊是将乳糖单水合物填充至相同的空胶囊中制成，服药方案与GP组相同。

二 专家述评（针灸学专家，临床研究方法学及卫生统计学专家）

1. 述评一

（1）选题分析

聚焦热点中的某一问题：乳腺癌是中国女性最常见的恶性肿瘤之一，其发病率位列女性恶性肿瘤之首，呈逐年上升且有年轻化趋势，但是本文并不是研究乳腺癌这一疾病，而是聚焦在乳腺癌患者潮热这一特定症状，选题小而精准，且符合针刺的优势疾病。

基础研究支撑：本文在研究背景中指出，针刺是一种非药物疗法，可能有助于改善潮热。特别是EA已被证明会影响内啡肽和其他中枢神经肽，为治疗潮热提供了生物学上的合理性。既往有基础研究作为支撑，为临床研究提供了证据。

针刺的安慰剂效应：针刺的安慰剂效应是一个多维度、复杂的现象，涉及患者的心理、生理反应以及研究方法学等多个方面。针刺的安慰剂效应是一个复杂且值得深入探讨的现象，本文没有逃避，而是证实了其安慰剂效应和反安慰剂效应。

（2）针刺干预的实施

治疗频次：本文中，前2周每周进行2次干预，后6周每周进行1次，8周内共进行10次治疗。这样的治疗频次较少，周期太长，如果频次增加，能否有更好的结果。

治疗师的背景：本研究为单中心试验，由2名分别具有8年和20年经验的针灸师操作，执业年限差距较大，需考虑操作是否存在差异。

2. 述评二

这项研究采用了四臂随机对照试验设计，将受试者随机分为EA、SA、GP和PP组。研究的主要目的是比较SA与PP在缓解乳腺癌幸存者潮热症状方面的效果差异，以评估非药物治疗的安慰剂效应及反安慰剂效应。基于这一明确假设进行的样本量计算确保了统计设计的合理性和充足的统计效能，同时有效控制了多重检验中的Ⅰ类错误。研究将受试者分为4组，旨在更全面地探索不同治疗方法的效果。通过加入EA和GP组可以深入探索真实治疗与安慰剂之间的差异。尽管这两组的样本量不足以支持评估其疗效，但可为未来大规模研究提供重要的初步证据支持。

研究设计中的随机化和盲法设计有效提高了研究质量，减少了偏倚风险。受试者的分配是通过计算机生成的随机数据来进行，并根据激素治疗状态进行分层，确保了组间均衡。不透明信封和不固定区组设计增加了随机化过程的不可预测性，从而降低了选择偏倚的风险。研究还对受试者、主要研究人员及统计人员进行了分组盲法，减少了信息偏倚。在统计分析方面，研究采用混合线性模型分析重复测量数据，这一方法充分利用了不同时间点的数据，提高了统计效能，并且能够评估个体差异的影响。

综上所述，该研究通过合理的设计和随机化方法验证了主要假设，并分析了有关不同治疗效果的差异。研究为非药物治疗方法在乳腺癌幸存者潮热管理中的应用提供了重要的临床证据。

第五十二节 "Alexander Technique Lessons or Acupuncture Sessions for Persons With Chronic Neck Pain: A Randomized Trial" 相关介绍和述评

一 论文介绍

1. 中文题目：亚历山大技术课程或针刺课程治疗慢性颈痛患者：一项随机试验

2. 作者：Hugh MacPherson, Helen Tilbrook, Stewart Richmond, Julia Woodman, Kathleen Ballard, Karl Atkin, Martin Bland, Janet Eldred, Holly Essex, Catherine Hewitt, Ann Hopton, Ada Keding, Harriet Lansdown, Steve Parrott, David Torgerson, Aniela Wenham, Ian Watt

3. 主要单位：University of York, Society of Teachers of the Alexander Technique and British Acupuncture Council

4. 发表期刊：*Annals of Internal Medicine*

5. 发布日期：2015年11月3日

6. SCI源文献：MACPHERSON H, TILBROOK H, RICHMOND S, et al. Alexander Technique Lessons or Acupuncture Sessions for Persons With Chronic Neck Pain: A Randomized Trial [J]. Ann Intern Med, 2015, 163 (9): 653-662.

7. 内容简介：本研究为3组随机、对照临床试验。为了探索对于慢性非特异性颈痛患者，针刺或亚历山大技术课程在Northwick Park颈痛量表（neck pain questionnaire，NPQ）评分方面是否比常规治疗效果更好，将517例慢性非特异性颈痛患者随机分为针刺组、亚历山大技术课程组和常规治疗组分别进行干预，观察3组治疗前后NPQ评分变化。得出结论：在12个月后，与常规治疗相比，针刺治疗和亚历山大技术课程均显著降低慢性非特异性颈痛患者颈部疼痛程度，并减少相关残疾的发生。

3组均接受常规治疗，包括常规提供给初级保健患者的一般治疗和颈部疼痛特定治疗，如处方药物、物理治疗或其他保健方法等。在常规治疗基础上，针刺组接受针刺治疗，亚历山大技术课程组接受亚历山大技术课程干预，疗程均计划在5个月内完成。随访12个月。

针刺组最多接受12次，每次50 min的治疗（共600 min）。最初针刺疗程通常每周1次，之后每两周1次。针刺操作基于传统中医学理论，包括针刺特有诊断解释和相关生活方式建议。

亚历山大技术课程组最多接受20次一对一课程，每次50 min（共600 min）。课程通常每周1次，也可以选择最初每周2次、之后每两周1次。亚历山大技术课程老师使用与常规实践和英国国家职业标准指南一致的语言和实际操作指导。

常规治疗组仅给予常规治疗。

二、专家述评（针灸学专家，临床研究方法学及卫生统计学专家）

1. 述评一

本研究为一项在英国初级卫生保健中心开展的随机对照临床试验，系统评估了亚历山大技术训练或针刺疗法（alexander technique lessons or acupuncture sessions，ATLAS）对于慢性非特异性颈痛患者的临床疗效。其贡献不仅在于为ATLAS治疗慢性颈痛提供了有效证据，还强调了心理因素对于临床疗效的重要性，对于指导临床实践、优化治疗方案及提高患者生活质量具有重要意义。

该研究方案设计较为严谨，将517例慢性非特异性颈痛患者随机分为3组分别干预：针刺加常规治疗、亚历山大技术训练加常规治疗、单独常规治疗，前两者在常规治疗的基础上分别给予12次、每次50 min的针刺治疗和20次一对一的亚历山大技术训练，主要评价指标为NPQ评分，次要指标包括当前疼痛强度、简版生活质量量表第2版（short form 12，version 2，SF 12v2）以及患者的自我效能感。其优点在于采用了大样本、平行随机对照试验，评价指标科学合理，且随访周期长达12个月，为评估长期疗效提供了有力支持。研究结果表明，ATLAS能有效缓解慢性颈痛患者的症状，提高生活质量，同时显著提升了患者的自我效能感，揭示了心理层面的积极变化在持续缓解慢性颈痛中的重要作用。该研究也预示着针刺作为一种非侵入性、低风险的干预措施，有望成为慢性疼痛治疗的重要补充及替代手段。

2. 述评二

这项实用性随机对照试验旨在评估ATLAS相较于常规治疗，在慢性颈痛患者中的长期临床疗效。研究采用了较广泛的纳入标准，以增强结果的普适性。受试者被随机分为3组，在常规治疗基础上分别接受针刺、亚历山大技术课程、单独常规治疗。这一设计旨在评估在现有常规治疗之上，额外的干预是否能够带来显著的临床改善。

试验通过安全的随机化系统实施动态区组随机化，确保了分组的严谨性和不可预测性。针灸师和课程教师均为专业协会成员，这在一定程度上保证了干预措施的标准化和一致性。统计分析遵循意向性治疗分析原则，确保所有随机分配的受试者均纳入分析，以减少选择偏倚。为处理数据缺失，研究使用了重复测量混合效应模型分析主要结局即12个月时的NPQ评分，并进行了多项敏感性分析，以确保结果的稳健性。虽然研究进行了两次主要假设检验以比较两种不同干预的效果，但未提及多重检验校正，这可能是一个不足之处。然而，由于两项假设检验均达到统计学显著性，研究结果的解读可能未受实质性影响。

尽管由于干预本身特性难以实现盲法，研究在设计、实施和统计分析阶段采取了一系列措施，有效降低了潜在偏倚，提高了研究结果的可靠性和有效性。

第三章

《研究者发起的中医药临床研究天津共识》内容与解读

第一节 研究者发起的中医药临床研究天津共识

为进一步规范中医药临床研究的选题立项、设计评价、过程管理及质量控制，提升中医药临床研究的质量，促进其健康发展，并增强中医医疗卫生机构在疾病诊断、治疗和预防方面的能力，特制定《研究者发起的中医药临床研究天津共识》。

一、研究者发起的临床研究是指医疗卫生机构开展的，以个体或群体（包括医疗健康信息）为研究对象，不以药品、医疗器械（含体外诊断试剂）等产品注册为目的的研究活动，重点关注疾病的诊断、治疗、康复、预后、病因、预防及健康维护等方面。

二、依托天津中医药大学第一附属医院，充分发挥世界针灸学会联合会、世界中医药学会联合会、中国针灸学会、中华中医药学会等组织的指导作用，成立中医药临床研究中心。该中心将采用创新开放的管理机制和运行模式，建立多学科融合的专业化临床研究方法学团队，构建临床研究评价技术平台，组织开展研究者发起的中医药临床研究，形成高质量的临床证据，提升并彰显中医药的临床价值。

三、完善和修订《针灸临床研究管理规范》《中医药临床研究管理规范》，以规范中医药临床研究过程中各项行为，保障研究对象的权益，确保研究结果的真实性和研究结论的可靠性，为中医药的安全有效使用提供科学依据。

四、依托中医药临床研究中心，组织国内外研究力量，聚焦中风、痴呆、高血压、疼痛及抑郁症等重大疾病和常见病的难点，发挥针灸的优势，明确其治疗适应范围，弥补药物疗法的不足，形成中西医优势互补、体现中国诊疗能力和水平的针灸临床诊疗方案及高质量的临床证据，并通过临床指南等方式在国内外推广应用。同时，运用现代科学技术明确阐述针灸治疗疾病的原理，创新并发展针灸理论，研发智能针灸诊疗设备，力求取得原创性成果。以国际标准为引领，推动全球针灸学术的发展，提升针灸在防病治病中的临床价值，助力针灸走向世界。

五、由天津中医药大学第一附属医院提供专项经费，并争取国内外各方面的支持，建立多方经费筹措机制，保障研究者发起的临床研究的持续开展。

疾病索引（ICD-11）

表1 本书中所涉及的国际疾病分类（ICD-11）

疾病种类	节（第二章）
02　肿瘤	
未特指的直肠乙状结肠交界处恶性肿瘤（2B91.Z）	第十一节
乳腺癌，特指类型（2C60）	第二十二节、第三十四节、第四十节、第四十七节、第五十一节
未特指的述及或假定为原发性的特指部位恶性肿瘤，除外淋巴、造血、中枢神经系统或相关组织（2D3Z）	第三节、第三十八节
未特指部位未特指的癌（2D41）	第三十九节
05　内分泌、营养或代谢疾病	
多囊卵巢综合征（5A80.1）	第四十三节
未特指的抑郁障碍（6A7Z）	第十五节、第十八节
其他特指的焦虑或恐惧相关性障碍（6B0Y）	第四十六节
创伤后应激障碍（6B40）	第一节
阿片类物质使用所致障碍（6C43）	第十三节
阿片类物质依赖，目前使用（6C43.20）	第五节
08　神经系统疾病	
帕金森病（8A00.0）	第二节、第十二节、第十九节
无先兆偏头痛（8A80.0）	第三十二节
未特指的偏头痛（8A80.Z）	第四十四节
腕管综合征（8C10.0）	第四十五节
11　循环系统疾病	
稳定型心绞痛（BA40.1）	第三十七节
未特指的心房颤动（BC81.3Z）	第二十八节
13　消化系统疾病	
颞下颌关节疾患（DA0E.8）	第七节
大肠粘连伴梗阻（DB30.2）	第十六节
未特指部位的克罗恩病（DD70.Z）	第十七节
功能性消化不良（DD90.3）	第三十三节
腹泻型肠易激综合征（DD91.01）	第二十一节
功能性便秘（DD91.1）	第三十一节、第四十八节

突出的头部医疗单位或科研机构，主要职责包括顶层设计、整体协调、监督运行实施与质量控制、数据汇总与分析及成果发布。二级单位由各地区具有较强科研能力的医疗机构或高校组成，主要负责协助一级单位实现上下联通，参与研究方案与规划，并承担伦理审查、实施方案及样本和数据采集等任务。三级单位则由市级医院、基层医疗机构或小型研究机构构成，其主要任务为参与数据收集和成果推广。通过三级网络架构的建立，实现资源的优化配置与高效利用，形成从顶层设计到基层实践的完整科研链条。

4. 规范研究过程及行为

完善和修订相关管理规范是确保中医药临床研究质量的关键步骤。这些规范不仅重视研究结果的真实性和可靠性，还强调对研究对象权益的保护。通过规范研究过程中各个环节，防止研究偏差和不当行为的发生，确保中医药临床研究的规范性和科学性，为中医药的安全有效使用提供依据，有助于提升公众对中医药的信任度和接受度。《天津共识》明确提出，中医药临床研究应聚焦重大疾病和常见病的难点，并强调发挥针灸等中医特色疗法的优势，集中力量攻克中医药领域的关键技术和临床难题。通过中西医结合、优势互补的方式，形成更具针对性和有效性的中国诊疗方案，提升中医药的临床价值与国际影响力。运用现代科学技术揭示针灸等疗法的治病原理，推动理论创新与技术进步，提升中医药的科学性与可信度，为中医药的国际化奠定基础。

5. 构建多元化经费筹措体系

经费是保障中医药临床研究持续开展的重要条件之一。《天津共识》提出，应努力争取国内外多方面的资源支持，构建多元化的经费筹措体系，并加强对经费使用的监管与评估，以确保由研究者发起的临床研究的持续性和稳定性。同时，加强临床研究结果的转化与应用，确保研究成果能够有效服务于临床，为患者带来实质性益处。这种机制有助于缓解研究经费紧张的问题，为中医药临床研究的深入开展提供必要的物质保障。

综上所述，大力发展"研究者发起的中医药临床研究"对提升中医药的国际地位、推动其现代化与国际化具有重要意义。通过集中资源、建立特色评价体系、增加研究经费及组建多学科人才团队等措施，为中医药的长远发展奠定基础，推动中医药在全球范围内得到更广泛的应用和价值体现，为人类健康事业作出更大贡献。

执笔人：石江伟、沈燕、庄朋伟、杨常泉（天津中医药大学第一附属医院，国家中医针灸临床医学研究中心）

主审：张艳军、王金贵、樊官伟（天津中医药大学第一附属医院，国家中医针灸临床医学研究中心）；刘保延、刘志顺、何丽云（中国中医科学院）

表，充分证明了中医药的临床有效性，并推动了中国方案纳入国际临床实践指南。随着中医药在国际上的影响力不断增强，加之现代科技的助力及多学科的深度融合，其现代化进程也在加速。全球对健康生活方式的追求，使得中医药所蕴含的独特理念和治疗方法愈加受到青睐。预计在不久的将来，中医药将在全球健康领域发挥更加重要的作用。

研究者发起的临床研究是指医疗卫生机构开展的，以个体或群体（包括医疗健康信息）为研究对象，且不以药品或医疗器械注册为目的，旨在研究疾病的诊断、治疗、康复、预后、病因、预防及健康维护等活动。为推动中医药的创新发展，研究者发起的中医药临床研究的重要性愈发凸显，并得到广泛认可。

研究者发起的中医药临床研究仍然面临诸多问题：①"分散作战"现象普遍，组织化程度明显不足。各单位往往独立开展研究，缺乏统一的规划与协调，导致大量低水平的临床研究重复出现，影响科研进展，造成资源浪费，并可能对临床实践产生误导。②缺乏符合中医药自身特色的临床研究评价体系。目前，现有的评价体系无法准确衡量中医药临床研究的价值与疗效，限制了其深入发展。③面临经费不足的困境。科研经费是保障科研活动顺利进行的前提，缺乏充足且持续的研究资金已成为影响临床研究的重要瓶颈问题。

因此，如何解决这些问题，提高中医药临床研究的组织化程度，建立科学的评价体系，并确保充足的研究经费，成为当前亟待解决的重要课题。

二 《天津共识》的内容解读

1. 争取政策支持

国家和地方主管部门在"研究者发起的中医药临床研究"中扮演着至关重要的角色。中医药临床研究亟需争取多方位的政策支持，并通过行业力量推动行动计划的实施，以为中医药临床研究创造更加有利的发展环境与条件。

2. 构建研究平台与组建人才团队

本着资源整合与协同创新的理念，通过构建多学科融合的专业化团队和技术平台，为中医药临床研究提供有力支撑。汇聚多学科科研力量，组建临床研究专业团队，广泛吸引国内外知名院校、医疗机构、科研院所及研发型企业的积极参与，共同构建医-学-研-产-政深度协作的创新体系，建立多学科融合的专业化临床研究方法学团队，涵盖研究设计、质量控制及数据管理等领域的专业人才。通过科学有效的组织架构，形成中医药临床研究共同体，集中优势资源，开展大样本、多中心、高质量的临床研究。

3. 形成临床研究共同体的运行机制

构建高效的全国中医药临床研究共同体的三级网络架构，其中一级单位为科研实力

六、积极争取国家和地方各主管部门的指导、帮助及支持,为推进中医药的现代化和走向国际作出更大贡献。

执笔人:刘保延　张艳军　王金贵

共识制定专家组(按照姓名拼音排序):杜宇征(天津中医药大学第一附属医院)、杜元灏(天津中医药大学第一附属医院)、樊官伟(天津中医药大学第一附属医院)、费宇彤(北京中医药大学)、符文彬(广东省中医院)、岗卫娟(中国中医科学院)、郭义(天津中医药大学)、郝重耀(山西中医药大学)、胡思源(天津中医药大学第一附属医院)、黄宇虹(天津中医药大学第二附属医院)、孔凡铭(天津中医药大学第一附属医院)、李华南(天津中医药大学第一附属医院)、刘保延(中国中医科学院)、刘存志(北京中医药大学)、刘国正(中医杂志社)、陆丽明(广州中医药大学)、毛钧(美国纪念斯隆-凯特琳癌症中心)、倪光夏(南京中医药大学)、荣培晶(中国中医科学院)、孙鑫(华西医院)、王保和(天津中医药大学第一附属医院)、王斌(天津中医药大学第一附属医院)、王金贵(天津中医药大学第一附属医院)、王舒(天津市中医药研究院附属医院)、王贤良(天津中医药大学第一附属医院)、武晓冬(中国中医科学院)、张虹(成都中医药大学)、张艳军(天津中医药大学第一附属医院)、赵凌(成都中医药大学)、庄朋伟(天津中医药大学第一附属医院)

第二节 《研究者发起的中医药临床研究天津共识》解读

2023年11月11日,中国·天津第十六届国际针灸学术研讨会在天津召开。本次会议由天津中医药大学第一附属医院、世界针灸学会联合会等主办,国家中医针灸临床医学研究中心等承办。会议期间,邀请了30位中医药、方法学等领域的专家,以"研究者发起的中医药临床研究体系建设"为主题召开闭门会议。与会专家围绕研究者发起的中医药临床研究的组织架构、保障机制、研究重点等方面进行深入探讨,最终形成《研究者发起的中医药临床研究天津共识》(以下简称《天津共识》)。

一 《天津共识》的形成背景

中医药以其独特的特色和优势正日益受到国际社会的广泛关注,临床研究的重要性也愈发凸显。临床实践的决策转化需要高质量的循证来源,近年来,中医药在治疗心脑血管疾病、癌症、代谢性疾病、疼痛症状及胃肠功能障碍等重大疾病和常见病的临床及机制研究方面取得显著进展。这些研究成果已在 *JAMA*、*The Lancet*、*The New England Journal of Medicine*、*Annals of Internal Medicine*、*The BMJ* 等国际权威期刊上发

疾病索引（ICD-11）

（续表）

疾病种类	节（第二章）
14　皮肤疾病	
慢性荨麻疹（EB00.1）	第九节
15　肌肉骨骼系统或结缔组织疾病	
未特指的炎性关节炎 & 膝关节（FA2Z&XA8RL1）	第八节、第三十节
未特指的脊柱退行性病变（FA8Z）	第五十二节
16　泌尿生殖系统疾病	
更年期潮热（GA30.4）	第四十九节
未特指的上尿路结石（GB70.Z）	第二十三节
与盆腔脏器脱垂相关的压力性尿失禁（GC40.50）	第四十二节
18　妊娠、分娩或产褥期	
未特指的妊娠期剧吐（JA60.Z）	第十节
其他特指的产褥期并发症（JB44.Y）	第二十四节
21　症状、体征或临床所见，不可归类在他处者	
椎间盘水平的神经管狭窄，腰部（ME93.43）	第六节
慢性原发性内脏痛（MG30.00）	第二十六节
慢性广泛疼痛（MG30.01）	第二十九节
慢性原发性肌肉骨骼痛（MG30.02）	第二十七节、第三十六节
慢性癌痛（MG30.10）	第十四节、第二十五节
慢性周围神经性疼痛（MG30.51）	第三十五节
急性术后疼痛，不可归类在他处者（MG31.2）	第二十节、第五十节
语言困难和失语（MA80.1）	第四节
24　影响健康状态或与保健机构接触的因素	
为辅助生殖技术而与保健机构接触（QA30.1）	第四十一节

2. 述评二

（1）研究设计和过程实施

该项研究采用了多中心、随机、对照设计，主要有以下几方面特点：①研究采用了真针刺组、假针刺组、等待治疗组3组设计，是针刺临床研究中的经典设计。同时，研究提前明确了将进行真针刺与假针刺及真针刺与等待治疗的两次比较，采用这种设计除了可以评价针刺的特异性效应之外，还可以通过真针刺与等待治疗的比较来评价真针刺的整体效应。已经有研究表明针刺具有较强的安慰剂效应，且由于针刺疗法的特点，目前常用的假针刺通常并不是完全无治疗效应的空白对照，因此，假针刺通常也具有一定的效应，这对于以假针刺为对照的研究而言，有一定的影响。本研究增加了等待治疗组，可以较好地弥补该问题。②研究采用2∶1∶1的组间比例，可以使更多的受试者进入真针刺组，更加符合伦理学要求。③假针刺组的设计采用了非穴位浅刺的方式；同时，在假针刺组还提供了非耳穴位置的假耳穴治疗；两种假干预方式的叠加，有可能会增加假针刺组的效应。④研究事先定义了最小临床意义差值为BPI-SF减少2分，并基于该差值进行了样本量估计和确定最终的结论。

（2）临床研究方法学及统计学方法的选择及应用

整体上看，本项研究的统计学方法较为规范。①样本量计算：样本量计算过程基于事先确定的两次比较进行了检验水准α的调整，并考虑了不依从的比例和脱落率，以及可能发生沾染的比例，但研究并未给出基于上述考虑后，最终确定的样本量是多少例。②统计分析：统计分析以多因素分析方法为主，充分考虑了研究过程中可能的影响因素。同时，对于复杂的混合效应模型的细节报告较为全面，给出具体的协方差矩阵、随机效应及固定效应因素，有利于读者全面了解分析的细节。对缺失数据的处理及检验水准的调整等关键内容也进行了明确的报告。对于盲法评价，真针刺组和假针刺组虽然猜测正确的比例差异有统计学意义，但经过交互作用分析后，表明猜测结果对于研究结果没有影响。对于针灸研究来说，由于针刺疗法的特殊性，实现真正的盲法较为困难，因此，即使实施了假针刺，也有必要评价盲法是否成功。

第四十一节 "Effect of Acupuncture vs Sham Acupuncture on Live Births Among Women Undergoing in Vitro Fertilization: A Randomized Clinical Trial" 相关介绍和述评

一 论文介绍

1. 中文题目：针刺与假针刺对体外受精妇女活产的影响：一项随机临床试验

2. 作者：Caroline A. Smith, Sheryl de Lacey, Michael Chapman, Julie Ratcliffe, Robert J. Norman, Neil P. Johnson, Clare Boothroyd, Paul Fahey

3. 主要单位：NICM Health Research Institute, Western Sydney Universit; College of Nursing and Health Sciences, Flinders University; School of Women's & Children Health, University of New South Wales

4. 发表期刊：*JAMA*

5. 发布日期：2018年5月15日

6. SCI源文献：SMITH C A, de LACEY S, CHAPMAN M, et al. Effect of Acupuncture vs Sham Acupuncture on Live Births Among Women Undergoing in Vitro Fertilization: A Randomized Clinical Trial [J]. JAMA, 2018, 319 (19): 1990-1998.

7. 内容简介：本研究为单盲、平行组随机临床试验，旨在确定针刺与假针刺对体外受精（in vitro fertilization，IVF）活产率的影响差异。女性在决定接受IVF或胞质内单精子注射周期时被招募，并在卵泡刺激方案开始之前进行随机化。本研究将848名准备接受新IVF周期的孕妇随机分为针刺组和假针刺组，观察两组活产的情况（活产定义为在妊娠20周以上分娩1个或更多活产婴儿，且出生婴儿体质量至少为400 g）。得出结论：在接受IVF的女性中，在卵巢刺激和胚胎移植时，针刺与假针刺的使用对活产率的影响没有显著性差异。

针刺组和假针刺组均在卵巢刺激的第6～8天进行第1次针刺，胚胎移植当天进行2次针刺，共针刺3次，每次持续25 min。

针刺组的针刺方案采用德尔菲（Delphi）法制定，在达到80%的小组成员同意某个针刺治疗方案（穴位、深度、频率等）时，方案才会被保留下来。治疗策略基于传统中医方案。所选穴位位于腹部和腿部的子宫和卵巢的神经支配区域，以刺激子宫血流；位于手臂和腿部的区域，以抑制中枢神经系统传递信号到身体其他部分和生物应激反应。第1次治疗使用的核心穴位包括归来（ST29）、关元（CV4）、气海（CV6）、三阴交（SP6）和血海（SP10）。此外，根据中医诊断，从标准化方案中选取最多5个其他穴位。采用手法针刺，达到得气针刺感。在胚胎移植当天，首次针刺在胚胎移植前1 h内进行，选用穴位包括归来（ST29）、地机（SP8）、血海（SP10）、太冲（LR3）、关元（CV4），神门（HT7）、内关（PC6）或印堂（EX-HN3）中的1个穴位，以及耳穴子宫。胚胎移植后进行第2次针刺，穴位包括百会（GV20）、太溪（KI3）、足三里（ST36）、三阴交（SP6）、内关（PC6）和耳穴神门（TF4）。针刺使用Park装置进行，以确保参与者的盲法操作。

假针刺组使用Park装置支持的Park假针头行非插入式针刺。这种针具有可伸缩的针杆和钝尖。针灸师被指示将假针轻轻地放置在皮肤表面，而不对针进行任何操作，以尽量减少生理效应。为了尽量减少生理影响，以远离已知穴位且没有已知功能的位置作为假穴位。假穴位与解剖标志相关。每次治疗选择6个假穴位进行假针刺。

二 专家述评（针灸学专家，临床研究方法学及卫生统计学专家）

1. 述评一

该研究是一项具有多个研究中心、随机分配、平行对照、单盲、假针刺对照的试验。研究设计涵盖了在促排卵的第6～8天、胚胎移植前后的针刺治疗，每次针刺持续25 min，共计3次。

研究结果显示，针刺与假针刺对于接受IVF女性的活产率影响差异并无统计学意义，因此不支持使用针刺作为提高接受IVF女性活产率的辅助手段。作为一项多中心、大样本的随机对照试验，该研究在设计上表现出较高的严谨性。然而，在适宜人群的选择、针刺方案的设计及操作等方面仍需深入研究。

首先，针刺的效果不仅取决于针刺方案（如取穴、刺激量及介入时机等），也和患者的身体状况紧密相关。因此，在临床研究中，需要设定合理的纳入和排除标准，以探索适合接受针刺治疗的IVF人群，进一步明确针刺在IVF中的疗效及作用机制。

其次，IVF的针刺方案主要包括选穴方案、刺激量和介入时机等。刺激量是影响针刺疗效的主要因素之一，正确把握量效关系并进行深入探索始终是临床研究的核心。由于本试验仅进行了3次针刺治疗，刺激量可能不足，因此得出的阴性结论可能与未能达到所需针刺治疗量有关。

最后，该试验的针刺方案是基于"德尔菲法"确定的，这与临床实践存在一定差距；穴位配伍与前期研究方案不一致，其合理性仍有待商榷。因此，实施严格并符合循证医学要求的研究设计是提高针刺辅助IVF临床研究质量及结论可信度的关键。

未来针刺辅助IVF的临床研究应当遵循严格的循证医学研究模式。选择经过临床初步观察有效的研究方案进行病例序列研究或小样本独立随机对照试验，并根据试验结果不断优化和完善研究方案。在积累了大量的可靠研究数据和成熟的研究方案之后，再开展多中心、大样本的随机对照试验研究。

2. 述评二

（1）研究设计和过程实施

该研究为单盲、平行组随机对照试验，旨在评估针刺对接受IVF女性的活产率的影响。研究在澳大利亚和新西兰的16个IVF中心进行，最终纳入样本量为848名女性。该研究设计的优势在于样本量大，能够提供更具统计显著性的结果，同时多中心的设置增强了结果的外部有效性。此外，研究通过基于胚胎移植周期数、年龄和研究地点的分层随机化，有效减少了潜在的混杂因素。然而，研究也存在一定的局限性。例如，针刺组与假针刺组间的胚胎移植阶段存在不平衡，这可能影响结果的可靠性。此外，由于越来越多的女性在社区接受针刺治疗，因此拒绝参加研究，导致样本量未达到预期目标，这可能影响研究结果的普遍性和代表性。

（2）临床研究方法学及统计学方法的选择及应用

在临床研究方法学方面，该研究严格遵循了随机对照试验的设计规范，包括随机化、分层和单盲法等，这些方法在控制偏倚和提高结果可信度方面起到了重要作用。主要分析采用了意向性治疗原则，并通过敏感性分析进一步验证了结果的稳健性，显示出研究在数据分析上的科学严谨性。然而，统计学方法上仍有改进空间。首先，虽然研究主要依赖风险差和相对风险进行组间比较，但没有对多重比较进行调整，这可能增加了发现假阳性的风险。其次，在面对样本量不足的问题时，虽然研究进行了灵敏度分析，但未能严格遵循样本量估算的初衷，导致结果的解释可能存在一定的不确定性。此外，研究中的不均衡现象，如假针刺组中胚胎移植阶段的差异，未能充分解释其潜在影响，这在一定程度上削弱了结论的严谨性。

综上所述，该研究在设计和执行过程中展现出诸多优点，如大样本量、多中心研究和严谨的随机化流程，但同时也存在一些需要进一步探讨的问题，如样本量未达预期、多重比较调整不足及胚胎移植阶段不均衡对结果的潜在影响。尽管如此，研究结果仍为针刺在IVF中的应用提供了重要的临床证据，但在解读和推广结论时需保持谨慎。

第四十二节 "Effect of Electroacupuncture on Urinary Leakage Among Women With Stress Urinary Incontinence: A Randomized Clinical Trial" 相关介绍和述评

一 论文介绍

1. 中文题目：电针对压力性尿失禁女性患者漏尿的影响：一项随机临床试验

2. 作者：Zhishun Liu, Yan Liu, Huanfang Xu, Liyun He, Yuelai Chen, Lixin Fu, Ning Li, Yonghui Lu, Tongsheng Su, Jianhua Sun, Jie Wang, Zenghui Yue, Wei Zhang, Jiping Zhao, Zhongyu Zhou, Jiani Wu, Kehua Zhou, Yanke Ai, Jing Zhou, Ran Pang, Yang Wang, Zongshi Qin, Shiyan Yan, Hongjiao Li, Lin Luo, Baoyan Liu

3. 主要单位：中国中医科学院广安门医院，中国中医科学院中医临床医学基础研究所，中国中医科学院针灸研究所等

4. 发表期刊：*JAMA*

5. 发布日期：2017年6月27日

6. SCI源文献：LIU Z, LIU Y, XU H, et al. Effect of Electroacupuncture on Urinary Leakage Among Women With Stress Urinary Incontinence: A Randomized Clinical Trial [J].

JAMA, 2017, 317 (24): 2493-2501.

7. 内容简介：本研究为多中心、随机临床试验，为了评估电针与假电针对压力性尿失禁（stress urinary incontinence，SUI）女性患者的影响，将504例女性SUI患者随机分为电针组和假电针组，观察两组从基线到第6周的漏尿量变化。得出结论：在SUI女性患者中，与假电针组相比，腰骶区域电针治疗后漏尿量更少。

电针组和假电针组治疗频次均为每周3次（理想情况下每隔1天1次），每次30 min，连续6周，共18次。

电针组皮肤消毒后，在双侧中髎（BL33）和会阳（BL35）穴位放置无菌胶垫，将一次性针刺针通过胶垫刺入皮肤50～60 mm。中髎的针刺方向为30°～45°，会阳的针刺方向略微上外侧。进针后，对所有针进行小而均匀的捻转、提插操作，以达到得气。将电针仪的配对电极横向连接到双侧中髎和会阳的针柄上。电针刺激持续30 min，连续波频率50 Hz，电流强度1～5 mA（以穴位周围的皮肤轻度颤抖而无疼痛感为宜）。

假电针组接受假电针干预，使用安慰针在假穴位上进行干预。假穴位分别位于中髎、会阳旁1寸（≈20 mm）。操作步骤、电极放置等均与电针组相同，但不穿透皮肤、无电流输出或针刺操作以得气。

二 专家述评（针灸学专家，临床研究方法学及卫生统计学专家）

1. 述评一

女性SUI是临床常见病。目前，现代医学尚无有效治愈SUI的方法，通常采用的盆底肌训练效果有限，而一些严重患者即使手术治疗，也面临较高复发风险。传统针刺疗法治疗SUI具有一定优势，但以往的研究普遍存在样本量小、设计缺陷、偏倚风险高等局限性，严重限制了其临床推广应用。刘保延、刘志顺研究团队基于该临床实际问题，通过纳入504例SUI女性患者的多中心随机对照研究设计，将患者分为电针组和假电针组，分别接受为期6周、每周3次的双侧中髎、会阳电针和假穴假电针治疗。研究结果发现，电针组在减少漏尿量、降低尿失禁次数等方面均明显优于假电针组，差异有统计学意义，停止治疗后疗效可以维持24周，治疗期间不良事件较少发生。该试验选题临床价值高，针刺干预措施细节披露完整，详细介绍了穴位的选择和定位、针刺的角度、针刺手法、电针的具体参数、治疗周期等具体细节，具有科学严谨的方法学设计，突破既往研究瓶颈，通过大样本多中心研究，为中医针刺治疗女性SUI的有效性和安全性提供了高质量循证证据。当然，该研究假针刺对照组采用无皮肤穿透和电流输出的方式，如何保障盲法的效果？需要更多的细节进行评估，未来研究如果采用刺入性针刺结合无电流输出的方式进行安慰对照，盲法可能更有保障。

2. 述评二

（1）研究设计和过程实施

该研究是一项为期30周的多中心、随机、假电针刺对照试验，在中国12家医院进行，纳入504例SUI女性患者。研究采用固定区组分层随机方法，通过中央化随机系统将患者按照1∶1比例分配，分别接受电针与假电针治疗，保证了组间均衡性。使用假电针设计对患者实施盲法，并进行了盲法效果测评，尽可能减少期望效应与主观判断对结果的影响。主要结局为基线到第6周的漏尿量变化，通过1h尿垫试验测试，指标客观、可测量，能有效评估针刺治疗SUI效果，具有重要临床意义。该研究设计与实施严谨。

（2）临床研究方法学及统计学方法的选择及应用

该研究进行样本量估算考虑了20%失访与预先设定的亚组分析，最终纳入504例40~75岁SUI女性患者。该研究遵循意向治疗分析原则，拟合混合效应模型，使用漏尿量基线值作为协变量，治疗作为固定效应，中心之间、中心与治疗之间的相互作用作为考虑中心差异的随机效应，该分析方法充分考虑重复测量数据，并调整重要协变量，能有效处理不同患者间的变异性。在随机缺失假设下，使用多重填补法对主要结局进行填补，相较于单一填补方法，可减少偏倚。研究进行4次敏感性分析（1次预先设定、3次事后分析）评估缺失数据对结果的影响，验证结果的稳健性；开展1次事后亚组分析观察电针对不同严重程度SUI的影响。研究充分讨论了试验中存在的局限性，该临床研究方法学及统计学方法的选择与应用合理且恰当。

第四十三节 "*Effect of Acupuncture and Clomiphene in Chinese Women With Polycystic Ovary Syndrome: A Randomized Clinical Trial*" 相关介绍和述评

一 论文介绍

1. 中文题目：针刺和克罗米芬对中国妇女多囊卵巢综合征患者疗效的随机临床试验

2. 作者：Xiao-Ke Wu, Elisabet Stener-Victorin, Hong-Ying Kuang, Hong-Li Ma, Jing-Shu Gao, Liang-Zhen Xie, Li-Hui Hou, Zhen-Xing Hu, Xiao-Guang Shao, Jun Ge, Jin-Feng Zhang, Hui-Ying Xue, Xiao-Feng Xu, Rui-Ning Liang, Hong-Xia Ma, Hong-Wei Yang, Wei-Li Li, Dong-Mei Huang, Yun Sun, Cui-Fang Hao, Shao-Min Du, Zheng-Wang Yang, Xin Wang, Ying Yan, Xiu-Hua Chen, Ping Fu, Cai-Fei Ding, Ya-Qin Gao, Zhong-Ming Zhou, Chi Chiu Wang, Tai-Xiang Wu, Jian-Ping Liu, Ernest H. Y. Ng, Richard S. Legro, Heping Zhang, PCOSAct Study Group

3. 主要单位：世界中医药学会联合会生殖医学专业委员会，黑龙江中医药大学第一附属医院妇产科，徐州市妇幼保健院门诊部

4. 发表期刊：*JAMA*

5. 发布日期：2017年7月27日

6. SCI源文献：WU X K, STENER-VICTORIN E, KUANG H Y, et al. Effect of Acupuncture and Clomiphene in Chinese Women With Polycystic Ovary Syndrome: A Randomized Clinical Trial [J]. JAMA, 2017, 317 (24): 2502-2514.

7. 内容简介：本研究为双盲（克罗米芬对比安慰剂）、单盲（真针刺对比假针刺）析因试验。分析针对多囊卵巢综合征（polycystic ovary syndrome，PCOS）患者，单用针刺或与克罗米芬联用，针刺是否增加PCOS患者分娩活产儿的可能性。将1000例PCOS患者按1∶1∶1∶1的比例随机分为4组（针刺+克罗米芬组，针刺+安慰剂组，假针刺+克罗米芬组，假针刺+安慰剂组），分别进行干预，观察4组受试者妊娠20周或更晚时的活产率。得出结论：单独针刺或联合克罗米芬并未增加PCOS活产率。

针刺治疗采用标准化方案。所有受试者每周接受2次针刺治疗，每次30 min，最多治疗32次。

针刺（针刺+克罗米芬组，针刺+安慰剂组）采用深刺针配合手法和低频电刺激，采用2套针刺穴位交替使用以避免针刺局部酸痛。针刺穴位位于腹部和腿部肌肉、手部和头部。针刺后，所有针具均施以捻转直至得气产生酸麻感，即产生针感。针感反映了在脊髓与中枢水平投射至中枢神经系统的传入神经纤维被激活。手部和头部针刺每10 min行针1次。腹部和腿部穴位行捻转手法并连接低频电刺激。

假针刺对照（假针刺+克罗米芬组，假针刺+安慰剂组）采用浅针刺+模拟电刺激，无手法刺激。浅刺深度小于5 mm，选取双侧肩部和上臂的非经非穴，刺入后不行针。连接电极，打开电针仪以模仿真针刺，但刺激量为0，即无电流刺激。

克罗米芬或安慰剂于每个月经周期服用5天，连用4个月经周期。受试者在月经周期第3～7天开始每日口服1片（50 mg）克罗米芬或等量安慰剂。如无排卵，口服药物增加1片（50 mg），如出现排卵则维持原剂量。克罗米芬或安慰剂最大剂量每日不超过150 mg或每个月经周期不超过750 mg。

二　专家述评（针灸学专家，临床研究方法学及卫生统计学专家）

1. 述评一

PCOS是影响女性不孕的常见原因。临床上单用克罗米芬治疗PCOS的失败率（无排卵）高达23.4%。本项研究采用随机对照试验设计评估针刺联合克罗米芬改善PCOS患者活产率的效果，具有很高的临床价值。此外，该项研究创新性地使用了2×2析因设计来分析克罗米芬和针刺的总体效应及独立成分效应，能帮助临床医师更准确地判定针刺和克罗米芬各自的效果及联合效果。但在针刺干预措施的设计当中，有几个方面值得深入思考，以便开展进一步的研究。第一，针刺的穴位选择和干预方案更多地考虑了针刺对神经系统刺激。PCOS作为一种复杂疾病，如果按照中医诊断不孕症进行治疗，应该考虑以任脉、足少阴肾经取穴为主。未来研究如果基于传统辨证循经取穴开展治疗，是否能取得更好的疗效值得思考。第二，针刺方案以腹部和下肢部位取穴为主，假针刺对照则以上肢取穴为主。这种设计是否会导致盲法效果不佳，也值得深入思考。未来研究可以考虑真针刺的穴位与假针刺部位相邻以获得更好的盲法效果。第三，PCOS作为一种同时影响生殖系统和内分泌系统的疾病，记录患者改善内分泌紊乱症状的合并用药情况很有必要。未来研究可以设计表格采集患者合并用药信息，并做相关统计分析。

总体而言，该研究的临床选题价值高，采用的临床设计方法新颖，为针刺辅助治疗PCOS提供了高质量证据。

2. 述评二

该研究在国际上具有较大影响力，在国内也广受关注。该研究在中国21个中心进行，采用了4组的2×2析因设计，共纳入1000例PCOS患者，评估了针刺和克罗米芬的效果及其相互作用，每周针刺2次。研究发现，无论针刺联合克罗米芬还是联合安慰剂均没有提高活产率，也没有增加受孕率、双胞胎率和排卵率。

研究的大样本及析因设计是其非常显著的特征，提高了其科学价值和临床价值。试验脱落率较低，报告严谨规范，统计分析深入，为临床合理治疗PCOS不孕症提供了明确的指引。研究的析因设计统计分析方案较之试验开始之前有较大改动，是本研究在文中自我报告的一个重要局限。研究立论依据强调了针刺治疗PCOS及相关不孕症的前期研究证据及临床现状，提供了9篇国际临床现状研究及少量小样本随机对照试验作为支持，但如果能够有来自中国的前期临床调研或试验作为在国内开展上千例大样本临床研究的支持则会更有说服力。此外，研究的纳入标准没有规定入组受试者均有妊娠意愿，也没有规定是否为育龄期妇女，而研究的主要结局是活产率。治疗选穴、假针的穴位设置、疗程、针刺频率、随访疗程设计等如果能够提供更为有力的前期临床、基础研究证据和理论依据则可以使得研究方案更有说服力；研究中提到了针灸师的背景为中医专业研究生，并强调了专门为此研究方案对其进行了培训，如果能更详细描述其资质和临床经验则会更加符合国际报告规范。

第四十四节 "The Long-Term Effect of Acupuncture for Migraine Prophylaxis: A Randomized Clinical Trial" 相关介绍和述评

一 论文介绍

1. 中文题目：针刺预防偏头痛的远期疗效：一项随机临床试验

2. 作者：Ling Zhao, Jiao Chen, Ying Li, Xin Sun, Xiaorong Chang, Hui Zheng, Biao Gong, Yinlan Huang, Mingxiao Yang, Xi Wu, Xuezhi Li, Fanrong Liang

3．主要单位：成都中医药大学针灸推拿学院，四川大学华西医院中国循证医学中心，湖南中医药大学针灸推拿学院

4．发表期刊：*JAMA Internal Medicine*

5．发布日期：2017年2月20日

6．SCI源文献：ZHAO L, CHEN J, LI Y, et al. The Long-Term Effect of Acupuncture for Migraine Prophylaxis: A Randomized Clinical Trial [J]. JAMA Intern Med, 2017, 177 (4): 508-515.

7．内容简介：本研究是为期24周的随机临床试验，为了探索针刺在减少偏头痛患者头痛发作频率及在偏头痛预防上的远期疗效，将249例无先兆偏头痛患者随机分为针刺组、假针刺组及等待治疗组分别进行干预，观察3组受试者基线至第16周偏头痛发作频率。得出结论：在无先兆偏头痛患者中，与假针刺或等待治疗相比，针刺可能在减少偏头痛发作方面存在长期疗效。

针刺组、假针刺组均接受20次电针治疗（每日1次，连续治疗5天，休息2天），每次30 min，共持续4周。

针刺组每次选4穴，固定选取风池（GB20）、率谷（GB8），另外两穴依据头痛部位经络辨证选取，在外关（TE5）、阳陵泉（GB34）、昆仑（BL60）、后溪（SI3）、合谷（LI4）、内庭（ST44）、太冲（LR3）、丘墟（GB40）中选取。除上述穴位外，不允许使用其他穴位。使用长25～40 mm，直径0.25 mm的一次性无菌针灸针。针灸师每次选取单侧治疗，双侧交替。针刺得气后接电针仪。刺激频率2/100 Hz，刺激强度0.1～1.0 mA（以患者耐受为度）。

假针刺组基于前期研究选取4个非经非穴，除针刺后不施行手法诱导得气感以外，其余操作及参数均与针刺组保持一致。

等待治疗组在试验开始时不接受针刺治疗，但24周后可免费获得20次针刺治疗。

二 专家述评（针灸学专家，临床研究方法学及卫生统计学专家）

1．述评一

（1）选题分析

25%～38%的偏头痛患者需要预防性治疗和药物干预，但这类治疗常伴有不良反应，且过度使用止痛药或接受特异性抗偏头痛治疗可能导致药物过度使用性头痛。针灸在国内外被广泛用于治疗偏头痛，尤其适用于药物难治性患者。既往研究发现，针刺在减轻偏头痛疼痛强度、发作频率和持续时间方面有效，但研究样本量小，存在一定的局限性。本临床试验在扩大样本量的同时，还聚焦针刺的长期效果，这一研究对于成功预防和减少偏头痛发作至关重要。

（2）针刺干预的实施

针刺干预具有合理性，因为针刺可缓解偏头痛发作时的疼痛（急性效应）和预防

偏头痛发作（长期效应）；关于针刺干预，选用风池、率谷为主穴，并根据头痛区经络辨证各选取2个穴位，交替使用左右穴位进行单侧治疗。在针刺实际操作中和论文描述中，对针具规格、针法操作、得气和电针刺激参数（电针刺激仪）等都有明确交代；关于治疗方案，共治疗20次（每天1次，每次30 min，连续5天，休息2天），时长共4周，总体干预时间适宜；本试验没有采用其他辅助干预措施；关于针灸师的背景，所有针灸师均接受了至少5年培训并具有4年临床经验；对照设置采用假针刺方法，即选4个非穴位点，不得气，电刺激和治疗时间与真针刺组相同，方法简单实用。

2. 述评二

本项临床研究的设计和实施体现了高度的科学性和严谨性。研究在中国开展，采用了多中心、随机对照的试验设计，增强了研究结果的科学性和可推广性。研究方案提前注册并顺利实施。研究的实施过程中，对于参与者的筛选、分组、治疗和随访等各个环节都制定了详细的操作标准和质量控制措施。此外，研究中所用的针刺方案都有较好的临床和理论基础，并对加减用穴、针刺次数、是否得气等都有明确的指导和要求。研究对针灸师的资质和经验也进行了明确要求。一系列举措良好地保障了针刺治疗的标准化、个性化和质量控制。

研究既采用了假针刺对照又采用了等待治疗（空白组）进行对照。这样的对照形式有利于观察到假针刺的效应，对于针刺疗效的构成分析奠定了基础；但这也使得等待治疗组患者没有被完全施盲，针灸师及其他与患者有接触的研究工作人员的盲法也不可能完全做到。而且，本研究的主要结局是第13~16周（共4周）中偏头痛发作的累积频次较之基线（入组前4周偏头痛发作的累积频次）的差值。该结局及次要结局通过患者日记采集，这是典型的患者自报告结局。此类结局，特别是症状类结局，受患者主观影响较大，对使用盲法来克服信息偏倚的需求较为明显。此外，文中对主要结局的英文描述容易引起误解，读者可能难以理解这是指4周内的累积数据。该研究的讨论比较充分，特别是关于等待治疗组在观察过程中病情减轻现象及基线病情数据可靠性方面的讨论。如果能进一步增加对假针刺组与等待治疗组设置目的及结果异同的比较，将有助于提升研究的意义和价值。

第四十五节 "Rewiring the Primary Somatosensory Cortex in Carpal Tunnel Syndrome With Acupuncture" 相关介绍和述评

一 论文介绍

1. 中文题目：针刺重建腕管综合征患者的初级躯体感觉皮质
2. 作者：Yumi Maeda, Hyungjun Kim, Norman Kettner, Jieun Kim, Stephen Cina, Cristina Malatesta, Jessica Gerber, Claire McManus, Rebecca Ong-Sutherland, Pia

Mezzacappa, Alexandra Libby, Ishtiaq Mawla, Leslie R. Morse, Ted J. Kaptchuk, Joseph Audette, Vitaly Napadow

3．主要单位：Athinoula A. Martinos Center for Biomedical Imaging, Department of Radiology, Massachusetts General Hospita; Department of Radiology, Logan Universit; Department of Physical Medicine and Rehabilitation, Harvard Medical School

4．发表期刊：*Brain*

5．发布日期：2017年3月2日

6．SCI源文献：MAEDA Y, KIM H, KETTNER N, et al. Rewiring the primary somatosensory cortex in carpal tunnel syndrome with acupuncture [J]. Brain, 2017, 140 (4): 914-927.

7．内容简介：本研究为单中心、盲法、安慰剂对照、随机平行组纵向神经影像学研究，旨在探讨针刺是否在减少腕管综合征（carpal tunnel syndrome，CTS）患者症状严重程度方面优于假针刺。研究共招募了79例CTS患者，随机分为局部针刺组、远端针刺组和假针刺组，分别进行干预，比较3组受试者治疗前后症状严重程度量表评分。得出结论：虽然真针刺和假针刺都能减轻CTS症状，但真针刺在改善周围神经系统和中枢神经系统功能方面优于假针刺；在针刺治疗后，大脑初级躯体感觉皮层（S1）发生了可塑性变化（即适应性或调整），而这种变化可以用来预测患者长期症状的缓解效果。

3组受试者均在门诊接受16次针刺治疗，共8周；治疗频次依次减少，前3周每周治疗3次，中间2周每周治疗2次，最后3周每周治疗1次。患者取仰卧位，采用标准化针刺与个体化针刺相结合的方式。

局部针刺组：选取患侧外关（TE5）、大陵（PC7），将电极置于穴位，使用恒定电流电针仪，刺激频率2 Hz，刺激时间20 min。刺激强度为患者感到中等强度但无痛感为宜。此外，依据患者具体情况，在患侧少海（SI8）、曲泽（PC3）、腕骨（SI4）、阳溪（LI5）、蠡沟（LR5）、尺泽（LU5）中选取3个穴位，所有穴位均得气。

远端针刺组：电针置于健侧三阴交（SP6）、太冲（LR3）、阳陵泉（GB34）、太溪（KI3）、商丘（SP5），进针10~30 mm。为了增加过程可信度，将一个非刺入式假针刺针置于患侧前臂非穴SH1。

假针刺组：将刺入式假针刺Streitberger针置于患侧前臂尺侧非穴（SH1、SH2）。与上述针刺组相似，连接电极，打开电针仪，但电极未插入有效端口。受试者被告知他们可能感到或无法感到电流刺激。同时，另取3个假针刺针置于患侧前臂桡侧非穴SH3，健侧下肢非穴SH4、SH5。

二 专家述评（针灸学专家，临床研究方法学及卫生统计学专家）

1．述评一

CTS是正中神经在腕管受压而表现出的一组症状和体征，属于周围神经卡压综合征中最常见的一种。CTS在成人中的患病率为2.7%~5.8%，并且其终身发病率高达10%~15%。该项试验采用安慰剂对照、随机平行组纵向神经影像学研究的设计，评估针刺治疗CTS的疗效，具有较高的临床价值。但在针刺干预措施的设计中，有几个方面值得进一步思考，以便开展更深入的研究。第一，CTS在不同年龄、性别、职业的人群中易患程度、严重程度等明显不同。CTS通常发生在36~60岁人群；女性与男性的比例为2∶1至5∶1；长期从事重复性手腕运动的人群，如计算机程序员、维修工人、画家等更易发病。本研究可在已获得研究结果的基础上做进一步分析，观察不同年龄阶段、性别、职业是否会存在不同的治疗效果。第二，本研究对针刺疗效的评估仅设立治疗前、治疗结束及随访结束3个时间点，在治疗过程中设立评估时间点能更好地反映针刺疗效随针刺时间及剂量的变化，从而更好地指导临床以选取最佳疗程。第三，两组针刺治疗取穴分别位于上肢、下肢，假针刺组则是上肢与下肢均有，取穴位置明显不同，这种设计是否会导致盲法效果不佳，值得思考。未来研究可以考虑双模拟设计，如针刺组分别采用上肢针刺取穴联合下肢假针刺取穴、上肢假针刺取穴联合下肢针刺取穴的取穴方案，使患者无法通过取穴位置判断治疗组别，以获得更好的盲法效果。

总体而言，该研究的临床选题价值高，采用的临床设计方法新颖，为针刺治疗CTS的有效性提供了高质量证据。

2. 述评二

（1）研究设计

本研究观察针刺治疗CTS对初级躯体感觉皮层（S1）可塑性的影响，采用随机（采用置换区组随机化）、对照（采用安慰剂即"假针刺"对照）、单盲（患者不知情而医师知情）的平行组纵向神经影像研究设计，有效控制了潜在的混杂因素，通过对比针刺与假针刺的疗效，确保了研究结果的可靠性和科学性。同样提前定义结局变量，对于症状严重程度的评价指标为波士顿腕管量表（Boston carpal tunnel questionnaire，BCTQ），测量时间为治疗开始时、治疗后和治疗后3个月随访。对于神经传导研究评价指标为中位感觉神经传导潜伏期，评价时间为治疗前和治疗后。对于手指分离距离评价指标为D2/D3分离，评价时间为治疗前和治疗后。

（2）过程实施

在实施过程中，采用3种干预方法，即局部针刺、远端针刺及假针刺，通过计算机生成的随机区组分配，确保了各组间的均衡性。针刺治疗由经验丰富的针灸师执行，减少了操作变异性。此外，采用了多种评价工具，包括以BCTQ评估症状，神经传导研究评估腕部神经功能，以及功能性MRI评估大脑皮层的可塑性，覆盖了主观和客观指标，确保了研究的多维度性。

（3）临床研究方法学及统计学方法的选择及应用

在统计分析阶段，采用重复测量方差分析观察BCTQ评分、神经传导功能和手指

第二章 SCI源期刊高质量针灸临床研究述评

分离距离的变化,并且进行了事后检验,以处理纵向数据和多组比较问题。但是仍然存在一些问题,对于BCTQ评分,文章中重复测量方差分析得到组别(真针刺、假针刺)与时间(基线、治疗后、3个月随访)交互作用具有趋势显著性($P=0.098$),但结果无统计学意义;此外,针对事后检验,文中实际应用的方法是针对指标(如BCTQ评分)变化量进行分析,即应用了新的统计学方法(如独立样本t检验),因此在统计学上用事后检验这个术语可能不准确。

总体而言,该研究结合传统的临床评估方法和先进的神经影像技术,深入探讨了针刺对CTS的治疗机制,在设计和实施过程中严格遵循了临床研究方法学的标准,确保了结果的科学性和可靠性。通过多层次、多维度的评估方法,以及严谨的统计分析,揭示了针刺治疗CTS的神经生理机制。然而,研究也存在一些不足,如没有事先进行样本量估计、样本量相对较小、长期随访的数据有限等;此外,论文在应用重复测量方差分析时,并没有进行前提假设,即正态方差齐性检验。未来研究可考虑增加样本量,延长随访时间,以进一步验证和拓展现有发现。

第四十六节 "A Randomised Controlled Trial Examining the Effect of Acupuncture at the EX-HN3 (Yintang) Point on Pre-operative Anxiety Levels in Neurosurgical Patients"相关介绍和述评

一 论文介绍

1. 中文题目:一项随机对照试验研究针刺印堂穴对神经外科患者术前焦虑水平的影响

2. 作者:M. D. Wiles, J. Mamdani, M. Pullman, J.C. Andrzejowski

3. 主要单位:Sheffield Teaching Hospitals NHS Foundation Trust, University of Sheffield Medical School

4. 发表期刊:*Anaesthesia*

5. 发布日期:2017年1月16日

6. SCI源文献:Wiles M D, Mamdani J, Pullman M, et al. A randomised controlled trial examining the effect of acupuncture at the EX-HN3 (Yintang) point on pre-operative anxiety levels in neurosurgical patients [J]. Anaesthesia, 2017, 72 (3): 335-342.

7. 内容简介:本研究为单中心、前瞻性、随机对照试验,旨在探讨针刺印堂(EX-HN3)对神经外科患者术前焦虑水平的影响。研究纳入128例患者,随机分为针刺组(接受针刺印堂穴)和对照组(不干预),观察两组患者治疗前后焦虑水平的变化。主要结局采用状态-特质焦虑量表(state trait anxiety inventory, STAI-S6)作为评估标准，次要结局采用阿姆斯特丹术前焦虑与信息量表-焦虑部分（Amsterdam preoperative anxiety and information scale，APAISa）评估焦虑水平的变化、麻醉恢复室（postanesthesia care unit，PACU）报告术后疼痛评分（分为无/轻度或中度/重度疼痛）、阿片类药物需求、术后恶心呕吐（postoperative nausea and vomiting，PONV）的发生率。得出结论：与对照组相比，针刺印堂穴可有效降低等待神经外科手术患者的术前焦虑水平。

针刺组接受1次针刺治疗（于印堂穴刺入揿针）。针刺过程中不追求得气感。受试者被要求每10 min按揉揿针，留针30 min后取下，随后完成第二次STAI-S6问卷和APAISa问卷。手术前无进一步干预，所有治疗均在患者床边进行。术中管理（包括提供镇痛药和止吐药）由麻醉师根据临床需要决定。

对照组未接受针刺干预，仅在床边等待30 min，之后完成第二次STAI-S6问卷和APAISa问卷。手术前无进一步干预，所有治疗同样在患者床边进行。术中管理（包括提供镇痛药和止吐药）均由麻醉师根据临床需要决定。

二　专家述评（针灸学专家，临床研究方法学及卫生统计学专家）

1. 述评一

（1）选题分析

选题着眼于如何解决临床中的难点和热点问题，分析关键临床问题的提炼与构建，体现其价值意义。

这项单中心、前瞻性的随机对照试验针对神经外科患者普遍存在的"术前焦虑"这一临床实际问题，使用揿针刺激按压印堂穴的方法，并与对照组进行对比，主要结局是测量30 min后的焦虑水平（STAI-S6评分），次要结局包括焦虑水平的变化（APAISa评分）、PACU报告的术后疼痛评分、阿片类药物需求及PONV的发生率。研究表明，针刺组STAI-S6问卷得分显著低于对照组，且两组患者均未发生不良事件，从而证实了针刺印堂穴可降低神经外科患者的术前焦虑水平。

近年来，加速术后康复（enhanced recovery after surgery，ERAS）理念备受关注。其核心在于通过在围手术期采取一系列基于循证医学证据的措施，旨在减少手术创伤与应激反应，加速患者康复进程。将针刺疗法融入快速康复外科领域，可望在围手术期管理中发挥重要作用。该研究抓住神经外科患者的临床痛点，巧妙融合中医外治手段，研究目标明确，研究思路清晰，操作简便可行，有较好的临床指导意义。

（2）针刺干预的实施

该研究针刺干预方案采用揿针施于印堂穴，并每10 min施以旋按手法，操作简便，易学易用，无需其他辅助措施，便于临床推广。但其方案是否为既贴合针刺临床实际又能获得最佳疗效？可进一步开展研究。一是穴位选择，印堂是否为最佳效穴？是否有更好的协同穴组？二是刺激量，揿针（0.2 mm×1.5 mm）每10 min按压，在皮部的刺激量较小。与针刺比较疗效如何？每10 min刺激有无依据？揿针使用的频次、配穴的设计、按压手法的操作力度等方面可进一步细化。三是对照组选择，等待手术是一种临床实际状态，较难除外安慰剂效应，可设计假揿针组等。

2. 述评二

该研究采用随机对照试验设计，旨在评价针刺印堂穴对缓解神经外科患者术前焦虑的效果。研究采用了严谨的随机分组方法——随机排列区组法，将患者分为针刺组和对照组，但未描述患者招募过程，因此不清楚分配患者时随机序列是否会被破坏。针刺疗法临床研究对研究人员和受试者进行盲法极具挑战，但在招募患者时采用分配隐藏可有效降低偏倚。同时，通过采用假针刺作为对照，也可有效消除患者因未接收到针刺治疗而产生的主观影响。在人群方面，排除了精神疾病、先前接受针刺治疗和针刺用于预防呕心呕吐的患者，可以有效避免患者对焦虑量表理解能力的问题，以及因为曾经接受过针刺疗法的心理抗拒或安慰。在统计分析时，研究还应考虑不同人群的疗效差异，例如，纳入患者中有50%左右患有严重焦虑，应该探讨效应修饰因子（如焦虑严重程度）对针刺效果的影响。该研究在方法学部分明确了具有临床意义的焦虑水平改善程度（评分降低30%），但在结果部分却未对其进行分析究竟有多大比例的患者获得临床意义的改善。总的来说，研究设计还可进一步完善，尤其在隐蔽分组、采用假针刺对照、亚组分析和结果报告方面，从而深层次挖掘针刺的优势人群，为针刺缓解神经外科患者术前焦虑提供更高质量的循证医学证据。

第四十七节 "Acupuncture as an Integrative Approach for the Treatment of Hot Flashes in Women With Breast Cancer: A Prospective Multicenter Randomized Controlled Trial (AcCliMaT)" 相关介绍和述评

一、论文介绍

1. 中文题目：针刺作为治疗女性乳腺癌患者潮热的综合方法：一项前瞻性多中心随机对照试验

2. 作者：Grazia Lesi, Giorgia Razzini, Muriel Assunta Musti, Elisa Stivanello, Chiara Petrucci, Benedetta Benedetti, Ermanno Rondini, Maria Bernadette Ligabue, Laura Scaltriti, Alberto Botti, Fabrizio Artioli, Pamela Mancuso, Francesco Cardini, Paolo Pandolfi

3. 主要单位：Bologna Local Health Authority; Civil Hospital, Carpi

4. 发表期刊：*Journal of Clinical Oncology*

5. 发布日期：2016年3月28日

6. SCI源文献：LESI G, RAZZINI G, MUSTI M A, et al. Acupuncture as an Integrative Approach for the Treatment of Hot Flashes in Women With Breast Cancer: A Prospective Multicenter Randomized Controlled Trial (AcCliMaT) [J]. J Clin Oncol, 2016, 34 (15): 1795-1802.

7. 内容简介：本研究采用双臂、实用、多中心、随机对照试验，旨在探讨针刺治疗女性乳腺癌患者潮热的有效性。研究纳入190例女性乳腺癌患者，根据是否接受激素治疗进行分层随机分配，分为针刺组及强化自我管理组，观察两组受试者在第12周时每日平均潮热评分。得出结论：与单纯强化自我护理相比，针刺联合强化自我护理是治疗女性乳腺癌患者潮热、提高生活质量的有效综合干预措施。

针刺组在强化自我护理基础上，接受10次传统针刺治疗，每周1次，共12周。治疗方案确定了6种中医更年期证候，每次在针刺治疗前，根据受试者舌脉辨证取穴，在三阴交（SP6）、曲池（LI11）、关元（CV4）三穴基础上，可以使用补充穴位，但最多不超过11个，采用0.30 mm×0.40 mm无菌一次性针灸针，臀部以外的腧穴针刺深度为0.5～1.0 cm，臀部腧穴针刺深度则为1.0～2.0 cm，行针得气，不允许弹针或捻转针具，每次针刺20 min。适当根据中医诊断提供艾灸治疗。治疗在5家癌症专科医院和3家健康中心进行。

对照设置组：强化自我护理，自我护理的指导手册是由研究团队达成共识后编写，包括有关潮热、癌症的相关信息和针对饮食、锻炼和心理支持的详尽指导。

二 专家述评（针灸学专家，临床研究方法学及卫生统计学专家）

1. 述评一

（1）选题分析

乳腺癌作为女性最常见的恶性肿瘤之一，其治疗过程常伴随着多种不良反应，其中潮热是乳腺癌患者在接受化疗或激素治疗时最常见的症状之一。本研究着力于解决针刺结合强化自我护理在治疗乳腺癌女性潮热和改善生活质量方面的综合疗效，研究设计充分考虑患者的个体差异和疾病特点，采用多中心、随机对照试验，确保研究结果的可靠性和可重复性。针刺结合强化自我护理为乳腺癌潮热患者提供一种非药物、低成本且有效的治疗选择，有助于缓解潮热症状、改善生活质量，减轻患者的身心负担。

（2）针刺干预的实施

研究中有辨证取穴，不同证型的标准是什么？是否可能出现主观性？选穴方面，每次治疗使用的穴位不超过11个，不同证型之间的穴位个数差异太大。评价的时候，不同证型、不同选穴也可以进行亚组分析，结果可能会更加严谨。一般临床试验针刺频率为1周3次或隔天1次，本研究每周1次，进行10次针刺治疗是否存在针刺频次过低不太符合临床实际的嫌疑。

2. 述评二

（1）研究设计和过程实施

该项研究采用了多中心、随机、对照设计，属于实用性随机对照试验。主要有以下几方面特点：对比了针刺与强化自我护理的综合疗法相对于单纯强化自我护理对治疗女性乳腺癌患者潮热的有效性，而不是采用安慰对照进行特异性效应的评估；试验组采用了针刺与艾灸结合的治疗措施，并且考虑了患者的证型，辨证选择针刺穴位和艾灸治疗，更接近临床实际。

研究实施过程严谨。由于缺乏关于有乳腺癌病史的女性更年期综合征管理的指南，强化自我护理的方案是基于团队专家共识形成；在定期访视中，研究人员还评估了患者对强化自我护理建议的执行情况。

针灸师与患者之间的交谈尽量减少，以限制非特异性治疗效果。

（2）临床研究方法学及统计学方法的选择及应用

整体上看，本项研究的统计学方法较为规范。①随机化：按是否进行了激素治疗（促性腺激素释放激素激动剂）进行分层，较好地控制了激素对研究结果的影响。②样本量计算：基于前期预试验结果进行样本量估计，可以提高准确性；尽管研究未按照预期设计完成全部患者入组而提前终止，但对研究结果影响不大。③统计分析：整体上较为规范，但有几处可进行更优化处理，如采用是否进行激素治疗作为分层因素进行随机，但实际上几乎所有患者都接受激素治疗，且近一半参与者正在接受促性腺激素释放激素类似物联合治疗，这可能会影响到分层随机的实施，甚至导致试验随机化方法的调整，但文章并未对此细节进行交代。主要疗效指标采用 t 检验进行统计分析，未考虑基线及其他可能影响因素对结果的影响。

第四十八节 "Acupuncture for Chronic Severe Functional Constipation: A Randomized Trial" 相关介绍和述评

一 论文介绍

1. 中文题目：针刺治疗慢性重度功能性便秘：一项随机试验

2. 作者：Zhishun Liu, Shiyan Yan, Jiani Wu, Liyun He, Ning Li, Guirong Dong, Jianqiao Fang, Wenbin Fu, Lixin Fu, Jianhua Sun, Linpeng Wang, Shun Wang, Jun Yang, Hongxing Zhang, Jianbin Zhang, Jiping Zhao, Wei Zhou, Zhongyu Zhou, Yanke Ai, Kehua Zhou, Jia Liu, Huanfang Xu, Yuying Cai, Baoyan Liu

3. 主要单位：中国中医科学院广安门医院，中国中医科学院中医临床基础医学研

究所，四川大学华西医院

4. 发表期刊：*Annals of Internal Medicine*

5. 发布日期：2016年9月13日

6. SCI源文献：LIU Z, YAN S, WU J, et al. Acupuncture for chronic severe functional constipation: a randomized trial [J]. Ann Intern Med, 2016, 165 (11): 761-769.

7. 内容简介：本研究为随机、平行、假针刺对照试验，旨在探讨电针治疗慢性重度功能性便秘（chronic severe functional constipation，CSFC）的疗效。研究纳入1075例CSFC患者，随机分为电针组与假电针组，分别进行干预，主要结局是观察两组患者第1～8周平均每周完整自主排便次数（complete spontaneous bowel move-ments，CSBMs）较基线的变化。得出结论：8周的电针治疗增加了CSBMs，且对CSFC的治疗是安全的。

两组均接受28次治疗，每次治疗30 min，在8周内完成（前两周每周5次治疗，剩余6周每周3次治疗）。

电针组取穴双侧天枢（ST25）、腹结（SP14）、上巨虚（ST37）。患者取仰卧位，采用0.30 mm×50 mm或0.35 mm×75 mm一次性针灸针直刺天枢、腹结，进针深度为30～70 mm，不行针直至针刺入腹壁肌层。将电针仪弹簧夹连接双侧天枢、腹结，电针刺激30 min，电针参数设置为疏密波10/50 Hz、0.1～1.0 mA，刺激强度以受试者感觉舒适为度。此外，采用0.30 mm×40 mm一次性针灸针直刺上巨虚，进针深度约为30 mm，行提插、捻转平补平泻3次（每10 min操作1次）至得气。

假电针组受试者在双侧假天枢、假腹结和假上巨虚浅刺。将0.30 mm×25 mm针灸针刺入非穴3～5 mm深，不行针。与电针组相似，将特殊构造的电针仪弹簧夹连接双侧假天枢、假腹结。通电时，假电针组电针仪的指示灯和声音开启，但无实际电流输出。

二 专家述评（针灸学专家，临床研究方法学及卫生统计学专家）

1. 述评一

（1）选题贴合临床实际问题

本研究的选题聚焦CSFC。这一疾病在全球范围内的发病率高达16%，患者生活质量显著下降。便秘患者通常面临长期的症状困扰，传统药物如泻药和促动力药虽然常用，但其疗效有限，且伴随复发性强、依从性差等问题。因此，寻找一种有效且安全的替代疗法成为当务之急。本研究通过将电针引入CSFC的治疗中，填补了非药物治疗便秘的研究空白，也为针刺治疗该疾病提供了强有力的临床证据支持，体现了其在选题上的临床价值和社会意义。

在本研究中，电针作为选题的核心干预措施，得益于其在中医理论和现代医学研究中的双重支持。穴位选择基于中医"脾胃为后天之本"的理论，强调通过调理脾胃

中相对普遍且影响生活质量。通过对这一特定人群的研究，能够为癌症疼痛管理提供新的思路和方法。

（2）研究设计

本研究提出明确的研究假说，与假针刺组或等待治疗组相比，真针刺组在治疗6周时AI相关关节疼痛程度降低（根据BPI-WP）。根据以往研究结果，将BPI-WP评分减少2分确定为有临床意义的变化。采用等待治疗组的设计，旨在应对以往研究中对安慰剂效应的担忧。这一设计能够更好地评估真实针刺与假针刺的效果差异，为结果的解读提供更为可靠的依据。研究中特别注意了针刺操作者的培训和掌握程度的评估，保证了针刺效果。

（3）局限性分析

文中清晰列出了多项局限性，例如患者随机分配到等待治疗组时无法实现盲法，且真针刺组患者对治疗的信念可能影响结果。主要结局基于相对短期的观察，缺乏12个月以上的长期跟踪数据，尚需要进一步的研究来评估治疗效果的持续性。

（4）社区参与及可及性问题

研究提到的参与者招募缓慢及干预费用等问题，反映了在实际临床环境中推广针刺治疗的挑战，这些因素在今后的研究中需要被重视并解决。

（5）未来研究方向

由于该研究未能评估疗效的维持和耐久性，未来的研究应当关注这一方面，以及探讨不同患者群体对针刺的反应差异。

（6）统计分析

①使用Poisson回归：为了估计风险差异和相对风险，研究中采用了Poisson回归模型，并使用了稳健标准误差。这种方法适用于计数数据的分析，能够更好地处理事件发生的频率。②混合模型分析：统计分析中使用了线性混合模型，这表明研究者考虑到了个体间的变异性和重复测量的结构，从而提高了模型的准确性。③多重比较校正：在主要结局的比较中，研究者采用了Bonferroni调整来控制多重比较的错误率，设定显著性水平为$\alpha=0.025$。这一措施有助于减少假阳性结果的可能性。④数据完整性：在分析中，研究者关注了不同组别的随访数据的可用性，结果表明各组的数据报告率相似（$P=0.93$），这降低了由于组间差异导致的偏差。⑤临床重要性评估：虽然统计学结果显示真针刺组在减轻关节疼痛方面与假针刺组和等待治疗组存在显著差异，但研究者指出观察到的改善在临床重要性上仍不确定，这反映了统计与临床意义之间的区别。

综上所述，本研究在选题上具有重要的临床意义，设计较为严谨，但也存在一定的局限性，未来研究可在此基础上进行更深入的探索。本文的统计分析方法严谨，充分考虑了数据的特性和研究设计的需求。

2018, 320 (2): 167-176.

7. 内容简介：本研究为随机临床试验，旨在观察针刺对减少芳香化酶抑制剂（aromatase inhibitor，AI）相关关节疼痛的效果。受试者为服用AI的绝经后乳腺癌患者，简明疼痛量表最疼痛项目（brief pain inventory worst pain，BPI-WP）评分最低为3分（评分范围0～10，分数越高表示疼痛越严重）。226例受试者按照2∶1∶1随机分为真针刺组（$n=110$）、假针刺组（$n=59$）和等待治疗组（$n=57$）。主要结局是治疗6周的BPI-WP评分，使用线性回归比较平均6周的BPI-WP评分，将BPI-WP评分减少2分定义为有临床意义。得出结论：对于服用AI的绝经后乳腺癌患者，与假针刺或等待治疗患者比较，针刺治疗6周可以显著降低AI相关关节疼痛程度。

真针刺组和假针刺组治疗频次均为每周2次，每次30～45 min，共6周（12次）；然后每周1次，每次30～45 min，共6周。治疗方案是针对患者最疼痛的3个关节区域量身定制。每次治疗期间，都会施行手法重新刺激。

真针刺组使用不锈钢、一次性、无菌和可抛弃型针头，并以传统的深度和角度插入。全身穴：外关（TE5）、合谷（LI4）、足临泣（GB41）、解溪（ST41）、太溪（KI3）；耳穴：神门（TF4）、肾（CO10）、肝（CO12）、上肺（CO14）、交感（AH6a）；肩关节相关穴：肩髃（LI15）、肩髎（TE14）、臑俞（SI10）；手腕部穴：阳谷（SI5）、阳池（TE4）、阳溪（LI5）；手指穴：后溪（SI3）、八邪（EX-UE9）、三间（LI3）；腰部穴：腰阳关（GV3）、筋缩（GV8）、肾俞（BL23）；臀部穴：环跳（GB30）、悬钟（GB39）；膝部穴：阴陵泉（SP9）、血海（SP10）、梁丘（ST34）。

假针刺组是在非针刺穴位使用细短针进行浅刺。假针方案包括针对关节的治疗和耳穴假压疗法，即在耳朵上的非针刺穴位上涂抹黏合剂。假穴1、2，分别位于左、右前臂外侧，靠近肘部，肩胛骨下方3寸、向小肠经前方0.5寸；假穴3、4，分别位于左、右胫骨内侧髁下缘，肝经的膝关（LR7）前上方1寸。假耳穴1，在耳郭的螺旋点5号和6号之间；假耳穴2，在耳郭的螺旋点4号和3号之间；假耳穴3，耳尖和螺旋点1之间的耳郭螺旋上。关节特异性假穴：膝盖，分别在假穴3或4上2寸；臀部，在大腿髌骨上约4寸，距胆经前1寸；肩部，两侧手臂外侧，腋窝前皱襞下方5寸，肺经前方1寸；腰椎，在第8胸椎水平，距脊柱中心5寸，距膀胱经外侧2寸；手指/手腕，在两侧前臂外侧，靠近肘部，距肘尖5寸，向小肠经前方0.5寸。

等待治疗组患者接受24周标准随访护理，24周后接受10次针刺治疗。

二 专家述评（针灸学专家，临床研究方法学及卫生统计学专家）

1. 述评一

（1）研究背景与重要性

本研究关注的是乳腺癌患者在使用AI时出现的关节疼痛，这一问题在乳腺癌患者

研究在干预过程中详细记录了不良事件，提供了全面的安全性数据。对治疗预期的评估和对睡眠药物使用情况的跟踪进一步增加了研究结果的全面性和可信度。

（3）临床研究方法学及统计学方法的选择及应用

在试验初期，本研究根据预试验的参数进行样本量估算，有助于节省时间和成本。在统计分析时，本研究采用了线性混合效应模型分析主要和次要结局，适当考虑了重复测量数据的相关性。这种方法能有效处理缺失数据，并通过调整基线预期值进一步验证结果的稳健性。使用Cohen's d解释效应大小，使结果的临床意义更加清晰。在主分析之外，研究还进行了基于性别、种族、教育水平和基线疼痛状况的亚组分析，这有助于发现不同亚组间的差异，并为个体化治疗提供依据。然而，研究者也明确指出，由于研究样本量较小，这些亚组分析结果仅具有探索性意义，未来需要更大规模的研究来验证。

综上所述，这篇文献在研究设计、过程实施、方法学选择及统计分析方面均表现出较高的科学性和严谨性，结果可靠且具有临床应用价值。然而，这篇文献也指出选择的人群不是完全随机的，仍然具有潜在的选择偏倚，即所有受试者都接受过高等教育，未来可以进一步扩展到更加多元化的样本人群。

第四十节 "Effect of Acupuncture vs Sham Acupuncture or Waitlist Control on Joint Pain Related to Aromatase Inhibitors Among Women With Early-Stage Breast Cancer: A Randomized Clinical Trial" 相关介绍和述评

一 论文介绍

1. 中文题目：针刺、假针刺或等待对照对早期乳腺癌女性芳香化酶抑制剂相关关节疼痛的影响：一项随机临床试验

2. 作者：Dawn L. Hershman, Joseph M. Unger, Heather Greenlee, Jillian L. Capodice, Danika L. Lew, Amy K. Darke, Alice T. Kengla, Marianne K. Melnik, Carla W. Jorgensen, William H. Kreisle, Lori M. Minasian, Michael J. Fisch, N. Lynn Henry, Katherine D. Crew

3. 主要单位：Columbia University Medical Center, Fred Hutchinson Cancer Research Center, SWOG Statistics and Data Management Center

4. 发表期刊：*JAMA*

5. 发布日期：2018年6月6日

6. SCI源文献：HERSHMAN D L, UNGER J M, GREENLEE H, et al. Effect of Acupuncture vs Sham Acupuncture or Waitlist Control on Joint Pain Related to Aromatase Inhibitors Among Women With Early-Stage Breast Cancer: A Randomized Clinical Trial [J]. JAMA,

症状方面的潜力日益受到关注。然而，令人遗憾的是，尽管这两种疗法展现出了积极的治疗前景，但临床医师对其的认知仍显不足，实际应用中也未能给予充分的重视与利用。这既反映了当前临床领域在失眠治疗策略上的局限性，也揭示了提升临床医师对新疗法认知与接受度的紧迫性。

本选题正是针对这一临床难点与热点问题，作者通过深入剖析当前的临床现状，精准提炼出阻碍失眠治疗进展的关键性挑战与潜在的发展机遇。旨在通过系统的研究与探讨，展现这些非药物治疗手段在改善患者睡眠质量、提升整体健康水平方面的深远价值与重要意义。

本研究在选题设计上尤为注重创新性与可行性的平衡，力求在理论探索与实践应用之间架起一座坚实的"桥梁"。通过深入的理论研究与实践验证，作者期待能够推动针刺疗法与CBT-I在临床中的广泛应用与持续优化，为临床实践的持续改进提供坚实的理论支撑与实践指导。同时，该选题也重点关注了针刺干预在治疗过程中的合理性与科学性，以及针刺细节的标准性把控。通过进一步细化针刺治疗方案、规范治疗操作手法等措施，来提升针刺治疗的效果与安全性。此外，治疗方案的规划与治疗师的资质也是影响治疗效果的重要因素。因此，建议在治疗师的选择上应优先考虑具有丰富失眠治疗经验的专业人士，以确保患者能够获得最佳的治疗效果。

本选题不仅具有重要的理论价值与实践意义，还将在推动临床研究的进一步深化与拓展、促进医疗水平的全面提升方面发挥积极作用。期待通过本选题的研究与探讨，能够为临床癌症患者失眠的治疗领域带来新的思路与突破。

2. 述评二

（1）研究设计

本研究为一项随机对照试验，旨在比较针刺与CBT-I对癌症幸存者失眠的治疗效果。采用双中心、平行组的随机对照有效性试验，通过随机化分配受试者至针刺组和CBT-I组，避免了选择偏倚，增加了结果的内在有效性。研究通过置换区组随机化按研究地点分层，并使用密封信封法进行分配，确保了随机化过程的隐蔽性，有助于减少选择偏倚。盲法的设置针对主要研究者、共同研究者和统计人员等主要研究人员，防止偏见影响研究结果，确保数据分析更加客观。此外，该研究详细描述了受试者的纳入和排除标准，确保了研究人群的同质性。纳入标准包括对失眠严重程度和治疗完成时间的明确定义，排除标准则考虑了其他睡眠障碍和精神疾病的影响，保证了研究结果的可靠性和可解释性。本研究提前定义结局指标分为主要结局和次要结局，主要结局为失眠严重程度指数（主要时间点为治疗结束后的8周，次要时间点为治疗结束后的20周）；次要结局为匹兹堡睡眠质量指数，确保研究设计的严谨性，提高研究结果的质量。

（2）过程实施

两组干预的实施均由经过培训的专业人员进行，进一步提高了研究的内部效度。

of Medicine at the University of Pennsylvania; Department of Psychiatry and Behavioral Sciences

4. 发表期刊：*Journal of the National Cancer Institute*

5. 发布日期：2019年4月9日

6. SCI源文献：GARLAND S N, XIE S X, DUHAMEL K, et al. Acupuncture Versus Cognitive Behavioral Therapy for Insomnia in Cancer Survivors: A Randomized Clinical Trial [J]. J Natl Cancer Inst, 2019, 111 (12): 1323-1331.

7. 内容简介：本研究为随机对照临床试验，为了探究针刺与失眠认知行为疗法（cognitive behavioral therapy for insomnia，CBT-I）治疗癌症幸存者失眠的疗效，将160例受试者随机分为针刺组和CBT-I组，观察两组治疗后的失眠严重程度指数（insomnia severity index，ISI）、疼痛、疲劳、情绪和生活质量等。得出结论：虽然这两种治疗方法都产生了有意义和持久的改善，但CBT-I更有效，应该作为一线治疗方案。

针刺组每周接受2次针刺治疗，为期2周，随后每周接受1次治疗，为期6周，共接受10次治疗。针刺组的治疗方案包括体针和耳穴治疗，体针方案包括双侧神门（HT7）、三阴交（SP6）及中线上的百会（GV20）、神庭（GV24），每次治疗30 min。耳穴治疗选用单侧神门（TF4）、交感（AH6a）。每周治疗2次，持续2周。首次针刺还包括详细病史陈述和检查，长达60 min，之后每次治疗30 min，总时长330 min（与针灸师总接触时间约150 min）。由4名具有11~14年经验的持证针灸师提供干预措施。

CBT-I是一种人工多元干预，包括睡眠限制、刺激控制、认知重构、放松训练和教育。睡眠限制和刺激控制旨在通过限制在床上的时间和活动来打破床与非睡眠之间的条件关联。认知重构可解决与睡眠相关的焦虑。放松训练则针对生理唤醒。此外，还提供了健康睡眠行为方面的教育。CBT-I组首先每周接受1次CBT-I治疗（共5次），随后每2周接受1次治疗（共2次），共治疗7次，持续8周。首次CBT-I治疗时间为60 min，其余疗程每次30 min，总接触时间为240 min。由4位持证治疗师和5位心理学实习生负责完成CBT-I测试。所有治疗师均接受CBT-I培训，研究人员负责监督研究方案，并填写研究检查表，以确保治疗真实性。

二 专家述评（针灸学专家，临床研究方法学及卫生统计学专家）

1. 述评一

癌症患者在面对疾病带来的重重挑战时，失眠症的发病率高达60%，这一数据无疑突显了癌症患者群体在心理健康与睡眠质量上的严峻形势。若未能及时采取有效措施进行干预，失眠很可能转化为一种顽固且难以根治的慢性病态，进而引发一系列连锁反应，如焦虑、抑郁加剧，以及生理机能衰退，对患者的整体健康构成不容忽视的双重威胁。

在此背景下，针刺疗法与CBT-I作为两种备受瞩目的非药物治疗手段，在缓解失眠

①研究对象：为接受放疗的头颈癌患者，但需注意中国的患者为住院患者，美国的患者为门诊患者，既往均未接受过针刺治疗。②干预措施：每周3次针刺，持续6～7周，细节见述评一。③对照设置：安慰对照采用假针刺，标准对照采用标准治疗（如刷牙，使用含氟牙膏、牙线等口腔护理）。④终点事件：主要结局选择患者自报的口腔干燥得分。⑤研究场景：中美癌症专科医院。⑥随机方法：采用中心随机分组，整合了适应性随机化（最小化法）和分层随机化（按疾病分期、年龄、性别、平均计划腮腺剂量、有无诱导治疗、是否联合化学治疗）两种协变量适应性随机化策略。协变量适应性随机化策略在临床试验中被广泛用于平衡协变量，保持随机化，尤其适用于有许多重要的预后因素需要处理时，本案例刚好符合。⑦盲法：对患者和评价者均采用盲法，但患者可能并未被严格实施盲法，但研究者未对患者的知晓情况进行调查。⑧分配隐匿：未明确报告。⑨样本量计算：尽管前期没有预试验或文献数据支持样本量计算，但研究者充分发挥了临床背景优势，界定了有临床意义的效应值大小，按照0.5标准差测算（此处有文献支持），每组100例患者即可满足需求。进一步考虑25%的失访率，最终对399例患者进行了随机化。

（2）临床研究方法学及统计学方法的选择及应用

统计分析中针对3组间的效果比较部分较为简单直接，但以下两点需注意。①协方差分析：在分析主要终点事件（放疗1年后的口腔干燥得分）时，研究者为了更好地控制基线口腔干燥得分、中心效应，采用了协方差分析，这一操作在随机临床试验中较为常见，尤其样本量相对较小时，主要是为了解决即便采用了协变量适应性随机化但依然可能存在基线协变量不均衡的风险问题。②混合模型分析：在分析口腔干燥得分变化时，由于每例患者均测量了5个时间点的口腔干燥得分（包括基线，第7周放疗结束时，放疗结束后3、6、12个月），故研究者采用混合模型分析处理个体多个时间点数值之间相关性的问题。

第三十九节 "Acupuncture Versus Cognitive Behavioral Therapy for Insomnia in Cancer Survivors: A Randomized Clinical Trial" 相关介绍和述评

一 论文介绍

1. 中文题目：针刺与失眠认知行为疗法治疗癌症幸存者失眠：一项随机临床试验

2. 作者：Sheila N. Garland, Sharon X. Xie, Kate DuHamel, Ting Bao, Qing Li, Frances K. Barg, Sarah Song, Philip Kantoff, Philip Gehrman, Jun J. Mao

3. 主要单位：Departments of Psychology and Oncology, Memorial University of Newfoundland; Department of Biostatistics, Epidemiology, and Informatics, Perelman School

种不会引起得气感觉的刺激。选择的耳穴是神门（TF4）、零点、唾液腺2和喉，使用0.16 mm×15 mm的耳针进行针刺。承浆和右侧的中渚为中线/单侧取穴，其他均双侧取穴。本研究中唯一使用的面部穴位是承浆。

SA组设置的方案包括真针刺激不治疗口干症的腧穴、真针刺激非腧穴和安慰针刺激非腧穴。Park系统是一种经过验证的、不破皮的、可伸缩的装置，有一个独立的装置将其附着在皮肤上，用于安慰针刺。所选位置包含：①承浆下方0.5寸和外侧0.5寸的非穴位（对于有胡须的受试者）；②支沟（TE6）径向0.5寸和近端0.5寸（双上肢）的非穴位处；③足三里（ST36）下方1.0寸，外侧0.5寸处（双侧下肢）。在右膝上方中渎穴处使用1根0.25 mm×40 mm的针进行针刺，以引起得气感。这个穴位不适用于口干症。最后，在每只耳朵上使用4根0.16 mm×15 mm耳针进行针刺（双侧共8个耳穴）。SA组按照与TA组相同的时间表进行针刺治疗。

SCC组患者接受标准治疗，包括口腔卫生（每日使用含氟牙膏刷牙、使用牙线和含氟托盘）。

二 专家述评（针灸学专家，临床研究方法学及卫生统计学专家）

1. 述评一

该论文选题着眼于解决临床中的难点和热点问题，即头颈癌患者接受放疗后常见的不良反应——RIX。RIX严重影响患者的生活质量，现有治疗方法效果有限。该研究通过设置随机对照试验系统地比较真针刺与假针刺及标准护理在预防RIX中的效果，探索一种安全有效的非药物治疗途径，具有较高的临床应用价值。

针刺干预实施科学合理，研究采用标准化、经过验证的针刺方案和穴位，确保治疗的一致性和可重复性，每次治疗均由经验丰富的针灸师进行，确保了操作的专业性和安全性。尽管研究设计合理，但仍存在一些局限性：①中美两国的治疗环境存在差异，可能影响研究结果的一致性。②对照组设置合理，但缺乏对不同对照组之间疗效差异的深入分析，即SA组与SCC组之间的对比，可能影响对针刺真实效果的准确评估。③在针刺细节方面，虽然描述了针刺的深度和得气感，但未提及个体差异对针刺效果的可能影响，如患者体质、对针刺的敏感程度等。④研究未充分考虑辅助治疗措施（如口腔保湿剂、唾液替代品等）对针刺疗效的可能影响，也未对这些措施与针刺疗法的联合应用进行探讨。

2. 述评二

（1）研究设计和过程实施

研究采用了两中心、多臂、双盲随机对照试验，设计相关的9个要素考量如下。

第三十八节 "Effect of True and Sham Acupuncture on Radiation-Induced Xerostomia Among Patients With Head and Neck Cancer: A Randomized Clinical Trial" 相关介绍和述评

一 论文介绍

1. 中文题目：真针刺和假针刺对头颈癌患者放射诱导口干症的疗效：一项随机临床试验

2. 作者：M. Kay Garcia, Zhiqiang Meng, David I. Rosenthal, Yehua Shen, Mark Chambers, Peiying Yang, Qi Wei, Chaosu Hu, Caijun Wu, Wenying Bei, Sarah Prinsloo, Joseph Chiang, Gabriel Lopez, Lorenzo Cohen

3. 主要单位：Department of Palliative, Rehabilitation, and Integrative Medicine, University of Texas MD Anderson Cancer Center；复旦大学上海肿瘤防治中心综合肿瘤科；Department of Radiation Oncology, University of Texas MD Anderson Cancer Center

4. 发表期刊：*JAMA Network Open*

5. 发布日期：2019年12月6日

6. SCI源文献：GARCIA M K, MENG Z, ROSENTHAL D I, et al. Effect of True and Sham Acupuncture on Radiation-Induced Xerostomia Among Patients With Head and Neck Cancer: A Randomized Clinical Trial [J]. JAMA Netw Open, 2019, 2 (12): e1916910.

7. 内容简介：本研究为一项多中心、3期随机临床试验，为了确定针刺是否可以预防接受放射治疗（简称"放疗"）的头颈癌患者放射诱导性口干症（radiation-induced xerostomia，RIX）的发生，将399例受试者随机分为标准治疗对照（standard care control，SCC）组、真针刺（true acupuncture，TA）组和假针刺（sham acupuncture，SA）组，观察3组治疗开始时，放疗结束时，放疗结束后3、6、12个月的患者的RIX（由口干问卷确定）、临床上显著的口腔干燥（口干问卷得分＞30）的发生率、唾液流量、生活质量、唾液成分等。得出结论：与SCC组相比，治疗1年后的TA组患者的RIX症状更轻且明显减少。

为了确保所有组的放疗条件相等，评估针刺方案的有效性，所有患者均接受每周3次的头颈癌放疗，放射剂量和方式相同，为期6~7周。在放疗6~7周期间，TA组和SA组每周分别接受3次针刺治疗（与放疗同一天进行）。

TA组根据中医经典理论、当前对于每个穴位相关的解剖位置和神经血管组织及其适应证的理解选择穴位。本方案选择的体穴是承浆（CV24）、双侧列缺（LU7）和双侧照海（KI6）。一根安慰针被放置在右侧的中渎（GB32），旨在为TA组患者提供一

1∶1∶1∶1比例分配到DAM、NAM、SA和WL组，保证了组间均衡性，所有患者均按照指南推荐接受16周的抗心绞痛基础治疗。对DAM、NAM与SA组的患者施盲，尽可能减少期望效应和主观判断对结果的影响。主要结局为基线到第16周心绞痛发作频率变化，指标客观可测量，能有效评估针刺治疗心绞痛症状的效果，结果具有重要临床意义。该研究设计与实施严谨。

（2）临床研究方法学及统计学方法的选择及应用

该研究在估算样本量时考虑了15%的患者失访，最终招募404例35~80岁患者。研究使用意向性治疗（intention to treat，ITT）分析原则，采用Kruskal-Wallis方法进行统计分析，发现针刺16周可有效降低心绞痛的发作频率，并进一步探索该获益可能与穴位特异性有关。研究讨论了试验中存在的一些局限性，但仍存在其他不足：①6例患者因失访等原因被排除在外，未纳入ITT分析，且未进行预先设定的敏感性分析来评估被排除在外的患者对结果的影响；②未对可能影响结局的重要协变量进行预先设定的调整分析；③采用最后观察值结转法填补缺失数据，该方法简单易实施，但可能引入偏倚，低估治疗效果。

三 作者谈

发表在 JAMA Internal Medicine 杂志的 Acupuncture as Adjunctive Therapy for Chronic Stable Angina: A Randomized Clinical Trial 是基于梁繁荣教授团队的第二个973计划"经穴效应循经特异性规律及关键影响因素基础研究"完成的。首先，一切的科研选题应来源于临床问题。在临床上许多CSA患者虽然经过西医治疗后部分症状得到改善，但心绞痛这一主要症状却仍然存在，于是很多患者在西医治疗无果后，转而寻求针刺辅助干预。我们在理论研究及临床实践中均发现针刺经穴可以减少CSA患者的心绞痛发作次数及疼痛强度。然而，当时针刺经穴干预心绞痛的相关研究存在基础研究多、临床研究少、临床样本小、检验效能低等问题，这导致临床证据质量低、临床推广难。因此，为了解决这些问题，我们围绕经穴效应循经特异性设计了本项研究。其次，合理的研究设计应重视前期准备。在开始研究前我们团队一直在思考：患者接受针刺治疗的意愿如何？我们应该纳入什么类型、什么病情程度的患者进行研究？基于此，我们进行了详细的文献检索、广泛的问卷调查及反复的专家论证，最终完成了研究设计。最后，严谨的临床实施应依赖于质量控制。本研究从2012年10月到2015年9月在全国5个地区的分中心同步展开，由于中心分散，保持各中心研究一致性尤为重要。因此，我们参照高质量的随机对照研究的管理方式与方法，制定了标准化操作流程，并委托第三方公司来进行项目的整体管理。

赵凌

成都中医药大学

SA组选取两个固定假穴位，针刺针插入双侧假穴位，留针30 min，但不产生得气感；针刺手法和电刺激的参数与DAM、NAM组相同。

WL组患者未接受针刺，但在16周研究结束后可免费安排12次针刺治疗。

二　专家述评（针灸学专家，临床研究方法学及卫生统计学专家）

1. 述评一

本研究选择针刺作为辅助治疗手段，以降低CSA患者心绞痛发作频率为主要研究目的，致力于提升CSA患者的生活质量，而非单纯关注指标数值的变化。这恰好是祖国医学整体观思想的体现。对于患者而言，他们需要的不仅是延长生命的长度，更需要的是改善自身的生活质量。

在针刺方式的选择上，研究团队考虑十分全面。从临床研究方法学的角度来看，通过针刺治疗组和空白对照组的结果对比，可以验证针刺的有效性。从中医辨证论治的角度来看，研究中的DAM、NAM、SA组可以进一步探讨不同经络、不同穴位方案对于心绞痛治疗的疗效，可以很好地展示经络腧穴的治疗效果。这3个组别的设置既尊重了国际上对于临床研究设计的要求，也保持了中医学特色。

针对目前的医学治疗模式，制定符合伦理同时具有临床意义的针刺辅助治疗CSA的研究方案是本研究的最大意义之一。在本研究中，不同组别的样本量设置合理，如果仅设置1∶1的针刺组和空白对照组，不仅浪费样本量，得出的结论也难以延伸后续的研究。

研究选取的穴位是一大亮点：选穴精简、目的明确，为针刺临床研究的选穴方面提供了新的思路。该方案不仅可以通过DAM组中的内关和通里验证针刺的安全性，还可以验证中医经络理论中心包经和心经对于心系病症的疗效。在以往的针刺临床试验中，选穴常囿于临床治疗经验，将主穴、配穴结合作为选穴方案，但在某种程度上，使用的穴位越多，给研究带来的干扰信息也就越多。例如同样是温补的配穴，在阳盛体热和阳虚体寒之人可能会引起两种不同的效果。这是中医治疗理论的特点，却也是中医临床研究中难以忽视的混杂因素来源。从本研究中可以看到，只选取主穴可在一定程度上减少穴位和证型之间带来的混杂因素，使研究结果更加集中在"针刺对改善心绞痛发作频率确实有效"上。

2. 述评二

（1）研究设计和过程实施

该研究是一项多中心、随机对照试验，该试验在中国5家医院进行，共纳入404例CSA患者。研究采用可变区组分层随机方法，通过中央化随机系统将患者按照

第三十七节 "Acupuncture as Adjunctive Therapy for Chronic Stable Angina: A Randomized Clinical Trial" 相关介绍和述评

一 论文介绍

1. 中文题目：针刺辅助治疗慢性稳定型心绞痛的随机临床试验

2. 作者：Ling Zhao, Dehua Li, Hui Zheng, Xiaorong Chang, Jin Cui, Ruihui Wang, Jing Shi, Hailong Fan, Ying Li, Xin Sun, Fuwen Zhang, Xi Wu, Fanrong Liang

3. 主要单位：成都中医药大学针灸推拿学院，成都中医药大学附属医院针灸科，湖南中医药大学针灸推拿学院

4. 发表期刊：JAMA Internal Medicine

5. 发布日期：2019年7月29日

6. SCI源文献：ZHAO L, LI D, ZHENG H, et al. Acupuncture as Adjunctive Therapy for Chronic Stable Angina: A Randomized Clinical Trial [J]. JAMA Intern Med, 2019, 179 (10): 1388-1397.

7. 内容简介：本研究为随机临床试验，为了研究针刺作为抗心绞痛疗法的辅助疗法在减少慢性稳定型心绞痛（chronic stable angina，CSA）患者心绞痛发作频率方面的疗效和安全性，将404例患者随机分配到循经取穴（disease-affected meridian，DAM）组、他经取穴（acupoints on the nonaffected meridian，NAM）组、假针刺（sham acupuncture，SA）组和等待治疗（wait list，WL）组，观察4组从基线到第20周期间心绞痛发作频率每4周的变化。得出结论：与NAM、SA、WL相比，DAM作为抗心绞痛辅助疗法在缓解心绞痛方面表现出更好的疗效。

DAM、NAM、SA和WL组的所有患者均接受抗心绞痛药物治疗（推荐），包括β受体阻滞剂、阿司匹林或氯吡格雷、他汀类药物及血管紧张素转换酶抑制剂。

除WL组，DAM、NAM、SA组均接受12次针刺治疗（每周3次，持续4周），每次治疗持续30 min。

DAM组选取双侧内关（PC6）和通里（HT5），NAM组选取双侧孔最（LU6）和太渊（LU9）。两组均不允许使用研究方案以外的穴位。针刺治疗使用一次性不锈钢针灸针并加电。进针后行提插捻转，产生得气感（酸、麻、胀或放射性的感觉），每次针刺治疗持续30 min。此外，将辅助针刺入每个穴位外侧2 mm，深度为2 mm，无须手法刺激。这种方法可以确保对局部穴位起电刺激的作用。针刺后，使用HANS电针仪（型号LH 200A；HANS Therapy Co）施加于辅助针上，刺激频率为2 Hz，刺激强度为0.1～2.0 mA，以患者舒适为度。

2. 述评二

（1）研究设计和过程实施

研究采用了经典的单中心平行随机对照试验，对于设计相关的9个要素考量如下：①研究对象，是慢性腰痛患者，其亮点是纳入及排除标准流程图，来龙去脉均清晰地呈现出来。②干预措施，干预组患者在6周内接受12次电针治疗，每次持续时间45 min。③对照设置，安慰剂对照（假电针）最为推荐。④终点事件，主要终点事件选择治疗前后疼痛强度评分的变化值，这是公认的且本研究提供了文献依据。需注意附件的研究方案中，研究者明确提及在研究开始后对终点事件进行了调整，但提供的理由较为牵强。⑤研究场景，本研究选择在居民便捷可及的社区诊所，增加了结论的外推性。⑥随机化，本研究应用区组随机（每个区组4例患者），并且为了增加各社区诊所入组的均衡性，特意在研究开始前将原计划的简单随机进行了修改。⑦盲法，对研究对象设置盲法，值得借鉴的是，本研究在完成12次治疗后，调查每个研究对象对于自己所在组别的判断，并同时将这一判断作为0/1变量纳入分析。⑧分配隐匿，本研究通过标准化流程尽可能不让研究对象明晰所在分组，此做法值得后续研究借鉴。⑨样本量计算，本研究同时回答两个问题，一是除了与安慰剂组相比，电针针刺到底有无效果，二是到底哪些因素影响患者电针针刺的效果。相应的样本量计算也包括两部分，作者先针对第二个问题进行了样本量计算，但计算依据选择的是相关系数（0.4），得到电针组需要50例患者。随后，研究者按照电针组和假电针组均为50例患者，测算了可以探查的两组相关系数差值约为0.5，在进一步考虑样本损耗的基础上将最终样本定为每组60例。样本量计算选择以相关系数而非关联强度作为依据的做法值得商榷，很少有研究目的仅仅定位为存在关联，而不去探究关联的大小，尤其是作为随机临床试验的样本量计算更要慎重参考，与研究声明的主要终点事件不符，尤其是作者自身在结果部分汇报的也是治疗前后疼痛强度评分的变化值。

（2）临床研究方法学及统计学方法的选择及应用

统计分析中针对两组间的效果比较部分较为简单直接，但以下两点需注意：①缺失值和异常值处理，研究可贵之处在于提到了缺失机制探索及缺失数据的处理，但遗憾的是，并未提供各个变量的缺失比例。相反，作者对于异常值的处理和报告更为全面，值得学习。②探索治疗效果的影响因素，对治疗效果影响因素的探索考虑了多变量分析是值得肯定的做法，但作者最初的样本量计算仅仅考虑了单一变量与终点事件的相关系数，难免存在样本量不足的问题。同时，在多变量分析选择哪些变量时，未明确当干预组和对照组的结果不一致时如何处置。再者，探索患者分组与其他影响因素的交互作用时，因变量选择基线变量的处理有待商榷，理论上选择主要终点事件更为妥当。

system，PROMIS）疼痛强度量表的变化在统计学上无显著性差异；相较于假电针疗法，电针疗法的次要结局RMDQ的治疗效果有统计学差异；白人种族与较差的PROMIS评分和RMDQ结局相关。

真电针组和假电针组的治疗频率均为每周2次，持续6周，共计12次。

真电针组每次治疗持续约45 min，体针方案包括局部治疗和远端治疗，其中局部治疗是在受累皮区的膀胱经背俞穴进行经皮电神经刺激（4 Hz），远端治疗选穴包括太溪（KI3）、复溜（KI7）、少海（HT3）、后溪（SI3）、委中（BL40）、腰阳关（GV3）和百会（GV20）。其中，同侧太溪（KI3，负极）和复溜（KI7，正极）成对进行电刺激（2 Hz），持续20～25 min。除了体针方案外，受试者还将接受标准化的腰部热疗和耳针治疗。其中，耳穴包括神门（TF4）、零点（HX1）、丘脑和腰椎（AH9）。

假电针组的体针方案为假针刺，同时配合假热疗和假耳针治疗。假热疗将热灯放置于不同位置（小腿），时间缩短至10 min，强度降低。假耳针治疗则采用非穿透性针具，在无特定治疗效果的位置贴上两个小方形胶带（3 mm×3 mm），以避免产生治疗效果。其余设置与真电针组相同。

二 专家述评（针灸学专家，临床研究方法学及卫生统计学专家）

1. 述评一

疼痛是全球范围内最常见的临床问题之一，严重影响患者的生活质量。针刺的镇痛效果确切，无成瘾性且相对安全，是近年来国内外研究的热点。尤其是临床前研究表明，电针可能比手针产生更强的镇痛效果。电针在镇痛方面的应用甚广。而安慰剂效应在针刺研究中备受争议。本研究为单中心、平行、随机临床试验，比较真电针和假电针治疗慢性腰痛的疗效，对电针镇痛疗效的验证或将对针刺疗法的国际评价和推广运用产生影响。

这篇文章为评估电针与假电针在患有慢性腰痛的成人的疼痛和残疾中的治疗效果，并利用疼痛减轻和残疾的变化作为临床结果来确定与治疗反应相关的因素。该研究对121例受试者进行为期6周、12次的电针/假电针治疗。在充分考虑了盲法评估后，电针在减少与慢性腰痛相关的残疾方面有显著的治疗效果。这项研究引入了单变量与多变量分析方法，捕捉患者特征与真电针组的临床结果之间的单变量关联。研究发现，种族的文化差异对研究结果的影响，即白人种族与疼痛和RMDQ评分的较差结果有关。在为期10周的观察中（干预前2周、干预6周和干预后2周），尽管最终临床试验发现真电针与假电针在疼痛评分变化上无显著差异，然而，这是一个在随机临床试验中证明电针对慢性腰痛相关残疾的治疗效果具有统计学和临床显著性意义的研究，并且有助于了解与电针治疗的临床反应相关的患者因素。

研究缺乏对混杂因素的探讨。这是非常关键的。如果各组在接受其他辅助干预等方面不可比，则很难将结果归因于疗法。

样本量问题：虽然文中提到"将每组的样本量设定为25例，这一样本量能够估计治疗效果对结果的单侧90%置信区间的上限"，但并未阐明当前样本量的具体测算依据。当前研究样本量较小，且存在单中心研究、随访期短等局限性，影响研究结果的推广和对真实效果的评估。

本文统计学方法基本合理，但是缺乏对混杂因素的思考。当混杂因素在组间不均衡时，组间比较的结果可信度不高，应该将多因素分析的结果作为主要结局。

第三十六节 "Effect of Electroacupuncture vs Sham Treatment on Change in Pain Severity Among Adults With Chronic Low Back Pain: A Randomized Clinical Trial" 相关介绍和述评

一 论文介绍

1. 中文题目：电针与假电针治疗对成人慢性腰痛患者疼痛严重程度变化的影响：一项随机临床试验

2. 作者：Jiang-Ti Kong, Chelcie Puetz, Lu Tian, Isaac Haynes, Eunyoung Lee, Randall S. Stafford, Rachel Manber, Sean Mackey

3. 主要单位：Division of Pain Medicine, Department of Anesthesiology, Perioperative and Pain Medicine, Stanford University School of Medicin; Department of Biomedical Data Science, Stanford University School of Medicine; Department of Medicine, Stanford University School of Medicine, Stanford

4. 发表期刊：*JAMA Network Open*

5. 发布日期：2020年10月27日

6. SCI源文献：KONG J T, PUETZ C, TIAN L, et al. Effect of Electroacupuncture vs Sham Treatment on Change in Pain Severity Among Adults With Chronic Low Back Pain: A Randomized Clinical Trial [J]. JAMA Netw Open, 2020, 3 (10): e2022787.

7. 内容简介：本研究为双盲随机临床试验，旨在评估电针疗法与安慰剂在缓解成人慢性腰痛疼痛和改善功能障碍方面的效果，并探索与电针治疗和安慰剂反应相关的心理物理、情感和人口学因素。将121例受试者随机分为真电针组和假电针组，观察两组从基线到治疗完成后2周疼痛严重程度的变化和罗兰-莫里斯残疾问卷（Roland-Morris disability questionnaire，RMDQ）的变化。得出结论：在真电针组与假电针组之间，患者报告结局测量信息系统（patient-reported outcomes-measurement information

二 专家述评（针灸学专家，临床研究方法学及卫生统计学专家）

1. 述评一

这是一篇2020年发表在 *JAMA Network Open* 的文章，是以假针刺和非治疗作为对照，评估针刺对CIPN影响的临床研究。该研究不但验证了以假针刺为对照的可行性，还明确了针刺对CIPN的特异性疗效。

本研究切实围绕临床需求，确定有意义的研究选题。根据世界卫生组织的统计，癌症是全球第二大死因，化疗是干预癌症最重要的临床手段之一，超过50%的肿瘤患者都需要化疗。但是随化疗而来的包括周围神经病变在内的种种不良反应给患者带来了极大痛苦，也影响了正常的化疗干预周期，不利于患者的治疗与预后。本研究瞄准重大疾病，选准研究切入点，依据小切口，剖析大问题，明确提出针刺治疗CIPN是否有效这一临床问题，进而精确锚定针刺的特异性疗效，开展有效性研究。本研究能定性回答针刺干预该病是否有效的硬问题。

该研究基于前期实践基础，制定了水平较高、科学严谨的研究方案。CIPN是一种复合型的全身症状，不是局部或孤立的症状。针刺组采用耳针和体针相结合的方案。耳穴选取神门、零点和皮肤电信号点，体穴选取合谷、内关、后溪、太冲、地五会、丰隆、八风2和八风3。中医考虑周围神经病变多属营卫运行受阻，治疗则需调和营卫，取穴应以调养气血、活血通络为主。本研究取穴基本为大经大穴，尽管选取丰隆和内关兼顾了血分、络脉的问题，但是调养气血、养血活血的力度仍不足，临床实际治疗过程中需考虑增加血海（SP10）、三阴交（SP6）等穴位，故而从中医针灸临床实践角度考虑，该研究的针刺方案并非最佳，选穴组方有待进一步优化。鉴于该研究是一个解释性随机对照试验，故而更应该从设计角度重点突出有利于针刺疗效显现的干预方案。

2. 述评二

本文属于短篇报道，无法提供较多细节以供评价。就当前论文而言，存在以下问题。

对照组设置问题：①虽然受试者接受随机分组，但是分组的效果如何？主要结局指标在基线期是否可比？本文未说明。②虽然插入式假针刺组的设置存在挑战，但并非不可能，前期已有研究选择与结局无关的穴位进行针刺。当然，这些穴位的选取需要研究者有非常扎实的中医理论。目前本研究采用非插入式假针刺，无法达到安慰剂效应。

观察期选择问题：①为何选定8周作为效应评估的最长周期？②为何忽略8周内各期的疗效探索？这是关键点，需要结合针刺起效的时间特征、疾病特点等进行综合分析。

辅助干预问题：本文未阐述有无实施其他辅助干预措施及其合理性，换言之，本

第三十五节 "Effect of Acupuncture vs Sham Procedure on Chemotherapy-Induced Peripheral Neuropathy Symptoms: A Randomized Clinical Trial"相关介绍和述评

一 论文介绍

1. 中文题目：针刺与假针刺对化疗诱导的周围神经病变症状的影响：一项随机临床试验

2. 作者：Ting Bao, Sujata Patil, Connie Chen, Iris W. Zhi, Qing S. Li, Lauren Piulson, Jun J. Mao

3. 主要单位：Integrative Medicine Service, Memorial Sloan Kettering Cancer Center, New York, New York; Department of Epidemiology and Biostatistics, Memorial Sloan Kettering Cancer Center, New York, New York; Breast Medicine Service, Memorial Sloan Kettering Cancer Center, New York, New York

4. 发表期刊：*JAMA Network Open*

5. 发布日期：2020年5月11日

6. SCI源文献：BAO T, PATIL S, CHEN C, et al. Effect of Acupuncture vs Sham Procedure on Chemotherapy-Induced Peripheral Neuropathy Symptoms: A Randomized Clinical Trial [J]. JAMA Netw Open, 2020, 3 (3): e200681.

7. 内容简介：本研究为随机临床试验，为了探究真针刺、假针刺或常规治疗对化疗诱导的周围神经病变（chemotherapy-induced peripheral neuropathy，CIPN）症状的影响，将75例受试者随机分为真针刺组、假针刺组和常规护理组，观察每组治疗后第8周通过数字评分量表（numeric rating scale，NRS）测量的麻木、刺痛或疼痛等CIPN症状的严重程度。得出结论：与常规护理相比，针刺显著改善了CIPN症状；观察到真针刺组与假针刺对照组之间的效应量，将为未来设计科学严谨且具备充分统计学效能的针刺治疗CIPN试验提供有力依据。

真针刺组、假针刺组和常规护理组均接受为期8周的治疗。

真针刺组进行耳针和体针治疗，耳穴包括神门（TF4）、零点及第三个皮肤电信号点，体穴包括合谷（LI4）、内关（PC6）、后溪（SI3）、太冲（LR3）、地五会（GB42）、丰隆（ST40）、八风2和八风3。此外，还对从太冲（负极）到地五会（正极）施加电针治疗，频率为2～5 Hz，持续20 min。

假针刺组患者在非腧穴上接受非刺入操作。

常规护理组患者在整个研究期间未接受任何干预。

在以往的研究中，用于癌症患者治疗的大多数穴位位于躯体上，并且通常仅通过手动操作来刺激。而该研究采用密集的前额穴位和身体穴位的组合，并进一步对前额穴位进行电刺激。前额穴位受三叉神经感觉通路支配，在针刺调节多种脑功能中起着关键作用，包括处理疼痛、情绪和认知信息。该研究提示，EA/TNS+BA，特别是对前额穴位的电刺激，可以通过广泛调节神经化学途径和大脑区域产生长期的叠加甚至协同作用。

该研究中，选择MAS作为对照具有合理性，更好地保持了盲法。研究为拓展针刺在肿瘤领域的应用提供了良好的证据，同时也为化疗期间和化疗后的乳腺癌患者提供了一种可供选择的有效干预措施，为针刺的研究提供了新的思路和研究方向，展示出广阔的前景。

2. 述评二

（1）方案阐述

试验正式开始后，具体执行是否与所注册的描述相一致？是否出现方法的重要变更以及原因？均未在正文中予以体现。

（2）纳入及排除标准

当前研究纳入正在接受化疗或化疗结束后未超过2周的患者；试验开始后，针刺效果评估持续8周。部分在整个评估期或相当部分时间处于化疗状态的受试者与在参与前即已结束化疗者是否具有同质性有待讨论。

（3）样本量

文中提到"每组46例的样本量足以在80%的统计功效和0.05的显著性水平下检测出两组之间认知障碍的患病率差异达到30%"，但并没有给出明确的样本量测算方法。而这对于一项临床研究而言是非常重要的。

（4）随机化

文中提到"基于简单、完整、非顺序的随机代码，这些代码是使用计算机生成的随机区块提前生成的"，但随机序列的产生方法尚不明确。

（5）统计学方法

未阐明协变量的选择依据和数据是否满足t检验的前提条件。

（6）结果及结论

①主结果表格描述不清，如将重复测量的评分值与基线评分相比以计算P值，那么基线评分本身为何也能产生一个P值？②只有一个结局评分在试验第2周和第8周出现有统计学意义的结果，说明当前的结果对于"EA/TNS+BA组效果更好"的支持强度非常有限。可能原因包括EA/TNS+BA组实际效果不佳、检验功效不足、针刺短期效果不明显等，而两个有意义的效应值可能是随机结果。

本研究总体设计和统计学方法是合理的，但是上述问题，有待进一步核查。

的研究。由于MoCA对注意力功能和工作记忆的细微变化不敏感，使用正向和反向数字广度测试作为检测注意力功能和工作记忆的次要结局。得出结论：EA/TNS+BA在减少化疗引起的工作记忆障碍，以及某些消化系统、神经系统与痛苦相关症状的发生率方面有益。它可以作为乳腺癌患者化疗期间和化疗后的有效干预手段。

EA/TNS+BA组和MAS组针刺干预均连续进行8周，每周进行2次。针灸师在患者第一次就诊时会为其简单地介绍针刺过程。为消除不同针灸师之间的差异，同一受试者的所有针刺治疗均由同一位针灸师进行。

EA/TNS+BA组仅使用手法刺激以下15个身体穴位，包括双侧的神门（HT7）、合谷（LI4）、外关（TE5）、足三里（ST36）、丰隆（ST40）和三阴交（SP6）共12个穴位，以及中线的中脘（CV12）、关元（CV4）和水沟（GV26）3个穴位。同时，对6对前额穴位进行电刺激，正（＋）负（－）电极线连接如下：百会（GV20，＋）和印堂（EX-HN3，－），左四神聪（EX-HN1，－）和左头临泣（GB15，＋），右四神聪（EX-HN1，－）和右头临泣（GB15，＋），双侧率谷（GB8，左侧＋，右侧－），双侧太阳（EX-HN5，左侧＋，右侧－），双侧头维（ST8，左侧＋，右侧－）。将一次性针灸针（直径0.30 mm，长度25~40 mm）垂直或倾斜刺入穴位，深度为10~30 mm。对所有穴位进行手动操作以引起针刺感。另外对6对额部穴位进行额外的电刺激。仪器（型号：ITO ES-360）的输出峰值电流和电压分别为6 V和48 mA，恒定波频率为2 Hz，相位持续时间为100 s，持续30 min。将刺激强度调整至患者感觉最舒适的水平。使用低频而非高频电刺激是因其可以以更有利的方式调节大脑的生化反应，从而改善认知功能。电刺激持续30 min。身体穴位留针30 min。

对照组使用以下6个穴位：双侧通天（BL7，左侧＋，右侧－），双侧手三里（LI10）和双侧跗阳（BL59）。电刺激仅在双侧通天进行，参数与EA/TNS+BA组相同，但将强度调整至患者刚开始感觉到刺激的水平。选择这种控制方案基于以下两方面原因：①根据传统中医理论，所用穴位与所治疗的症状无关或相关性较小；②所用穴位的数量和电刺激强度保持在最低水平，也是使患者意识到正在接受主动针刺治疗的最低水平。

二 专家述评（针灸学专家，临床研究方法学及卫生统计学专家）

1. 述评一

三叉神经电刺激作为一种新兴的、非侵入神经调控手段，在神经科学领域受到越来越多的关注。该方法通过在头部施加微弱电流来刺激三叉神经，从而影响与认知和意识有关的神经环路。张樟进等研究发现，EA/TNS+BA这种新型针刺模式可能特别有利于减少化疗引起的工作记忆障碍，以及某些消化系统、神经系统与痛苦相关的症状。

点数据，考虑了预期缓解率、消除率和组内相关系数，以确保足够的统计功效。主要分析采用广义线性混合模型，适合处理重复测量数据，并考虑了组、时间和中心的交互作用。对连续变量使用独立样本t检验，确保分析的准确性。针对缺失数据，采用多重插补法，并进行敏感性分析以验证结果的稳健性。同时，设计了幽门螺杆菌感染的亚组分析，探索针刺对不同亚组的疗效差异，增强了研究的临床意义。然而，研究未详细说明多重比较校正措施，可能在显著性结果的解释上存在局限。未来研究可在这些方面改进，以提升结果的可靠性和广泛性。

第三十四节 "Electroacupuncture Trigeminal Nerve Stimulation Plus Body Acupuncture for Chemotherapy-Induced Cognitive Impairment in Breast Cancer Patients: An Assessor-participant Blinded, Randomized Controlled Trial" 相关介绍和述评

一 论文介绍

1. 中文题目：电针刺激三叉神经结合体针治疗乳腺癌患者化疗所致的认知障碍：一项评估者-受试者盲法、随机对照试验

2. 作者：Zhang-Jin Zhang, Sui-Cheung Man, Lo-Lo Yam, Chui Ying Yiu, Roland Ching-Yu Leung, Zong-Shi Qin, Kit-Wa Sherry Chan, Victor Ho Fun Lee, Ava Kwong, Wing-Fai Yeung, Winnie K.W. So, Lai Ming Ho, Ying-Ying Dong

3. 主要单位：香港大学深圳医院中医科，香港大学李嘉诚医学院中医药学院，香港理工大学护理学院

4. 发表期刊：*Brain, Behavior, and Immunity*

5. 发布日期：2020年4月13日

6. SCI源文献：ZHANG Z J, MAN S C, YAM L L, et al. Electroacupuncture trigeminal nerve stimulation plus body acupuncture for chemotherapy-induced cognitive impairment in breast cancer patients: An assessor-participant blinded, randomized controlled trial [J]. Brain Behav Immun, 2020, 88: 88-96.

7. 内容简介：本研究为随机对照临床试验，为了确定与最小针刺刺激（minimum acupuncture stimulation，MAS）相比，电针刺激三叉神经加体针（electroacupuncture trigeminal nerve stimulation plus body acupuncture，EA/TNS+BA）是否能够在改善化疗期间和化疗后乳腺癌患者的认知障碍和其他相关症状方面产生更好的临床结果，将93例受试者随机分为EA/TNS+BA组和MAS组。主要结局使用蒙特利尔认知评估量表（Montreal cognitive assessment，MoCA）进行测量，该评估量表已被广泛用于认知障碍

（GB40）和解溪（ST41）中间。

二 专家述评（针灸学专家，临床研究方法学及卫生统计学专家）

1. 述评一

功能性消化不良是临床常见胃肠病，严重损害患者的身心健康和生活质量。该病目前尚无特效治疗方案，临床多采用促胃肠动力药治疗，其短期疗效较好，但长期使用不良反应明显。针对该病"发病率高""对患者危害大""有效干预方式缺失"的临床痛点，北京中医药大学刘存志教授团队以功能性消化不良的主要亚型——PDS患者为研究对象，开展了针刺治疗PDS的有效性和安全性的评价研究。

该试验设计严谨，在针刺方案设计、对照组设置、结局指标选择等方面为后续研究提供了参考。一是半定量针刺干预方案设计，兼顾治疗标准化和个体化。研究以全国名老中医处方为基础，根据中医证型加以辨证取穴，制定了半标准化的针刺治疗方案，既保留了中医辨证论治的诊疗思路，又确保了研究的标准化和可重复性。二是对照组设置，体现了针刺干预特点和盲法实施原则。研究以与干预组相同数量的非经非穴点浅刺作为对照，该方法具有有效刺激量小、临床可行性高、盲闭患者效果好的优点。三是双主要结局选择，审慎评判针刺疗效。研究采用总体应答率和症状消除率双结局指标综合评价，科学严谨地证实了针刺治疗PDS的短期（4周治疗）和长期（12周随访）有效性，肯定了针刺干预PDS的治疗优势。

2. 述评二

（1）研究设计和过程实施

该研究为多中心、随机、假对照试验，评估针刺对功能性消化不良中PDS的疗效，设计合理，采用分层区组随机化，确保随机分配的独立性和公正性。参与者通过多种途径招募，严格的纳入和排除标准减少了混杂因素的干扰，保障了研究对象的同质性。对患者、结果评估员和统计分析员均实施盲法，有效降低了观察者偏倚，但针灸师未盲化可能导致实施偏倚。干预措施详细区分了针刺和假针刺的操作方法，有助于明确特异性与非特异性效应的差异。研究在干预和随访期间通过多时间点使用验证过的工具评估主要和次要结局，数据收集具有系统性、连续性，但数据管理细节略显不足。伦理审查和知情同意确保了研究合规性。整体而言，研究设计严谨、过程实施规范，为评估针刺对PDS的疗效提供了有力支持。

（2）临床研究方法学及统计学方法的选择及应用

研究在临床方法学和统计学方法上表现出高度的科学性。通过多中心、随机、假对照设计和分层区组随机化，进一步提升了研究的内部效度。样本量计算基于先前试

第三十三节 "Effect of Acupuncture for Postprandial Distress Syndrome: A Randomized Clinical Trial" 相关介绍和述评

一 论文介绍

1. 中文题目：针刺治疗餐后不适综合征：一项随机临床试验
2. 作者：Jing-Wen Yang, Li-Qiong Wang, Xuan Zou, Shi-Yan Yan, Yu Wang, Jing-Jie Zhao, Jian-Feng Tu, Jun Wang, Guang-Xia Shi, Hui Hu, Wei Zhou, Yi Du, Cun-Zhi Liu
3. 主要单位：北京中医药大学针灸推拿学院，中国中医科学院临床医学基础研究所，首都医科大学附属北京中医医院
4. 发表期刊：Annals of Internal Medicine
5. 发布日期：2020年5月12日
6. SCI源文献：YANG J W, WANG L Q, ZOU X, et al. Effect of Acupuncture for Postprandial Distress Syndrome: A Randomized Clinical Trial [J]. Ann Intern Med, 2020, 172 (12): 777-785.
7. 内容简介：本研究为多中心、随机、假对照试验，为了评估针刺与假针刺在餐后不适综合征（postprandial distress syndrome，PDS）患者中的疗效，将278例受试者随机分为针刺组和假针刺组，观察两组治疗前后基于整体治疗效果的缓解率和所有3种基本症状（食后饱腹感、上腹部腹胀和治疗4周后早期饱腹感）的消除率。得出结论：在PDS患者中，与假针刺组相比，针刺组基于整体治疗效果的缓解率和所有3种基本症状的消除率均提高；在每周接受3次、持续4周针刺的患者中，疗效持续超过12周。

针刺组和假针刺组患者均接受每周3次、持续4周（共12次）的治疗（理想情况下每2个工作日进行1次），每次治疗时间为20 min。两组均由至少有3年经验的持证针灸师进行。治疗使用一次性无菌针灸针（长度25～40 mm，直径0.25 mm）。

针刺组的针刺方案有9个穴位，包括8个基本穴位和1个辨证选穴穴位。基本穴位包括百会（GV20）、膻中（CV17）、中脘（CV12）、天枢（ST25）、气海（CV6）、内关（PC6）、足三里（ST36）、公孙（SP4）；辨证选穴若脾胃气虚选太白（SP3），肝气郁结选太冲（LR3），胃湿热选内庭（ST44）。对每个穴位进行30 s的捻转、提插手法，使患者产生得气感（酸、麻、胀、重）。

假针刺组是在非穴位处进行浅表皮肤穿透（深度2～3 mm），未进行得气操作。非穴位1：在头维（ST8）和鱼腰（EX-HN4）中间；非穴位2：在髂前上棘上方2寸；非穴位3：在脐下2寸，前正中线外侧1寸；非穴位4：在肱骨内上髁和尺骨茎突中部；非穴位5：在阳陵泉（GB34）下方3寸，位于胆囊与膀胱经之间；非穴位6：在丘墟

护理组不针刺,另外两组针刺,很容易被猜测出5个区组长度内的分组结果,影响效果评估。因此,区组长度建议为10更为理想。另外,在分层设计考虑中,"研究中心"不能作为分层因素的考虑,因为研究中心不同带来的差异与实施质量有关,与疾病人群特征及干预措施分类无关。

(2)临床研究方法学及统计学方法的选择及应用

纳入标准问题:符合头痛的国际诊断标准,但是,因为主要疗效指标是2个,"随机分组后第1~20周与基线(随机分组前4周)相比,偏头痛发作天数和每4周周期偏头痛发作次数的平均变化"。纳入标准只定义了头痛发作的次数2~8次,没有定义头痛天数,可能带来选择性偏倚。

主要疗效指标选择问题:主要疗效指标没有选择疼痛的严重程度评分(如VAS评分),而将其作为次要疗效指标。对此,应深入讨论其背后的原因,并在后续研究中可以考虑将VAS评分结合临床最小意义差值作为疗效评价的重要指标。

三 作者谈

选题时应重点关注重大疾病防治策略。偏头痛是全球第二大致残性疾病,其患病人数已突破10亿大关。特别在15~49岁的青壮年中,偏头痛是女性第一大疾病负担,是男性第二大疾病负担。《柳叶刀》杂志报道关于全球疾病负担的论文中提到,尽管头痛疾病负担很重,但在全球卫生政策中得到的关注却很少。既往调查发现,偏头痛患者使用预防性药物的依从性差,存在镇痛药滥用的情况。尽管近年来出现了针对偏头痛的降钙素基因相关肽靶向药物,但由于其价格非常昂贵,临床上并没有广泛应用。因此,对于药物疗效欠佳、不能耐受药物不良反应、有药物使用禁忌证、服用多种药物担心药物潜在相互作用、不愿意药物治疗的偏头痛患者,临床上需要有可靠疗效的非药物疗法。

既往针灸RCT研究出现相当多的阴性结果,导致针灸疗效被许多学者认为是安慰剂效应,这限制了传统针灸精髓思想的传播和发扬,制约了针灸科学研究的进展。通过深入分析文献,我们发现既往RCT的针刺组没有强调得气而削弱了疗效,对照组使用穿透性针具和同神经节段施针而提高了疗效,从而导致出现阴性结果。因此,我们致力于优化方案设计。首先,招募无针刺经历的患者以利于盲法成功实施;其次,假针刺组使用国际认可的非穿透性安慰针具,并于不同神经节段区域施针;再者,设立标准化施针流程,以限制针刺组因为无法盲住施针者而导致的安慰剂效应;最后,在治疗结束后评价患者盲法是否成功,以确认盲法的作用。

王伟

华中科技大学同济医学院附属同济医院

境平和、鼓励患者倾诉头痛感受、确保充足睡眠以及进行规律运动。对于重度疼痛患者（定义为VAS评分＞8分），给予双氯芬酸钠肠溶片（25 mg/片，最大耐受剂量200 mg/d）作为抢救用药。

二 专家述评（针灸学专家，临床研究方法学及卫生统计学专家）

1. 述评一

（1）选题分析

该文针对临床高发的偏头痛疾病，针对针刺疗法的适宜性，开展了一项随机对照试验研究。鉴于既往几项随机临床试验发现手法针刺和假针刺之间无显著差异，本研究深入探究了这一现象，发现与安慰剂对照设置的不当有关。因此，本研究采用了非穿透假针刺作为对照，并结合盲法评估，旨在明确手法针刺的疗效，并量化预防无先兆发作性偏头痛的真正安慰剂反应。这一研究更能反映出针刺治疗偏头痛的实际效应，有利于推动针刺疗法应用的国际化。

（2）针刺干预的实施

在具体临床试验中，针刺组的选穴合理；针刺过程描述清晰、可操作性强；提供治疗的14名执业针灸师，均有5年以上的临床经验，并在招募前参加过集中培训。尽管总体治疗方案合理，能说明临床治疗效应，但由于研究周期较短，无法看到持久的效果，有些欠缺。此外，本试验中没有采用辅助干预措施。考虑到以往临床试验中使用涉及穿透针的假针刺存在的问题，本试验中使用非穿透假针刺对照，而且有很不错的依从性，这是本项研究最值得肯定之处。尽管本研究中为确保成功盲法，招募了未接受过针刺治疗的患者，使用非穿透针作为对照，并设计相同的程序，但由于所选穴位与真针刺完全不在一个区域，针刺形式也有较大区别，是否真正做到了成功的盲法仍值得商榷。

2. 述评二

该文章在研究设计中，研究团队考虑了很多影响研究结果的因素，按照随机对照试验（randomized controlled trial，RCT）的原则进行了严格的设计，研究结果验证了假说，统计学方法规范，图表文字表达基本准确。但仍然存在以下问题，可能降低了或者削弱了组间结果的差异性。

（1）研究设计和过程实施

随机化设计中，中心与区组设计为5的考虑不恰当，可能带来偏倚风险。该研究分组采用中心区组随机化方法，中央随机系统进行随机分配，"按照中心分层区组大小为5"，存在选择性偏倚或信息偏倚风险。因为在3组设计中，2∶2∶1的分组设计，常规

Fengxia Liang, Hua Wang, Wei Wang

3. 主要单位：华中科技大学同济医学院附属同济医院神经内科，武汉市第一医院/武汉市中西医结合医院神经内科，华中科技大学同济医学院附属同济医院中西医结合研究所

4. 发表期刊：The BMJ

5. 发布日期：2020年3月26日

6. SCI源文献：XU S, YU L, LUO X, et al. Manual Acupuncture Versus Sham Acupuncture and Usual Care for Prophylaxis of Episodic Migraine Without Aura: Multicentre, Randomised Clinical Trial [J]. BMJ, 2020, 368: m697.

7. 内容简介：本研究为多中心、随机、双盲、三臂对照临床试验，旨在评估手法针刺作为预防疗法治疗无先兆偏头痛的疗效。研究共纳入150例既往未接受过针刺治疗的无先兆发作性偏头痛患者，按2∶2∶1的比例随机分为手法针刺组、假针刺组和常规护理组，随机分配采用中央随机系统，中心分层区组大小为5。观察3组患者与基线水平（随机分组前4周）相比，随机分组后偏头痛发作天数和每4周周期偏头痛发作次数的平均变化。其他指标包括偏头痛平均发作天数或第17～20周偏头痛严重程度经视觉模拟量表（visual analogue scale，VAS）评分减少至少50%的患者比例；偏头痛特异性生活质量问卷，匹兹堡睡眠质量指数，偏头痛残疾评估评分，贝克焦虑量表及贝克抑郁问卷Ⅱ的评分变化，以及从基线到第20周抢救药物使用的平均剂量。得出结论：20次手法针刺治疗在预防无先兆发作性偏头痛方面优于假针刺和常规护理。

所有患者均接受20次的针刺治疗或常规护理，每隔1天接受1次治疗，当完成第10次治疗后，休息9天，随后再接受同样流程的10次治疗（手法针刺组及假针刺组将在随机分组后即启动针刺治疗，而常规护理组将在等待24周后启动针刺治疗）。

手法针刺组取穴方案为双侧合谷（LI4）、太冲（LR3）、太阳（EX-HN5）、风池（GB20）、率谷（GB8）10个必用穴位；并根据经络诊断及患者症状选择附加穴位：双侧阳明经头痛选头维（ST8），太阳经头痛选天柱（BL10），厥阴经头痛选百会（GV20）。经手法操作获得得气感。在留针的30 min内，对每个穴位进行手法操作，持续10 s，每隔10 min重复1次，共计4次。

假针刺组在背部选取4个双侧非穴位点进行非穿透性假针刺，这些点与头痛部位处于不同神经支配节段。假针刺组操作为：消毒后，使用安慰针具进行模拟针刺。该安慰针具设计为钝头，当针具通过塑料环接触皮肤时，能引发患者的刺痛感，但实际上针具并未刺破皮肤，而是回弹至其管轴内部。假针刺组与手法针刺组尽可能保持相同的施针仪式感。

常规护理组：接受常规护理。护理内容包括告知患者可能引发偏头痛频率增加的生活方式；指导患者通过记录头痛日记来明确头痛的诱发或激惹因素；让患者保持心

Rong Zhang, Nicola Robinson, Myeong Soo Lee, Jisheng Han, Fan Qu

3. 主要单位：浙江大学医学院附属妇产科医院中医科，浙江工商大学食品与生物工程学院，嘉兴市妇幼保健院产科

4. 发表期刊：*JAMA Network Open*

5. 发布日期：2022年5月23日

6. SCI源文献：ZHU Y, WANG F, ZHOU J, et al. Effect of Acupoint Hot Compress on Postpartum Urinary Retention after Vaginal Delivery: A Randomized Clinical Trial [J]. JAMA Netw Open, 2022, 5 (5): e2213261.

7. 内容简介：本研究为多中心随机临床试验。为评估穴位热敷能否降低产后尿潴留发生率，将1200名阴道分娩受试者以1∶1的比例随机分配到干预组和对照组，观察两组受试者产后尿潴留发生率，以及产后宫缩疼痛强度、抑郁症状、泌乳情况。得出结论：阴道分娩后穴位热敷可降低产后尿潴留发生率、子宫收缩疼痛程度、抑郁发生率，增加母乳量。穴位热敷可以作为产后护理的辅助干预措施。

干预组和对照组均接受常规产后护理，包括监测生命体征（血压、心率、呼吸、体温和血氧饱和度），观察阴道出血量和恶露排出量，触诊宫底，清洗外阴，以及与新生儿早期互动。

干预组在分娩后30 min（时间点1）、24 min（时间点2）和48 h（时间点3）各接受1次持续4 h、温度为（45±2）℃的穴位热敷。时间点1：在神阙（CV8）和膀胱经八髎［上髎（BL31）、次髎（BL32）、中髎（BL33）、下髎（BL34）］各放置两个热源（Model A）；在双侧涌泉（KI1）各放置两个热源（Model B）。时间点2和3：仅在神阙（CV8）放置1个热源（Model A）。

对照组只接受常规产后护理。

二 专家述评（针灸学专家，临床研究方法学及卫生统计学专家）

1. 述评一

产后尿潴留是常见的产后并发症，未及时治疗会对产妇的康复造成严重影响，是产科临床亟待解决的问题。本研究将1200名阴道分娩妇女随机分为干预组和对照组，1085名完成了研究，其中干预组537名、对照组548名。干预组在常规产后护理的基础上，于分娩后30 min、24 h、48 h在（45±2）℃的恒定温度下进行4 h穴位热敷。热敷选穴神阙、八髎、涌泉。对照组仅接受常规产后护理，不进行穴位热敷。结果表明，穴位热敷腹部、腰骶和足底区域可降低阴道分娩后尿潴留的发生率，减轻子宫收缩疼痛程度，改善抑郁症状，并增加母乳量。这种中医辅助干预产后护理，对产后并发症有显著的治疗作用，满足患者自我保健需求。

本研究结论为临床防治产后尿潴留提供了新的思路和方法，其严谨的设计、科学规范的研究过程、可靠的结论，为临床防治该病提供了高质量的循证医学证据。

2. 述评二

（1）研究设计和过程实施

该随机对照试验在12家医院进行，旨在评估穴位热敷对产后尿潴留及其他指标的影响。研究设计和实施有以下亮点：①研究采用了多中心设计，这增加了结果的外部效度和普适性。②随机化和盲法严格，区组随机将患者分为穴位热敷组（干预组）和常规产后护理组（对照组），确保了分配的公平性；尽管护理人员无法完全盲法，但数据分析由被设盲的统计学专家进行，减少了分析过程中的偏倚。③干预措施详细规范，使用了经过认证的医疗设备，确保了干预的一致性和可重复性。

（2）临床研究方法学及统计学方法的选择及应用

该研究的主要结局是产后尿潴留发生率，次要结局包括评估产后子宫收缩疼痛强度的视觉模拟量表评分、爱丁堡产后抑郁量表评分、母乳量、新生儿体质量和不良事件发生率等，全面评估了穴位热敷对产后恢复的影响。研究的样本量计算中的显著性水平设为0.025，检验效能设为80%，失访率设为20%，设定合理，样本量充足。对于主要结局，使用Fisher精确概率法比较干预组和对照组产后尿潴留的发生率，并计算了相对风险及95%置信区间；对于次要结局，根据数据类型选择了合适的统计学方法，包括Wilcoxon秩和检验、*t*检验等。然而，该研究没有使用意向治疗分析，这可能导致高估干预措施的疗效。此外，研究是在产后住院期间进行的，穴位热敷的长期效果尚不清楚。

第二十五节 "Effectiveness of Electroacupuncture or Auricular Acupuncture vs Usual Care for Chronic Musculoskeletal Pain Among Cancer Survivors: The PEACE Randomized Clinical Trial" 相关介绍和述评

一 论文介绍

1. 中文题目：电针或耳针对比常规护理对癌症幸存者慢性肌肉骨骼疼痛的有效性：PEACE随机临床试验

2. 作者：Jun J. Mao, Kevin T. Liou, Raymond E. Baser, Ting Bao, Katherine S. Panageas, Sally A. D. Romero, Q. Susan Li, Rollin M. Gallagher, Philip W. Kantoff

3. 主要单位：Integrative Medicine Service, Department of Medicine, Memorial Sloan Kettering Cancer Center, New York, New York; Department of Epidemiology and

Biostatistics, Memorial Sloan Kettering Cancer Center, New York, New York; Department of Family Medicine and Public Health, University of California, San Diego School of Medicine, San Diego

4. 发表期刊：*JAMA Oncology*

5. 发布日期：2021年3月18日

6. SCI源文献：MAO J J, LIOU K T, BASER R E, et al. Effectiveness of Electroacupuncture or Auricular Acupuncture vs Usual Care for Chronic Musculoskeletal Pain Among Cancer Survivors: The PEACE Randomized Clinical Trial [J]. JAMA Oncol, 2021, 7 (5): 720-727.

7. 内容简介：本研究为一项多中心、随机对照、多臂平行临床研究，旨在评估电针或耳针治疗癌症幸存者慢性肌肉骨骼疼痛的有效性。研究纳入360例患者，按2:2:1随机分为电针组（$n=145$）、耳针组（$n=143$）及常规治疗组（$n=72$），并分别实施相应干预措施，观察3组患者简明疼痛量表（brief pain inventory，BPI）从基线至第12周的平均疼痛严重程度评分变化。得出结论：在患有慢性肌肉骨骼疼痛的癌症患者中，电针和耳针相较于常规治疗更能有效减轻疼痛。然而，耳针与电针相比并未展现出非劣效性，且耳针组患者报告了更多的不良事件。

电针组在10周内进行共计10次的电针治疗，选取疼痛部位附近的4个穴位及其他部位至少4个穴位以治疗合并症，经过手法操作，使局部产生酸麻胀痛的感觉以实现得气。随后使用A3922 E-STIM Ⅱ设备以2 Hz频率对4个局部穴位进行电刺激。所有针留针30 min。

耳针组在10周内进行共计10次的耳针治疗。每次治疗中，针灸师会将针灸针插入患者一侧耳朵的扣带回穴，随后指导患者步行1 min。步行结束后，评估患者的慢性疼痛的严重程度。如果疼痛严重程度仍然大于1分（满分10分），针灸师会考虑将针刺入另一侧耳朵的扣带回穴。这一过程会依次对其余耳穴（丘脑穴、Ω2穴、零点穴、神门穴）进行重复操作。治疗会在以下任一情况发生时停止：①疼痛严重程度降低到1分或0分（满分10分）；②患者拒绝进一步接受针刺治疗；③观察到血管迷走神经反应等不良反应。每次最多施10根针，治疗持续时间为10～20 min，治疗的总时长取决于施针的数量，留针3～4天。

对照组采用常规治疗方案，即患者接受由医疗保健医师开具的标准疼痛管理，包括止痛药的使用、物理治疗和糖皮质激素注射。

二 专家述评（针灸学专家，临床研究方法学及卫生统计学专家）

1. 述评一

（1）选题分析

该研究聚焦慢性肌肉骨骼疼痛管理，特别针对癌症幸存者这一特殊群体展开。随着癌症幸存者数量的不断增加，长期疼痛成为显著影响他们生活质量的关键因素，而传统药物治疗的局限性在阿片类药物危机背景下更为凸显。该研究通过比较电针和耳针疗法与常规治疗对癌症幸存者慢性肌肉骨骼疼痛的有效性，旨在为非药物疗法在管理疼痛领域提供新的循证医学证据。此研究不仅符合一线临床的实际需求，更在国际上具有重大应用价值，有助于推动针灸疗法的国际化进程及其在肿瘤领域的广泛应用。

（2）针刺干预的实施

针刺干预的设计遵循了严谨的科学原则。研究采用电针和耳针两种形式，前者通过电流刺激增强内源性阿片肽释放，后者操作简便，易于推广。两种干预均设计为10周内的每周1次疗程，符合针灸治疗的常规频率，确保了干预方案的合理性。研究团队由经验丰富的针灸师组成，其专业背景强化了治疗效果的可靠性。

电针治疗由具备5年以上肿瘤治疗经验的针灸师执行，治疗过程中采用了特定的穴位选择、针刺角度、得气感的追求及精确的电刺激参数设定，体现了针灸治疗的专业性和个性化特点。而耳针疗法则基于美国军方开发的标准化方案——战地针灸，操作简单，适用于更广泛的临床环境，尤其适合非针灸专业人员实施。两种针刺干预均进行了10周的疗程，每周1次，形成了连贯的治疗方案。对照组采用常规治疗，包括药物治疗、物理治疗等，为评估针刺疗法的有效性提供了必要的参照基准。尽管缺乏假对照组可能带来一定的偏倚风险，但研究团队通过严谨的设计和严格的质量控制，力求减少这种影响。治疗师的专业背景和技能确保了针刺干预的质量，同时也凸显了治疗师资质对干预效果的影响。研究的针刺干预设计严谨，实施过程注重细节，为评估针刺疗法在慢性疼痛管理中的有效性提供了坚实的基础。

2. 述评二

本研究是一项分层区组随机、三臂平行对照、多中心临床试验，目的是验证电针或耳针治疗癌症幸存者慢性肌肉骨骼疼痛的有效性，以及比较耳针相对于电针的治疗效果。试验参与者根据2∶2∶1的比例随机分为电针组、耳针组或常规治疗组，干预组接受10周共10次电针或耳针治疗，以12周BPI疼痛严重程度评分较基线变化的平均值作为主要结局指标。试验由6家中心共同完成，参与筛选的参与者共676例，入选360例，其中358例纳入分析，包括电针组145例，耳针组142例，常规治疗组71例；另2例参与者，因各访视点数据均缺失而未纳入最终分析。

本试验的主要假设有二类：一是在减轻疼痛严重程度方面，电针组和耳针组均优于常规治疗组；二是在上述假设成立时，耳针组非劣于电针组。Ⅰ类错误的控制，采用了Dmitrienko的2步骤序贯把关策略。样本量计算充分考虑了假设检验的方向、Ⅰ类错误和Ⅱ类错误、效应值、界值等因素。对主要结局指标的分析采用了线性混合模型。这些统计学策略和方法，保证了研究结论的可靠性，即电针或耳针疗法均可有效减轻不同癌症幸存者群体的慢性肌肉骨骼疼痛严重程度，尚不能证明耳针的疗效非劣于电针。

第二十六节 "Efficacy of Acupuncture for Chronic Prostatitis/Chronic Pelvic Pain Syndrome: A Randomized Trial" 相关介绍和述评

一 论文介绍

1. 中文题目：针刺治疗慢性前列腺炎/慢性盆腔疼痛综合征疗效的随机对照试验

2. 作者：Yuanjie Sun, Yan Liu, Baoyan Liu, Kehua Zhou, Zenghui Yue, Wei Zhang, Wenbin Fu, Jun Yang, Ning Li, Liyun He, Zhiwei Zang, Tongsheng Su, Jianqiao Fang, Yulong Ding, Zongshi Qin, Hujie Song, Hui Hu, Hong Zhao, Qian Mo, Jing Zhou, Jiani Wu, Xiaoxu Liu, Weiming Wang, Ran Pang, Huan Chen, Xinlu Wang, Zhishun Liu

3. 主要单位：中国中医科学院广安门医院；北京中医药大学东直门医院中医内科学教育部重点实验室；ThedaCare Regional Medical Center-Appleton, Appleton, Wisconsin

4. 发表期刊：*Annals of Internal Medicine*

5. 发布日期：2021年8月17日

6. SCI源文献：SUN Y, LIU Y, LIU B, et al. Efficacy of Acupuncture for Chronic Prostatitis/Chronic Pelvic Pain Syndrome: A Randomized Trial [J]. Ann Intern Med, 2021, 174 (10): 1357-1366.

7. 内容简介：本研究为多中心、随机、假对照试验。旨在评估针刺治疗对慢性前列腺炎（chronic prostatitis，CP）/慢性盆腔疼痛综合征（chronic pelvic pain syndrome，CPPS）的远期疗效。研究纳入440例中重度CP/CPPS男性患者，随机分为针刺组和假针刺组分别进行干预，两组均接受为期8周、共20次的治疗，并在治疗后进行24周的随访。主要观察指标为应答者的比例，定义为在第8周和第32周时，美国国立卫生研究院慢性前列腺炎症状指数（national institutes of health chronic prostatitis symptom index，NIH-CPSI）评分较基线至少降低6分的参与者。得出结论：与假针刺治疗相比，8周内接受20次针刺治疗能更有效地改善中重度CP/CPPS患者的症状，并且在治疗后24周内疗效持续。

针刺组在连续8周内接受20次、每次30 min的治疗。前4周每周进行3次，后4周每周进行2次治疗，选穴双侧中髎（BL33）、会阳（BL35）、肾俞（BL23）和三阴交（SP6）。一次性无菌针具以30°～45°的角度刺入中髎和会阳，前者针刺方向为内下方，后者为略微朝外上方，两个穴位的针刺深度均为50～60 mm。在肾俞和三阴交则垂直刺入，深度为25～30 mm。针刺后，除中髎外的所有穴位进行行针手法（每10 min行针1次，每次持续30 s），包括提、插、捻、转等。

假针刺组在连续8周内同样接受20次、每次30 min的治疗，治疗频率与针刺组相同。在双侧非穴位处（肾俞、中髎和会阴两侧各约 15 mm 处，三阴交两侧各约 10 mm 处）插入 2~3 mm，但不进行实际的针刺操作。

二 专家述评（针灸学专家，临床研究方法学及卫生统计学专家）

1. 述评一

（1）选题分析

解决未满足的临床需求：临床研究的最终目的是服务于临床，解决实际问题。本文选用 CP/CPPS 为研究对象，在临床中，男性 CP/CPPS 发病率高，严重影响身心健康，药物治疗存在局限性，且医疗负担较重。针刺治疗疼痛效果显著，因此，该疾病的针刺治疗值得探索。

借鉴既往的研究成果：通过查阅该病相关研究论文，了解历史和当前研究领域的主要问题、热点和难点，发掘出未被深入研究的问题，从而为本文的选题提供思路。在已发表的文献中，一项关于 CP/CPPS 的 Cochrane 评价指出针灸疗法可能缓解症状并具有安全性。然而，另一项研究则发现，与假针灸相比，针灸的疗效差异并不显著，尽管该研究的证据质量非常低。此外，针灸疗效的持久性仍不清楚。所以，在既往的研究结果上，有必要实施该病的高质量临床研究。

研究结果存在价值意义：本文的研究结果显示，8 周的针刺对中度至重度 CP/CPPS 患者的症状有改善，并且在治疗后至少 24 周内持续有效。这一发现不仅显示了针刺治疗的长期疗效，还为临床实践和指南制定提供了高质量的证据支持。因此，针刺治疗无副作用，安全有效，成本低，值得推广。

（2）针刺干预的实施

治疗周期贴合临床：在本研究中，针刺治疗从随机分组当天开始，并在连续 8 周内共进行 20 次针刺，前 4 周每周进行 3 次（理想情况下是隔日 1 次），后 4 周每周进行 2 次（理想情况下每 2 或 3 天 1 次）。CP/CPPS 为慢性疼痛疾病，本次研究频次为每周治疗 2~3 次，比较贴近临床实际，也减少了患者就医次数。

注重针刺细节：本研究对针刺操作描述非常详细，包括针具的选择、进针后手法、行针间隔与持续时间、行针手法及效果等。共有 23 名针灸师实施治疗。他们具备同时进行针刺和假针刺的能力，并尽可能在整个试验期间优先考虑同一位针灸师为特定参与者提供治疗。唯一缺点是未提及针灸师的执业年限和职称等。

2. 述评二

本研究是一项分层区组随机、单盲、假针刺对照、多中心临床试验，目的是验证针刺治疗 CP/CPPS 在改善症状、缓解疼痛、改善排尿功能障碍和提高生活质量的长期持续疗效。试验将参与者按 1∶1 随机分为针刺组或假针刺组，两组均接受为期 8 周、

20次的针刺治疗，以第8周和第32周的NIH-CPSI评分应答率作为主要观察指标。本试验共10家中心参与，筛选参与者共735例，入选440例，针刺组、假针刺组各220例；414例完成试验，针刺组206例、假针刺组208例；440例均纳入意向性治疗分析集。

本试验根据既往文献估算样本量，并采用广义线性混合模型进行主要数据分析。为控制Ⅰ类错误，规定2个时点评价结果均为阳性才可判断针刺治疗具有长期持续疗效。结果显示，第8、32周时，针刺组的NIH-CPSI评分应答率分别为60.6%和61.5%，而假针刺组分别为36.8%和38.3%，差异均有统计学意义，表明针刺治疗可以显著改善CP/CPPS的症状，且具有长期持续效应。此外，研究还通过缺失数据的多重填补、排除在盲法评估期间回答接受过假针刺患者数据、将针灸师变量作为随机效应等3种方法，对主要分析结果进行敏感性分析，分析结论一致，保证了研究结果的稳健性。

第二十七节 "Effect of Briefing on Acupuncture Treatment Outcome Expectations, Pain, and Adverse Side Effects Among Patients With Chronic Low Back Pain: A Randomized Clinical Trial" 相关介绍和述评

一 论文介绍

1. 中文题目：简报对慢性腰痛患者针刺治疗结果预期、疼痛及不良反应的影响：一项随机临床试验

2. 作者：Jürgen Barth, Stefanie Muff, Alexandra Kern, Anja Zieger, Stefanie Keiser, Marco Zoller, Thomas Rosemann, Benno Brinkhaus, Leonhard Held, Claudia M. Witt

3. 主要单位：Institute for Complementary and Integrative Medicine, University Hospital Zurich and University of Zurich, Zurich, Switzerland; Department of Biostatistics at the Epidemiology, Biostatistics and Prevention Institute, University of Zurich, Zurich, Switzerland; Department of Mathematical Sciences, Norwegian University of Science and Technology, Trondheim, Norway

4. 发表期刊：*JAMA Network Open*

5. 发布日期：2021年9月10日

6. SCI源文献：BARTH J, MUFF S, KERN A, et al. Effect of Briefing on Acupuncture Treatment Outcome Expectations, Pain, and Adverse Side Effects Among Patients With Chronic Low Back Pain: A Randomized Clinical Trial [J]. JAMA Netw Open, 2021, 4 (9): e2121418.

7. 内容简介：本研究为随机、单盲、四臂临床试验。为了探讨在慢性腰痛患者接受最小量针刺治疗前，不同宣讲内容是否会影响治疗结果预期和报告的不良反应，采

用2×2析因设计，对152例受试者随机给予常规预期有效性简报或高预期有效性简报（有效性），常规不良反应简报或严重不良反应简报（不良反应），观察受试者治疗后针刺治疗效果预期、疼痛强度量表、不良反应评分。得出结论：关于治疗益处（安慰剂）和不良反应（反安慰剂）的建议并不影响治疗预期或不良反应。关于不良反应的信息可能需要更多的研究来理解反安慰剂的效应。

所有患者均免费接受相同的标准化最小针刺（每周2次，每次45 min，共8次），针刺穴位在左右两侧的6个预先定义的点进行浅表针刺，这些点不是传统的针刺穴位，在治疗开始和结束时对针刺部位进行轻微的手动刺激。针刺在前臂上保持3 min，在其他点上保持25 min。在针刺前，患者随机接受定期常规预期有效性简报或高预期有效性简报（有效性），常规不良反应简报或严重不良反应简报（不良反应），并在为期4周（8次）的针刺过程中提供额外的辅助信息电子邮件。

二　专家述评（针灸学专家，临床研究方法学及卫生统计学专家）

1. 述评一

积极或消极的建议可以引发安慰剂或反安慰剂效应的不同结果。在临床上，医师在咨询期间会向患者推荐针灸等治疗方法，并会告知患者其风险和益处。在这种沟通中，临床医师的目标是增加安慰剂效应并尽量减少反安慰剂效应。本研究立足于不同结果的告知对治疗结局的影响，具备一定的临床意义。

这一研究设计不同于以往寻求对针刺有效性与安全性的验证，而是以针刺作为非药物干预的研究模型，根据对150例接受针刺治疗的慢性腰痛患者在针刺治疗前接受不同侧重点信息来探索不同的信息告知在慢性腰痛患者的预期疗效、疼痛和不良反应方面的影响。该团队立足于安慰剂效应的角度，采用2×2析因设计，将患者随机分为被告知常规预期有效性简报组或高预期有效性简报组和常规不良反应简报组或严重不良反应简报组。干预信息均有关于针刺治疗慢性腰痛有效性和不良反应的证据支持。所有患者接受为期4周、共8次的针刺治疗，在针刺治疗前及治疗中会提供口头和书面的告知信息，并在期间提供额外的邮件说明。在盲法设置方面，对针灸师、患者、统计人员均施盲是这项研究的一大亮点。而这项研究的结果显示，关于治疗有效性或不良反应的信息告知并不影响治疗预期或不良反应。这一结果不同于既往所认为的观点，或许会影响将来医师的谈话方式。

2. 述评二

（1）研究设计和过程实施

这项研究通过随机、单盲、四臂试验探讨不同简报信息对患者期望和临床结果的影响。研究采用2×2析因设计，包含2个独立因素，划分为常规预期有效性简报组、高预期有效性简报组、常规不良反应简报组、严重不良反应简报组共4个小组，可以在同一研究中同时评估多个因素及其相互作用，可以更全面地理解每个因素的独立和组合效应，更加高效。严谨的随机化和单盲设计，有助于减少偏倚并提高结果的可信度。研究中采用的中央区组随机化和由独立统计人员生成的随机序列，可以提高组间均衡性。此外，所有患者接受相同的标准化针刺治疗，干预的一致性得到了保障。

（2）临床研究方法学及统计学方法的选择及应用

研究使用治疗预期量表测量患者的治疗预期、使用数字评分量表评估疼痛强度、使用13项自我报告问卷对不良反应进行评分。研究的样本量计算科学，显著性水平、检验效能等设置合理。此外，研究采用了多重插补处理缺失数据。对于治疗预期，研究采用协方差分析评估常规预期有效性简报组和高预期有效性简报组组间是否存在差异，将基线治疗预期量表评分和性别作为协变量，以控制混杂因素对结局的影响。对于疼痛强度，采用了协方差分析并调整基线疼痛强度、性别、基线乐观和悲观情绪等协变量。对于不良反应评分，研究采用了纵向零膨胀负二项回归评估每次针刺治疗后常规不良反应简报组和严重不良反应简报组的评分差异，零膨胀负二项回归可以处理过度离散和零膨胀问题。

第二十八节 "Effect of Acupuncture on Atrial Fibrillation Stratified by CHA₂DS₂-VASc Score—A Nationwide Cohort Investigation" 相关介绍和述评

一 论文介绍

1. 中文题目：评分分层探究针刺对心房颤动的影响：一项全国队列调查

2. 作者：W.-S. Hu, C.-L. Lin, C.Y. Hsu

3. 主要单位：中国医药大学医学院（中国台湾），中国医药大学附属医院医学系心血管内科（中国台湾），中国医药大学附属医院健康数据管理办公室（中国台湾）

4. 发表期刊：*QJM: An International Journal of Medicine*

5. 发表日期：2021年5月20日

6. SCI源文献：HU W S, LIN C L, HSU C Y. Effect of acupuncture on atrial fibrillation stratified by CHA₂DS₂-VASc score—a nationwide cohort investigation [J]. QJM, 2021, 114 (6): 398-402.

7. 内容简介：本研究为回顾性队列研究。为了通过CHA₂DS₂-VASc评分分层，阐述针刺降低心房颤动（atrial fibrillation，AF）风险的作用，采用乘积极限法计算各组结局的累积发生率，组间比较采用时序检验（Log-rank）。采用单因素比例风险回归模型（Cox）估计发病率和风险比（hazard ratio，HR），采用多因素Cox比例风险模型估计校正HR，包括人口统计学协变量和合并症状态。得出结论：针刺对AF具有保护作用，且对于合并症较少的患者效果更明显。

该研究基于纵向健康保险数据库。在该研究中，共有235 866例在索引日期内接受针刺治疗（病例组）。随机选择无针刺病例（对照组）并以1:1的比例与病例组匹配。

$CHA_2DS_2\text{-}VASc$评分的组成部分包括心力衰竭、糖尿病、脑血管意外或短暂性脑缺血发作、血管疾病和高血压。该研究中考虑的其他潜在疾病是高脂血症、慢性阻塞性肺疾病、慢性肾脏病、甲状腺功能亢进症、睡眠障碍和痛风。

二 专家述评（针灸学专家，临床研究方法学及卫生统计学专家）

1. 述评一

针灸疗法在国内应用病症广泛，但对多数病种的获益仍缺乏高质量证据。AF是临床常见的心律失常类问题，长时间发作的最大危害是造成心房内血栓形成和脱落，造成受累器官或脑组织血栓栓塞、供血减少，甚至中断。本研究通过回顾性队列设计发现针刺对AF可能存在保护作用，且对$CHA_2DS_2\text{-}VASc$评分较低（AF卒中风险低）的患者更为显著。这一发现与针刺通过激活内源性保护机制发挥作用的基本假设是一致的，当机体功能损伤程度相对较低时，则能更好地激发内源性保护机制的运行，当损伤程度高时，针刺可发挥的空间也势必受到影响。因此，后续若考虑设计验证性研究，可以考虑纳入针对针刺优势更明显的人群，以便得到确证性结论。

本项研究为基于诊疗数据的回顾性研究，但诊疗信息中缺乏对针刺方案的记录，因此无法支撑对不同针刺方案的获益对比分析。但是否存在有效针刺次数、针刺获益的剂量反应关系及针刺效应的持续性等依然是需要继续探讨的问题。

2. 述评二

（1）研究设计和过程实施

为了探讨按$CHA_2DS_2\text{-}VASc$评分分层后针刺治疗对AF发病风险的保护作用，该研究采用了队列研究设计。根据PICO原则，本研究的研究对象（Participant）为中国台湾的健康保险研究数据库中1995年3月1日至2013年12月31日纳入的患者；暴露（Intervention）为针刺治疗，暴露组以第一次接受针刺治疗作为入组时间；对照（Control）为非针刺治疗，按照1:1与暴露组匹配（但该研究并未说明采用的匹配方法这一关键问题）；结局（Outcome）为AF发病。针刺治疗和AF等信息来自健康保险数据库中居民就医时的处方和疾病诊断信息。最终，该研究共纳入暴露组和对照组研究对象各235 866例。

（2）临床研究方法学及统计学方法的选择及应用

该研究在探讨针刺治疗对AF发病风险的保护作用方面选择了生存分析的统计学方法，方法的选择与数据特点相匹配。在生存分析中，截至2013年12月31日，研究对象未发生AF、退出或死亡被定义为删失。按照CHA_2DS_2-VASc评分（0～1；2～3；4～5；>5）分层后，该研究使用Kaplan-Meier法计算每组的累积发生率，并使用Log-rank检验比较组间差异，使用Cox比例风险模型进行校正混杂因素的HR估计，校正混杂因素考虑了人口统计学特征（文中未明确具体变量）和合并的基础疾病（高脂血症、慢性阻塞性肺疾病、慢性肾脏病、甲状腺功能亢进症、睡眠障碍和痛风）。此外，研究使用受试者工作特征曲线下面积估计了在接受针刺治疗和未接受针刺治疗的研究对象中使用CHA_2DS_2-VASc评分预测AF的能力，但并未交代选用的预测模型。

第二十九节 "Greater Somatosensory Afference With Acupuncture Increases Primary Somatosensory Connectivity and Alleviates Fibromyalgia Pain via Insular γ-Aminobutyric Acid: A Randomized Neuroimaging Trial" 相关介绍和述评

一 论文介绍

1. 中文题目：更大的体感传入伴随针刺通过岛叶γ-氨基丁酸增加初级体感连接并减轻纤维肌痛：一项随机神经影像学试验

2. 作者：Ishtiaq Mawla, Eric Ichesco, Helge J Zöllner, Richard A E Edden, Thomas Chenevert, Henry Buchtel, Meagan D Bretz, Heather Sloan, Chelsea M Kaplan, Steven E Harte, George A Mashour, Daniel J Clauw, Vitaly Napadow, Richard E Harris

3. 主要单位：Neuroscience Graduate Program, University of Michigan, Ann Arbor, MI, USA; Chronic Pain and Fatigue Research Center, Department of Anesthesiology, University of Michigan, Ann Arbor, MI, USA; Russell H. Morgan Department of Radiology and Radiological Science, The Johns Hopkins University School of Medicine, Baltimore, MD, USA

4. 发表期刊：*Arthritis & Rheumatology*

5. 发布日期：2021年5月31日

6. SCI源文献：MAWLA I, ICHESCO E, ZÖLLNER H J, et al. Greater Somatosensory Afference With Acupuncture Increases Primary Somatosensory Connectivity and Alleviates Fibromyalgia Pain via Insular γ-Aminobutyric Acid: A Randomized Neuroimaging Trial [J]. Arthritis Rheumatol, 2021, 73 (7): 1318-1328.

7. 内容简介：本研究为单中心、盲法、随机、假对照临床试验。为了了解体感传入对临床疼痛改善的具体贡献及所涉及的特定脑回路，将76例纤维肌痛（fibromyalgia，FM）患者随机分为接受有体感影响的电针（electroacupuncture，EA）组和无体感影响的模拟激光针（mock laser acupuncture，ML）组，并分别进行干预，观察两组受试者治疗前后简明疼痛量表（brief pain inventory，BPI）评分，并用静息态功能性磁共振成像（resting state functional MRI，rs-fMRI）和氢质子磁共振波谱（proton magnetic resonance spectroscopy，^{1}H-MRS）评估脑功能网络连通性水平。得出结论：针刺产生的躯体感觉成分调节了与岛叶神经化学相关的初级躯体感觉功能连接，进而减轻了FM的疼痛程度。

EA组和ML组治疗方案：每周2次，每次25 min，共4周。

EA组在3组穴位上施加了低频EA。这3组穴位包括：右侧曲池（LI11）至合谷（LI4），左侧阳陵泉（GB34）至三阴交（SP6），以及双侧足三里（ST36）。同时针刺百会（GV20）、右侧耳穴神门（TF4）和左侧太冲（LR3），但不施加电流。使用恒定电流电针治疗仪施以低强度和频率刺激，灵活设置脉冲宽度（1 ms）、频率（2 Hz）和形状（双向矩形）参数。

对照组，即ML组，选用模拟激光针疗法。其选穴在EA组穴位上方约1~2 cm处。在放置设备之前不进行按压，设备与皮肤无直接接触。

二 专家述评（针灸学专家，临床研究方法学及卫生统计学专家）

1. 述评一

针刺在治疗FM方面有一定的临床疗效，然而可能是由于方法学问题及潜在作用机制尚未明确等原因，其临床疗效及调控机制亟待深入探究。本研究基于先前研究，提出与安慰针刺相比，EA会通过中枢神经系统中的体感通路产生更好的镇痛疗效。因此，本研究的目的在于探究针刺是否可通过体感传入通路特异性调控大脑环路及代谢物，从而产生镇痛作用。同时，本项研究采用了随机对照试验的方法，以体感传入方面为切入点采用ML作为安慰对照，以此评估EA干预FM的临床疗效，并通过神经影像技术血氧水平依赖fMRI（blood oxygenation level dependent fMRI，BOLD-fMRI）及MRS来观察针刺治疗前后大脑功能连接和γ-氨基丁酸（Gamma-aminobutyric acid，γ-GABA）水平的变化。

本文具有四大亮点：①研究设计，本文将临床研究与神经影像研究相结合，在明确针刺临床疗效的同时，还初步探究了其潜在的神经调控机制；②对照组选取，安慰针刺的选取尤为巧妙，不仅避开了穴位触诊和触觉刺激对于安慰针刺疗效的影响，同时也更好地探究了EA的神经调控途径；③多模态技术，研究通过多模态神经影像技术，即通过Bold-fMRI及MRS来综合探究针刺对于大脑功能连接和代谢物水平的影响；④临床调控机制研究有一共同的局限性，即缺乏直接因果证据支持针刺对于具体神经

小（差异：-0.01～-0.14）。主观感受是CSBM的主要构成，该研究中的受试者未采用盲法。因此，完全排空感可能是针刺的非特异性效应，比如针刺治疗中医师与患者的紧密互动，患者对针刺的更高期望等。然而，针刺的非特异性效应和特异性效应不可分割。

与此同时，本试验根据Rome Ⅲ标准区分肠易激综合征和服用泻药的功能性便秘患者存在显著困难，该研究中部分患者可能患有肠易激综合征。其次，正常传输型便秘、慢传输型便秘或排空障碍型便秘没有被区分，对相关亚型进行亚组分析，能更好地明确电针治疗的优势人群。

总之，电针在第3～8周增加每周CSBM≥3次的患者百分比方面不逊于普芦卡必利，且其具有更好的安全性。电针的效应在8周的治疗期间逐渐累积，持续24周。对于SCC患者，在缓解不适和改善生活质量方面电针和普芦卡必利的效果相近。因此，对于SCC而言，电针是一项颇具临床价值的治疗方法。

2. 述评二

采用集中式网络/电话随机系统以1∶1的比例对经过2周导入期且符合条件的受试者随机分为两组，随机化序列由独立第三方应用SAS 9.3生成，按地点分层，区组长度可变，满足随机化分组和分配隐藏要求。原文表1中作者未进行组间均衡性比较，但各组的基线特征类似。两组干预差别明显，该试验的受试者未设盲。除了要验证的干预措施外，各组接受的其他措施相同。主要结局的缺失采用基于随机缺失机制假设下的多重填补法，敏感性分析基于符合方案数据集进行，次要结局未采用填补。基线特征描述和主分析基于调整的意向性分析数据集。采用相同的方法对各组研究对象的结局指标进行测评。结果测评方法可信，资料分析方法恰当，研究设计合理。在实施研究和资料分析过程中基本符合标准的随机对照试验。综上，结论可靠。

第三十二节 "*Manual Acupuncture Versus Sham Acupuncture and Usual Care for Prophylaxis of Episodic Migraine Without Aura: Multicentre, Randomised Clinical Trial*"相关介绍和述评

一 论文介绍

1. 中文题目：手法针刺、假针刺与常规护理预防无先兆发作性偏头痛：一项多中心、随机临床试验

2. 作者：Shabei Xu, Lingling Yu, Xiang Luo, Minghuan Wang, Guohua Chen, Qing Zhang, Wenhua Liu, Zhongyu Zhou, Jinhui Song, Huitao Jing, Guangying Huang,

普芦卡必利对严重慢性便秘（severe chronic constipation，SCC）的有效性和安全性，将560例SCC患者随机分为电针组和普芦卡必利组分别进行干预，观察在第3~8周平均每周完全自发性排便（complete spontaneous bowel movement，CSBM）为3次的受试者比例；同时参与者将完成粪便日记，评估第11~32周指定时间区域期间平均每周CSBM为3次的参与者比例，干预后平均每周自发性排便（spontaneous bowel movement，SBM）、平均每周CSBM次数较基线增加1次的参与者比例；使用救急药物的参与者比例及便秘患者生活质量评估、布里斯托粪便性状量表平均分数对比基线变化。得出结论：电针在缓解SCC方面优于普芦卡必利，且具有良好的安全性。8周电针治疗后效果可持续24周。电针治疗SCC是一种较有前景的选择。

电针组共进行8周电针治疗，前两周每周5次，之后6周每周3次，每次30 min，共进行28次治疗。穴位包括双侧天枢（ST25）、腹结（SP14）、上巨虚（ST37）。严重排便困难（基于参与者的主诉和粪便次数）者加双侧中髎（BL33），伴焦虑、抑郁症状者加百会（GV20）和神庭（GV24）。

普芦卡必利组，每天早餐前口服琥珀酸普芦卡必利2 mg，连续服用32周。第8周时行心电图检查，与基线相比，心电图有明显变化的参与者可以随时停用普芦卡必利。

二 专家述评（针灸学专家，临床研究方法学及卫生统计学专家）

1. 述评一

本试验是刘保延、刘志顺教授团队在《内科学年鉴》发表高质量研究证实针刺治疗慢性严重功能性便秘患者内在真实性的基础上，在SCC患者中，对电针与普芦卡必利进行的大规模、设计严谨、头对头比较的研究，以明确针刺治疗SCC的外在真实性。在这项试验中，电针疗法在第3~8周平均每周CSBM≥3次的参与者百分比方面并不逊色于普芦卡必利，且具有持续效应和更好的安全性。该研究的优势在于采用国际公认的CSBM作为核心结局指标，并有前期试验作为研究基础，从针刺治疗SCC的内在真实性向外在真实性研究拓展，循序渐进，研究规范，可行性强。

该研究同时发现电针和普芦卡必利的一些特点。如电针具有更好的安全性，治疗效果随治疗时间累积，表现为疗效在第6~8周超过了普芦卡必利，在第8周达高峰，在整个随访期维持与普芦卡必利相似的效果；而普芦卡必利起效较快，2周内起效，在整个试验期间疗效稳定。电针组在治疗和随访期间效果稳定（平均每周CSBM≥3次的患者比例为36.2%，随访期间为37.6%）。此外，电针可较好缓解SCC患者的不完全排空感，表现为在第3~32周，平均每周SBM的基线变化在电针组与普芦卡必利组间差异较大（差异：−0.47~−0.74）；而平均每周CSBM次数的基线变化在组间差异变

2. 述评二

采用中央分层随机化系统以1∶1∶1的比例将符合条件的受试者随机分为3组，随机化序列由独立的统计人员应用SAS 9.3软件生成，按医院分层，区组长度为6或9，满足随机化分组和分配隐藏要求。表1中作者未进行组间均衡性比较，但各组的基线特征类似。除了针灸师以外，受试者、结果评估人员和统计人员都对分组情况不知情，满足盲法要求。除了要验证的干预措施外，各组接受的其他措施相同。数据存在缺失，主分析结果采用基线值填补法，敏感性分析采用末次结转法、删除法和多重填补法。主要结局和次要结局的分析基于调整的意向性分析数据集，采用相同的方法对各组研究对象的结局指标进行测评，结果测评方法可信，资料分析方法恰当。研究设计合理，在实施研究和资料分析过程中基本符合标准的随机对照试验。综上所述，结论可靠。

第三十一节 "Electroacupuncture vs Prucalopride for Severe Chronic Constipation: A Multicenter, Randomized, Controlled, Noninferiority Trial" 相关介绍和述评

一 论文介绍

1. 中文题目：电针与普芦卡必利治疗慢性严重便秘的非劣效性随机对照研究

2. 作者：Baoyan Liu, Jiani Wu, Shiyan Yan, Kehua Zhou, Liyun He, Jianqiao Fang, Wenbin Fu, Ning Li, Tongsheng Su, Jianhua Sun, Wei Zhang, Zenghui Yue, Hongxing Zhang, Jiping Zhao, Zhongyu Zhou, Hujie Song, Jian Wang, Li'an Liu, Linpeng Wang, Xiaoying Lv, Xiaofang Yang, Yan Liu, Yuanjie Sun, Yang Wang, Zongshi Qin, Jing Zhou, Zhishun Liu

3. 主要单位：中国中医科学院广安门医院针灸科；中国中医科学院中医临床医学基础研究所；Catholic Health System Internal Medicine Training Program, University at Buffalo

4. 发表期刊：*The American Journal of Gastroenterology*

5. 发布日期：2020年11月3日

6. SCI源文献：LIU B, WU J, YAN S, et al. Electroacupuncture vs Prucalopride for Severe Chronic Constipation: A Multicenter, Randomized, Controlled, Noninferiority Trial [J]. Am J Gastroenterol, 2021, 116 (5): 1024-1035.

7. 内容简介：本研究为多中心、随机、对照、非劣效性试验。为了比较电针与

焦强化针刺（电针）对KOA是否有效、电针和手针的远期疗效如何的问题，设计了电针组与假针刺组、手针组与假针刺组的对照，共纳入442例KOA患者。电针组和手针组采用相同的穴位（这些穴位的选择基本符合针刺临床实际情况，可视为有效针刺处方），假针刺组选取8个远离传统穴位或经络的非穴位。3组均为每周治疗3次，每次留针30 min，治疗8周，随访18周，共计26周的研究周期。在治疗的第4、6、8周和随访的第16、26周观察、记录结局指标的变化并进行统计学处理。

结果证明：①KOA患者对电针、手针、假针刺的干预均有不同程度的应答，以电针的应答率为最高。②在对疼痛的改善上，电针、手针的改善程度均优于假针刺，而且在第26周时，这一优势仍然存在。③在研究周期内，电针始终对WOMAC量表中膝关节功能和僵硬改善明显，而手针则与假针刺的差异无统计学意义。④对疗效的总体评价上，在第4、8、16周时，电针和手针组优于假针刺组。⑤在12项简明健康调查（12-item short form health survey，SF-12）评分中，无论是生理影响还是心理影响，3种干预均无有意义的变化，仅在第26周时，电针和手针比假针刺略优。

以上结果可能提示：①假针刺组的设计没有很好地起到剥离安慰针作用。尽管电针组与假针刺组、手针组与假针刺组之间的效应差异均有统计学意义，但也掩盖不了假针刺组的治疗效应。然而，假针刺组的治疗效应在随访期间下降得较快。按照针灸理论，浅刺也是一种治疗方式，可以起到治疗效果。本研究中，进行浅刺的点基本在能影响膝关节活动的肌肉或者关节处，也能对患膝产生一定的作用。因此这种假针刺设计，剥离针刺安慰剂作用的效果不是很明显，反而增加了假针刺的作用，结果是缩小了假针刺组与电针组、假针刺组与手针组的效应差异。②手针组的干预设计没有充分发挥针刺手法的作用。电针组、手针组对疼痛改善明显，均优于假针刺组，不仅NRS、WOMAC指标有改善，3组补充止痛剂的患者数量也说明这个问题。但是在对患膝僵硬和功能改善方面，电针组在各个时间段均优于假针刺组，而手针组则与假针刺组的差异较小，电针组可能优于手针组。这个现象可能与手针组的操作设计有关。本研究中手针组的操作除了追求得气感之外没有额外的手法操作，这与"手针"的命名不太相符。一般来说，手针还应该包括在留针过程中的一些手法操作，以便能更好地促进经气流行，达到更好的疗效。而且，在手针组增加手法操作与电针组不断进行的疏密波电刺激更加匹配（但是这样也许会影响到盲法的成功）。如果在手针组的操作中适当增加一些手法，则手针组的应答率有可能提高。

本研究亦有一个有趣的结论，"有无针灸经历对疗效没有有意义的影响"，这或许是对"中国患者多有针灸经历，对针灸的心理预期会更大"的反证。

本研究是近年来发表的优秀针灸临床研究之一。临床问题选择有意义，研究设计严谨，治疗及观察周期比较长，盲法成功率较高，多中心研究中注意到针灸师资质及统一培训操作，这些细节均较好地保证了研究质量。

2. 作者：Jian-Feng Tu, Jing-Wen Yang, Guang-Xia Shi, Zhang-Sheng Yu, Jin-Ling Li, Lu-Lu Lin, Yu-Zheng Du, Xiao-Gang Yu, Hui Hu, Zhi-Shun Liu, Chun-Sheng Jia, Li-Qiong Wang, Jing-Jie Zhao, Jun Wang, Tong Wang, Yang Wang, Tian-Qi Wang, Na Zhang, Xuan Zou, Yu Wang, Jia-Kai Shao MD, Cun-Zhi Liu

3. 主要单位：北京中医药大学针灸推拿学院，首都医科大学附属北京中医医院针灸科，上海交大-耶鲁大学生物统计和数据科学联合中心

4. 发表期刊：*Arthritis & Rheumatology*

5. 发布日期：2020年11月10日

6. SCI源文献：TU J F, YANG J W, SHI G X, et al. Efficacy of Intensive Acupuncture Versus Sham Acupuncture in Knee Osteoarthritis: A Randomized Controlled Trial [J]. Arthritis Rheutol, 2021, 73 (3): 448-458.

7. 内容简介：本研究为多中心、随机、假对照临床试验。为了评估强化针刺与假针刺治疗膝骨关节炎（knee osteoarthritis，KOA）的疗效，将480例KOA患者随机分为电针组、手针组和假针刺组分别进行干预，观察受试者治疗后反应率，即到第8周时同时在疼痛和功能方面取得最小临床重要改善受试者比例。疼痛维度使用数字评定量表（numeric rating scale，NRS）测评，功能维度使用美国Western Ontario和McMaster大学骨关节炎指数（Western Ontario and McMaster Universities osteoarthritis index，WOMAC）测评。得出结论：对于KOA患者，与假针刺相比，电针治疗在第8周时可减轻疼痛、改善功能，且效果可持续到第26周；手针治疗在随访中体现出效果，但在第8周时对KOA没有体现出明显效果。

电针、手针和假针刺组治疗频次均为每周3次，每次30 min，治疗8周，随访18周，共26周。

电针、手针组选穴处方均由5个必选穴和3个辅穴组成。5个必选穴为犊鼻（ST35）、内膝眼（EX-LE4）、曲泉（LR8）、膝阳关（GB33）及阿是穴（患者痛感最显著点）；3个辅穴由针灸师依据经络辨证从穴位库中选取，需要在针刺过程中达到"得气"。假针刺组选穴处方由8个远离常规穴/经络的非穴位点组成，针刺要求为透皮（刺入深度2～3 mm），不施手法、不"得气"。

电针、手针和假针刺组均使用电针仪。电针与手针组均选曲泉、膝阳关为一对夹电针，另一对由辅穴中挑选2穴组成；假针刺组则任选4个非穴点两两配对夹电针。电刺激调试方面，电针组选择2/100 Hz疏密波，调整强度至针体轻微振动；手针和假针刺组则调试为指示灯闪烁但无电流通过模式。

二 专家述评（针灸学专家，临床研究方法学及卫生统计学专家）

1. 述评一

这是一项在中国国内9家医院进行的针刺多中心临床随机对照研究。研究主要聚

通路的调控机制,虽然本项研究同样存在这一问题,但本项研究在相关性分析的基础上,进一步采用了中介分析,尽可能地说明针刺调控机制的方向性。

2. 述评二

(1)研究设计和过程实施

为了评估针刺的体感传入中枢神经系统的作用机制,以及这些机制如何在FM中产生镇痛反应,该研究采用了单中心、盲法、随机、假对照试验设计,其中采用了动态区组随机的随机化方法。而且论文未交代样本量估计的方法和参数设置。根据PICO原则,本研究的研究对象(Participant)为满足试验纳入、排除标准的FM患者;干预(Intervention)为EA;对照(Control)为ML。EA组和ML组的治疗次数(每周2次×4周)和每次治疗时长相同。结局(Outcome)包括多个:主要临床结局为BPI的严重程度分量表得分,机制结局包括初级体感皮层的rs-fMRI(研究中实际报告的变量为$S1_{leg}$连接性)和右前岛叶的Glx(谷氨酰胺和谷氨酸复合物)和GABA+(研究中实际报告的变量为GABA+/Cr)的^{1}H-MRS测量值,次要临床结局为患者报告结局测量信息系统(patient-reported outcomes measurement information system,PROMIS)焦虑和抑郁量表评分。所有结局均在试验前和试验后分别进行测量。

(2)临床研究方法学及统计学方法的选择及应用

研究一共纳入了79例受试者,其中试验组40例,对照组39例,数据分析基于符合方案集(试验组35例,对照组37例)。对于临床结局指标,该研究采用了重复测量方差分析,分析了处理和时间的交互作用、处理因素的主效应、时间的主效应及处理因素的单独效应。使用校正年龄的皮尔逊相关系数对试验前后S1leg连接性、GABA+和BPI严重程度的变化值进行关联分析。此外,研究者还使用了单侧检验的*Fisher Z*变换确定使用皮尔逊相关系数评估的关系在试验组和对照组中是否存在相关方向的差异。最后,为了评估试验组中GABA+/Cr是否对$S1_{leg}$连接性对BPI严重程度的效应有中介作用,研究者进行了中介分析,通过偏差矫正的Bootstrap百分位法计算校正年龄后的间接效应的95%置信区间。

第三十节 "*Efficacy of Intensive Acupuncture Versus Sham Acupuncture in Knee Osteoarthritis: A Randomized Controlled Trial*"相关介绍和述评

一 论文介绍

1. 中文题目:强化针刺与假针刺治疗膝骨关节炎的疗效比较:一项随机对照试验

（2）过程实施

研究开始前，研究方案提前注册，方案和统计分析计划提前公布，具备发表高水平临床研究的重要前提条件。

方案实施过程中，患者遵守分配隐藏和盲法的相关要求被随机分至针刺组和假针刺组。研究的盲法实施是使用密封的信封隐藏分组信息，由未参与招募、治疗或评估的研究助理保存。为有效实施盲法，研究者巧妙地使用了一种方便易行而科学合理的方案，较好地解决了针刺临床试验盲法实施较难的问题。未设盲的人员包括负责随机化模块的针灸师和研究助理。所有其他研究人员，包括患者、结果评估人员和统计人员均被设盲。

（3）临床研究方法学和统计学方法

样本量计算是研究者基于既往自身研究和临床经验所决定的。研究巧妙选择针刺后第 10 min 时 VAS 较基线下降≥50% 的患者比例（响应率）为主要结局指标。主要结局指标的选择基于临床实践，解决针刺是否能够治疗患者在接受镇痛治疗的 10 min 后仍感受到中重度疼痛的临床目标。统计分析过程中，对于基线特征，连续分布变量用平均值或中位数描述；离散变量用频率和百分比描述。分析基于意向性治疗分析原则，包括所有随机患者。评估了响应率、挽救性镇痛、再访和入院率及不良事件。通过混合效应模型对 VAS 评分进行组间比较；以各时间点的相应量表评分作为因变量，以治疗为主要因素，以时间与治疗为交互效应，基线值作为协变量，并使用随机截距来模拟受试者内相关性，进行重复测量分析；采用协方差分析校正基线 VAS 作为敏感性分析评估 10 min 时 VAS 的差异。研究的临床方法学严谨和统计方法得当。

第二十四节 "Effect of Acupoint Hot Compress on Postpartum Urinary Retention After Vaginal Delivery: A Randomized Clinical Trial" 相关介绍和述评

一 论文介绍

1. 中文题目：穴位热敷对阴道分娩后尿潴留的影响：一项随机临床试验

2. 作者：Yuhang Zhu, Fangfang Wang, Jue Zhou, Shuiqin Gu, Lianqing Gong, Yaoyao Lin, Xiaoli Hu, Wei Wang, Aihua Zhang, Dongmei Ma, Chunxiao Hu, Yan Wu, Lanzhong Guo, Limin Chen, Leiyin Cen, Yan He, Yuqing Cai, Enli Wang, Honglou Chen, Jing Jin, Jinhe Huang, Meiyuan Jin, Xiujuan Sun, Xiaojiao Ye, Linping Jiang, Ying Zhang, Jian Zhang, Junfei Lin, Chunping Zhang, Guofang Shen, Wei Jiang, Liuyan Zhong, Yuefang Zhou, Ruoya Wu, Shiqing Lu, Linlin Feng, Hong Guo, Shanhu Lin, Qiaosu Chen, Jinfang Kong, Xuan Yang, Mengling Tang, Chang Liu, Fang Wang, Xiao-Yang Mio Hu, Hye Won Lee, Xinfen Xu,

率方面未发现差异，可能是由于双氯芬酸后续强效镇痛引起的天花板效应。针刺可考虑作为缓解急性肾绞痛的一种辅助疗法。

受试者确诊肾绞痛后，均给予50 mg/2 ml双氯芬酸钠肌肉注射，随后进行30 min的针刺或假针刺治疗。

针刺组选取双侧腰痛点（EX-UE7），每例患者使用4根针（每侧手2个穴位），进针角度为90°，针刺深度为0.5寸（8～10 mm）。每个穴位进行捻转提插至少30 s，以达到得气（痛、麻、胀、沉）。

假针刺组选用假针刺疗法。根据相关文献，筛选出具有缓解急性肾绞痛作用的穴位。排除这些穴位后，选取前臂16个穴位，分为8个亚组，每组选择2个穴位，将其周围3 mm的区域定义为非穴位区域。假针刺组在双侧非穴位处进行浅表皮肤穿刺（深度为1～4 mm，每例4根针），但不进行得气针刺操作。

二 专家述评（针灸学专家，临床研究方法学及卫生统计学专家）

1. 述评一

肾绞痛为患者所能感受到的最严重的疼痛之一。因此，在尽可能短的时间内有效镇痛对肾绞痛的治疗至关重要。肌肉注射双氯芬酸钠后疼痛缓解的平均时间为18.64 min。然而，37.5%的患者在15 min时仍有中度或重度疼痛。因此，寻求有效和可行的治疗方法缓解疼痛，对于临床急诊缓解肾绞痛至关重要。本研究将针刺与肌肉注射双氯芬酸钠相结合，使用中西医结合的方法缓解肾绞痛。旨在探讨针刺作为镇痛药的辅助治疗能否加速急性肾绞痛患者的疼痛缓解。研究将80例泌尿系统结石引起的肾绞痛患者随机分为针刺组和假针刺组。针刺组患者接受"腰痛点针刺+双氯芬酸钠"镇痛治疗，假针刺组患者接受"非穴浅刺+双氯芬酸钠"镇痛治疗。结果表明，与假针刺组相比，针刺联合肌肉注射双氯芬酸钠在紧急情况下对肾绞痛患者是安全的，并能快速有效地缓解疼痛。针刺作为缓解急性肾绞痛的一种选择性辅助疗法，疗效显著。

该研究设计科学严谨、过程规范合理、结论可信，为中医针灸结合西医疗法运用于急诊科、快速缓解肾绞痛提供了高质量的循证医学证据，对临床治疗肾绞痛具有良好的推广价值。

2. 述评二

（1）研究设计

该研究是单中心、假针刺对照的随机临床试验。按照临床试验报告统一标准（consolidated standards of reporting trials，CONSORT）来报告研究结果，是发表高水平期刊的基本条件。

周后接受针刺。统计学方法上，采用多变量线性回归按组比较52周时的BPI-WP评分，调整基线评分和研究地点的指标变量，其中2个指标变量代表不同的干预组。该研究采用线性混合模型对截至第52周的每个患者报告结果领域的所有评估进行纵向分析，其中个体被视为随机效应；评估时间（作为线性和二次函数）及其与治疗的潜在相互作用被视为固定效应。回归分析包括对基线评分、研究地点的指标变量和干预组的2个指标变量的协变量调整。对各组在初始研究评估后停止使用AIs或使用任何止痛药（包括对乙酰氨基酚、布洛芬、其他非甾体抗炎药或麻醉药）的患者比例进行检验。研究统计方法严谨得当。

第二十三节 "Effect of Adjunctive Acupuncture on Pain Relief Among Emergency Department Patients With Acute Renal Colic Due to Urolithiasis: A Randomized Clinical Trial" 相关介绍和述评

一 论文介绍

1. 中文题目：针刺辅助治疗对泌尿系结石所致急性肾绞痛的急诊患者疼痛缓解的影响：一项随机临床试验

2. 作者：Jian-Feng Tu, Ying Cao, Li-Qiong Wang, Guang-Xia Shi, Lian-Cheng Jia, Bao-Li Liu, Wei-Hai Yao, Xiao-Lu Pei, Yan Cao, He-Wen Li, Shi-Yan Yan, Jing-Wen Yang, Zhi-Cheng Qu, Cun-Zhi Liu

3. 主要单位：北京中医药大学国际针灸创新研究院，北京中医药大学针灸推拿学院，首都医科大学附属北京中医医院急诊科

4. 发表期刊：*JAMA Network Open*

5. 发布日期：2022年8月9日

6. SCI源文献：TU J F, CAO Y, WANG L Q, et al. Effect of Adjunctive Acupuncture on Pain Relief Among Emergency Department Patients With Acute Renal Colic Due to Urolithiasis: A Randomized Clinical Trial [J]. JAMA Netw Open, 2022, 5 (8): e2225735.

7. 内容简介：本研究为单中心、假针刺对照、随机临床试验。为了探讨针刺作为镇痛药的辅助治疗能否加速急性肾绞痛患者的疼痛缓解。将80例因泌尿系结石导致急性肾绞痛的患者随机分为针刺组和假针刺组分别进行干预，观察两组受试者针刺后10 min（主要结局）及0、5、15、20、30、45、60 min的响应率[响应率定义为疼痛视觉模拟量表（visual analogue scale，VAS）评分较基线下降至少50%的受试者比例]，以及补救性镇痛和不良事件。得出结论：与假针刺组相比，针刺联合肌肉注射双氯芬酸在紧急情况下对肾绞痛患者是安全的，并能快速有效缓解疼痛；在减少镇痛药使用

二 专家述评（针灸学专家，临床研究方法学及卫生统计学专家）

1. 述评一

虽然AIs在临床乳腺癌治疗中的有效性已被证明，但是有50%的患者因其相关性关节痛而导致依从性降低。本文从此角度出发，报告了针刺疗法在此类患者中的持续益处。该研究将Ⅰ至Ⅲ期乳腺癌的绝经后妇女（使用芳香化酶抑制剂30天及以上）随机分为针刺组、假针刺组和等待对照组（针刺干预12周，共18次，每次30～45 min；假针刺执行非穴浅刺方案，以52周时的BPI-WP评分为主要结局指标，结果显示：在AIs相关关节痛的绝经后乳腺癌妇女中，与假针刺组或等待对照组相比，针刺干预在缓解关节疼痛方面展现了显著的统计学差异。本研究强调了1年内针刺反应的持久性，以及同时使用假针刺组和等待对照组充分评估针刺干预效果的重要性。鉴于目前药物疗法和非药物疗法治疗AIs相关关节痛的结果不一，且尚未对针刺干预效应的持久性进行观察，本研究的结果证实了针刺在AIs相关关节痛患者中的持续益处，该镇痛机制可能与先前Nature报道的针刺穴位激活迷走神经-肾上腺通路，产生抗炎效应有关。

2. 述评二

（1）研究设计

该研究是多中心、盲法假针刺和等待对照组随机临床试验。按照临床试验报告统一标准（consolidated standards of reporting trials，CONSORT）来报告研究结果，满足拟发表期刊的基本条件。

（2）过程实施

研究开始前，研究方案提前在Clinicaltrials.gov注册。研究方案于研究开始前公布。这是发表高水平临床研究的重要前提条件。

实施过程中，将受试者通过研究点动态平衡随机分为针刺组、假针刺组和等待对照组。针刺组使用不锈钢、一次性、无菌针灸针，并以传统的深度和角度插入。假针刺组的方案包括使用细短针在非传统针刺穴位进行微创、浅针刺的核心标准化处方等。等待对照组在研究参与的前24周内未接受针刺。该研究设置了两个对照组，通过对比，能更好地体现针刺的疗效。

（3）临床研究方法学和统计方法

该研究的主要结局指标是52周时的BPI-WP评分结果。样本量基于主要结局指标来确定。该研究的主要假设是与假针刺组或等待对照组相比，针刺能在52周时减轻AIs相关关节疼痛。所有次要分析或事后分析均未被视为探索性分析，进行多重比较调整。在意向治疗原则下，使用了所有可评估的52周评分结果，即使对照组患者在24

7. 内容简介：本研究为一项多中心、盲法假针刺和等待对照随机临床试验，旨在探讨对于芳香化酶抑制剂（aromatase inhibitors，AIs）相关关节疼痛的患者（原发性浸润性乳腺癌Ⅰ、Ⅱ、Ⅲ期），针刺疗法在减少疼痛方面是否比假针刺和等待对照组的治疗效果更佳。研究将226例患者按2∶1∶1随机分为针刺组、假针刺组和等待对照组分别进行干预，观察3组患者在第52周的简明疼痛量表-最严重疼痛（brief pain inventory-worst pain，BPI-WP）评分。得出结论：接受12周针刺治疗的患有AIs相关关节疼痛的女性，在52周时相比假针刺组和等待对照组的女性，其疼痛感有所减轻，表明针刺疗法对这类患者具有长期益处。

针刺组与假针刺组均接受为期12周干预，前6周每周进行2次治疗，随后的6周每周进行1次治疗。所有患者均获得了10次针刺治疗的优惠券（包括标准化的体针和耳穴治疗），可在第24～52周时使用。

针刺组针刺时，所有穴位均先用酒精擦拭消毒，随后根据标准穴位位置进行针刺，以产生"得气"感。留针时间为20～25 min，期间再次行针，重新产生"得气"感。对于仰卧位难以触及的关节特定穴位，可完成第一次针刺（对仰卧位状态下可施针的穴位行针）后，根据实际情况以适当的深度和角度再进行针刺，产生"得气"感，并留针10 min。治疗过程中不使用电刺激。体穴：外关（TE5）、足临泣（GB41）、阳陵泉（GB34）、合谷（LI4）、解溪（ST41）、太溪（KI3）。耳穴：神门（TF4）、肾（CO10）、肝（CO12）、肺（CO14）、交感（AH6a）。关节特定穴位：①膝，阴陵泉（SP9）、血海（SP10）、梁丘（ST34）；②手指，后溪（SI3）、八邪（EX-UE9）、三间（LI3）；③腰部，腰阳关（GV3）、筋缩（GV8）、肾俞（BL23）；④肩部，肩髃（LI15）、肩髎（TE14）、臑俞（SI10）；⑤臀部，环跳（GB30）、悬钟（GB39）；⑥手腕，阳谷（SI5）、阳池（TE4）、阳溪（LI5）。

假针刺为非传统穴位的浅层针刺。假针刺方案包括对身体、关节及耳部的假穴位进行浅层针刺干预。身体假穴方案：①假穴1，位于左前臂外侧，近肘部，当尺骨鹰嘴下3寸，小肠经前0.5寸；②假穴2，位于右前臂外侧，近肘部，当尺骨鹰嘴下3寸，小肠经前0.5寸；③假穴3，位于左胫骨内侧髁下方，肝经膝关（LR7）前上1寸；④假穴4，位于右胫骨内侧髁下方，肝经膝关（LR7）前上1寸。耳部假穴方案：①耳假穴1，位于耳郭5号点和6号点之间的耳郭上；②耳假穴2，位于耳郭4号点和3号点之间的耳郭上；③耳假穴3，位于耳郭耳轮上，耳尖与耳轮1号点之间。关节特定假穴方案：①膝，位于假穴3、假穴4上2寸；②手指/手腕，位于左、右前臂外侧，近肘部，当尺骨鹰嘴下5寸，小肠经前0.5寸处；③腰椎，位于背部，当胸椎第8节，脊椎正中5寸，膀胱经外经2寸（双侧进针）；④肩，位于左右臂外侧，肘上，尺骨鹰嘴上3寸，小肠经前0.5寸处；⑤臀部，位于大腿，髌骨上约4寸，胆经前1寸处。

等待对照组患者可根据需要，选择服用对乙酰氨基酚和非甾体抗炎药来缓解关节不适症状。这些用药情况将在预定的时间点进行记录，并填写在补充药物报告表中。

（2）临床研究方法学及统计学方法的选择及应用

该研究的主要结局是治疗第4周的有效应答率，次要结局包括其他时间点的综合缓解率、症状严重程度、生活质量、抑郁症状和不良反应等，提供了多维度的数据以全面评估针刺的疗效和安全性。采用了意向性治疗分析，且进行了符合研究方案分析，两种分析方法的结果具有一致性。此外，该研究采用了末次观测值结转法对缺失数据进行了填补。对于主要结局，研究采用了广义线性混合模型处理患者在不同时间点的重复测量数据，考虑了个体的变异性和时间效应；对于次要结局和盲法质量的评估，根据数据类型选择了适当的统计学方法，包括方差分析、卡方检验等。

该研究的研究设计和统计分析较为科学且严谨，然而，还有一些局限性需要注意。首先，该研究是预试验，样本量未经严格估计，研究结果可为今后大规模的研究提供参考数据，但可能无法得到确认性结果；其次，虽然包括了8周的随访，但针刺对IBS-D的长期疗效和持续性仍不明确；另外，研究参与者均为中国人，限制了结果在其他国家和种族中的普适性；最后，许多结局指标依赖患者自我报告，可能受到主观偏差和期望效应的影响。

第二十二节 "Comparison of Acupuncture vs Sham Acupuncture or Waiting List Control in the Treatment of Aromatase Inhibitor-Related Joint Pain: A Randomized Clinical Trial" 相关介绍和述评

一 论文介绍

1. 中文题目：针刺对比假针刺或等待对照组治疗芳香化酶抑制剂相关关节疼痛的随机临床试验

2. 作者：Dawn L. Hershman, Joseph M. Unger, Heather Greenlee, Jillian Capodice, Danika L. Lew, Amy Darke, Lori M. Minasian, Michael J. Fisch, N. Lynn Henry, Katherine D. Crew

3. 主要单位：Columbia University Irving Medical Center; Fred Hutchinson Cancer Center; SWOG Statistics and Data Management Center

4. 发表期刊：*JAMA Network Open*

5. 发布日期：2022年11月11日

6. SCI源文献：HERSHMAN D L, UNGER J M, GREENLEE H, et al. Comparison of Acupuncture vs Sham Acupuncture or Waiting List Control in the Treatment of Aromatase Inhibitor-related Joint Pain: A Randomized Clinical Trial [J]. JAMA Netw Open, 2022, 5 (11): e2241720.

位中的1个）进行针刺。固定穴位有天枢（ST25）、中脘（CV12）、关元（CV4）、足三里（ST36）、上巨虚（ST37）。针灸师再根据患者的中医辨证选择相应穴位，如肝郁脾虚证选用太冲（LR3），脾虚湿阻证选用三阴交（SP6），脾胃湿热证选用内庭（ST44）。

NSA组的6个固定穴位是水分（CV9）、梁门（ST21）、阴交（CV7）、条口（ST38）、阴市（ST33）、漏谷（SP7）。进针后，使用提插法和捻转法，使患者产生"得气感"（酸、麻、胀或放射的感觉）。

NA组使用钝头安慰针，其外观与传统针相似，选择5个远离经络或常规穴位的非穴位置，进行未穿透皮肤的假针刺操作。

二 专家述评（针灸学专家，临床研究方法学及卫生统计学专家）

1. 述评一

IBS是一种以腹痛、腹胀、排便习惯改变和（或）大便性状异常为主要临床表现的功能性胃肠疾病。IBS-D是临床最常见IBS亚型，多以止泻药和解痉药作为一线疗法。但是，服用药物仅能暂时缓解单一症状，且副作用频发，长期服药增加心血管疾病等不良事件的发生率，导致患者治疗满意度较低，很多患者选择停药。本研究采用下合穴、募穴等特定穴配伍，多中心随机对照临床研究，客观评价合募配穴治疗腑病的有效性和安全性，为针刺治疗肠腑病症的腧穴配伍原则提供循证医学证据，其技术可临床推广与应用。

该研究在针刺治疗IBS-D的临床研究中采用美国食品药品监督管理局（food and drug administration，FDA）推荐的有效应答率作为主要结局，在国内4家三甲医院进行多中心随机对照临床试验，将90例IBS-D患者按照1:1:1的比例随机分为3组，包括2个针刺组（SA组、NSA组）和1个假针刺组（NA组）。所有患者接受每周3次，连续4周，共计12次治疗。主要结局为第4周最严重腹痛评分至少减少30%，以及6型或7型大便天数减少50%以上的患者比例。结果显示，SA组（有效应答率为46.7%）与NSA组（有效应答率为46.7%）均显示具有临床意义的改善，但3组间差异无统计学意义；SA组患者整体症状缓解与生活质量提高等次要结局表现出更稳定的疗效趋势。

2. 述评二

（1）研究设计和过程实施

该研究是一项多中心、随机对照预试验，旨在检验采用FDA推荐的主要结局评价针刺治疗IBS-D疗效的可行性。研究设计严谨，采用了随机化、患者和评估者双盲、多组对照设计，确保了结果的可靠性，并减少了偏倚。患者被随机分配到3组（SA组、NSA组、NA组），并在4家三级医院进行，增强了结果的外部效度。干预措施详尽，每组的针刺方法和针刺点选择都有明确的说明，有助于研究的可重复性。

第二十一节 "Acupuncture for the Treatment of Diarrhea-Predominant Irritable Bowel Syndrome: A Pilot Randomized Clinical Trial" 相关介绍和述评

一、论文介绍

1. 中文题目：针刺治疗腹泻型肠易激综合征的随机对照临床预试验

2. 作者：Ling-Yu Qi, Jing-Wen Yang, Shi-Yan Yan, Jian-Feng Tu, Yan-Fen She, Ying Li, Li-Li Chi, Bang-Qi Wu, Cun-Zhi Liu

3. 主要单位：北京中医药大学针灸推拿学院，国际针灸创新研究院；河北中医药大学针灸推拿学院；成都中医药大学研究生院

4. 发表期刊：*JAMA Network Open*

5. 发布日期：2022年12月29日

6. SCI源文献：QI L Y, YANG J W, YAN S Y, et al. Acupuncture for the Treatment of Diarrhea-Predominant Irritable Bowel Syndrome: A Pilot Randomized Clinical Trial [J]. JAMA Netw Open, 2022, 5 (12): e2248817.

7. 内容简介：本研究为多中心随机临床试验。为了探索对于肠易激综合征（irritable bowel syndrome, IBS）患者，针刺在减少最严重腹痛评分方面是否比假针刺的效果好，将90例腹泻型IBS（diarrhea-predominant IBS, IBS-D）患者随机分为3组，包括2个针刺组［特异性穴位（specific acupoints, SA）组和非特异性穴位（nonspecific acupoints, NSA）组］和1个假针刺组［非经非穴（non-acupoints, NA）组］进行干预，观察3组有效应答率（最严重腹痛评分减少至少30%且6型或7型大便天数减少至少50%）。得出结论：SA组和NSA组均显示出对IBS-D症状有临床意义的改善，但3组间差异无统计学意义；提示针刺治疗IBS-D是可行的、安全的，但需要更大的、足够效能的试验来评估疗效。

3组治疗频次均为每周3次（理想情况下每隔1天1次），每次30 min，连续4周（12次）。治疗由具有5年针灸本科教育、至少3年临床经验的认证针灸师进行。每位针灸师都接受了为期2天的培训，可以对所有组进行治疗，并尽可能在整个试验过程中优先考虑同一位针灸师为固定患者提供治疗。洛哌丁胺被用作急救药物。鼓励患者在整个试验过程中避免使用药物或其他疗法来管理IBS。

针刺（SA组、NSA组）使用一次性无菌针（针长25～40 mm，直径0.30 mm）。所有受试者的穴位上都放置了胶垫，目的是帮助假针刺NA组患者最大限度地致盲并固定钝头安慰针。

SA组根据辨证诊断和特定穴位匹配原则，在6个穴位（5个固定穴位和3个可选穴

妇快速康复、提升生活质量及优化医疗资源分配具有重大意义。鉴于镇痛药物使用的严格限制，寻求非药物性镇痛手段显得尤为重要。

针刺疗法作为一种非药物、低风险的镇痛手段，其独特的优势在于能够减少药物依赖，降低不良反应的发生率，并促进机体自身的调节能力。近年来将针刺疗法应用于围手术期镇痛的各种临床研究层出不穷，针刺镇痛的疗效在国际上得到了广泛认可，并逐渐成为术后疼痛管理的重要一环。其非药物特性尤其契合对药物使用有严格限制或偏好的产妇群体，从而在剖宫产术后疼痛管理领域展现出独到的优势与高度的合理性。

在针刺疗法的临床研究中，安慰组的合理设置是确保研究结果科学性与准确性的关键环节。鉴于针刺治疗的复杂性和多样性，研究者需综合考虑安慰针刺的可操作性、安全性、盲法实现难度及治疗效应最小化等因素。本研究采用耳针与皮内针相结合的针刺方法，旨在通过其简便的操作流程、高安全性及持续稳定的刺激量实现干预的标准化与盲法的有效实施。同时，通过在安慰针刺操作前使用工具使受试者产生真实痛感以增强安慰剂效应，确保盲法的成功实施，从而更准确地评估针刺治疗的真实疗效。

2. 述评二

（1）研究设计和过程实施

该研究采用单中心、安慰剂对照、患者和评估者双盲设计，并包含一个额外的非随机对照组，确保了研究结果的可靠性和可重复性，且提供了对照常规治疗效果的基线比较。研究采用密封信封法进行随机分组，随机分组和干预实施由具有经验的3位针灸师负责。此设计保证了随机化的隐蔽性和结果的盲评，减少了选择偏倚和信息偏倚。针刺组和安慰剂组的干预措施设计严谨，使用了安慰针和神经笔，以确保对照组和实验组患者在感官体验上的一致性，从而有效控制安慰剂效应。

（2）临床研究方法学及统计学方法的选择及应用

该研究的主要结局是术后第一天运动时的疼痛强度，使用VRS-11进行测量，该量表简单易用，有效地量化了疼痛强度；次要结局包括多种疼痛和功能恢复指标及不良反应，全面评估了针刺的有效性和安全性。样本量计算基于功效分析和显著性水平，确保了统计效力。研究采用意向性治疗分析，即所有随机分组的患者均纳入最终分析，确保了随机化原则，减少偏倚。组间比较根据数据类型选择了适当的统计学检验方法，包括 t 检验、Mann-Whitney 检验等。这项研究在研究设计和统计学方法选择上均表现出较高的科学性和严谨性，随机分配、多组对照、双盲实施及意向性治疗分析等应用确保了研究结果的有效性和可靠性，但仍存在一些局限性，包括研究在单一医疗中心进行，可能限制了结果的外部效度和广泛应用；研究主要关注术后第一天的疼痛强度和其他短期结局，并未对长期效果进行评估等。

者术后第一天运动时的疼痛强度［采用11项口头评分量表（11-item verbal rating scale，VRS-11）进行测量］，术后第一天最大、最小疼痛强度及出院当天运动时疼痛强度，镇痛相关不良反应，镇痛药用量，活动时间和Foley导尿管拔除时间，患者随机分组的盲法质量和患者对疼痛治疗的满意度。得出结论：与安慰剂组和非随机常规护理组相比，针刺在减轻剖宫产术后疼痛和加速患者剖宫产术后活动方面是安全有效的；考虑人员和时间成本，针刺可以推荐作为择期剖宫产后患者疼痛控制的常规补充疗法。

针刺组患者均接受留置皮内针的耳穴和体针治疗，当一名医师向患者概述干预措施时，另一名医师根据试验方案对双侧4个耳穴和双侧6个体穴进行针刺。4个耳穴包括：神门（TF4）、肾（CO10）、肺（CO14）、皮质下（AT4）。耳穴针刺使用留置固定针（New Pyonex；Seirin Corp；长度1.5 mm，直径0.2 mm）。6个体穴包括：合谷（LI4）、足三里（ST36）、三阴交（SP6）、大肠俞（BL25）、关元俞（BL26）、小肠俞（BL27）。体针使用皮内针（长度6 mm，直径0.14 mm），使用和安慰剂组相同的针头覆盖和固定。这些针头似于耳针，但仅由塑料旋钮和没有针的自粘胶带组成，看起来与安慰剂组相同。医师指导患者通过按摩刺激耳针和合谷3~5 min，如果感到疼痛，则患者可要求额外的镇痛药物，这种疼痛强度必须在VRS-11评分中高于4分。

安慰剂组患者使用非穿透性安慰针治疗，将安慰针贴在特定穴位附近。为了模仿真实针刺的刺痛感，医师在使用安慰剂针时用SVESA神经笔（通常在针刺实践中用于识别皮肤阻力较低的区域）细的尖端对皮肤施加一定的压力，就会产生针刺感。医师会告诉患者神经笔是用来找穴位，但实际上是用笔尖产生压力。

针刺组的针刺针和安慰剂组的安慰针均在脊髓麻醉前放置，剖宫产术后针头仍在原位放置3天。所有干预措施需在剖宫产前20 min内完成，在使用针刺或安慰针后，患者立即被转移至手术室，接受标准治疗方案。

常规治疗组仅接受标准治疗方案、无额外干预。

标准治疗方案：剖宫产前接受标准化脊髓麻醉，即7.5 mg盐酸丁哌卡因+5 μg枸橼酸舒芬太尼，其可在术后最多4 h内提供足够的镇痛作用。根据当地临床指南制定的标准，术后镇痛方案为口服对乙酰氨基酚1 g，每天4次，必要时辅以双氯芬酸钾50 mg，口服，每天3次。在镇痛不足的情况下，皮下注射7.5 mg哌腈米特（一种阿片类药物，效力为吗啡的70%），每天最多6次。

二　专家述评（针灸学专家，临床研究方法学及卫生统计学专家）

1. 述评一

剖宫产术后疼痛管理因其对产妇康复进程、生活质量及医疗资源利用效率的深远影响，已成为临床实践中亟待解决的关键问题。实施有效的疼痛管理策略对于促进产

2. 述评二

在研究设计和过程实施方面，该研究采用单中心、随机、双盲设计，评估真针刺相较于假针刺对于缓解帕金森病患者焦虑症状的有效性。样本量计算基于预试验调查证据，样本量满足要求与试验设计的有效性，研究切实可行。研究结果报告流程同时遵循临床试验报告统一标准（consolidated standards of reporting trials，CONSORT）和针刺临床试验干预措施报告标准（standards for reporting interventions in clinical trials of acupuncture，STRICTA），确保了研究结论的可靠性。

在临床研究方法及统计学方法的选择及应用方面，本研究关注的主要结局为真针刺组和假针刺组关于HAMA得分在治疗后、治疗后随访8周的改变量的组间差异。分析策略上，该研究通过构建广义线性回归模型，引入组别与随访时间的交互项来检验两组HAMA得分在不同时期相较于基线的改变量是否存在组间差异，统计学方法可行、有效。此外，该研究除报告传统的组间均数差以外，也同时报告Cohen's d等量化组间差异的指标，从指标计算层面对研究结果的可靠性提供了双重保障。

第二十节 "Effectiveness of Acupuncture for Pain Control After Cesarean Delivery: A Randomized Clinical Trial" 相关介绍和述评

一 论文介绍

1．中文题目：针刺对剖宫产术后疼痛控制的有效性：一项随机临床试验

2．作者：Taras I. Usichenko, Berthold Johannes Henkel, Catharina Klausenitz, Thomas Hesse, Guillermo Pierdant, Mike Cummings, Klaus Hahnenkamp

3．主要单位：Department of Anesthesiology, University Medicine of Greifswald, Greifswald, Germany; Department of Anesthesia, McMaster University, Hamilton, Ontario, Canada; Department of Radiology, University Medicine of Greifswald, Greifswald, Germany

4．发表期刊：*JAMA Network Open*

5．发布日期：2022年2月28日

6．SCI源文献：USICHENKO T I, HENKEL B J, KLAUSENITZ C, et al. Effectiveness of Acupuncture for Pain Control After Cesarean Delivery: A Randomized Clinical Trial [J]. JAMA Netw Open, 2022, 5 (2): e220517.

7．内容简介：本研究为单中心、安慰剂对照、患者和评估者双盲的随机临床试验，为了探索针刺治疗剖宫产术后疼痛患者疼痛症状的有效性，将120例受试者随机分为针刺组、安慰剂组，另外非随机选择60例受试者作为常规治疗组，观察3组受试

刺组和假针刺组，分别治疗，观察两组受试者治疗前后汉密尔顿焦虑量表（Hamilton anxiety scale，HAMA）、统一帕金森病评定量表（unified Parkimson's disease rating scale，UPDRS）、39项帕金森病生存质量调查问卷（39-item Parkinson's disease questionnaire，PDQ-39）及血清促肾上腺皮质激素（adrenocorticotropic hormone，ACTH）和皮质醇（cortisol，CORT）水平。得出结论：与假针刺相比，针刺对帕金森病患者焦虑症有一定疗效，并可以改善患者的健康状况。

真针刺组和假针刺组治疗频次均为每周3次，每次30 min，持续8周。

真针刺组：根据中医理论和先前有关帕金森病和焦虑症的文献记录，选用固定处方，即神庭（GV24）、印堂（EX-HN3）、双侧神门（HT7）、双侧三阴交（SP6）和四神针。其中，四神针由百会（GV20）前、后、左、右各旁开1.5寸的4个穴位组成。使用一次性无菌不锈钢针（0.25 mm×25 mm，0.25 mm×40 mm）进行针刺，进针后，以180~200转/分的频率捻针1 min，随后留针30 min。

假针刺组：使用特殊的一次性、无菌不锈钢针，在与真针刺组相同的穴位上进行非刺入性模拟针刺，进针后，以180~200转/分的频率捻针1 min，随后留针30 min。

二 专家述评（针灸学专家，临床研究方法学及卫生统计学专家）

1. 述评一

帕金森病作为一种神经系统退行性疾病，可并发一系列相关症状，这些症状严重影响患者的生活质量，并促进病情的进展。如何发挥针刺优势，有效治疗这些并发症，得到业界肯定并推广应用意义重大。对此，广州中医药大学针灸研究团队取得了显著进展。

该团队研究聚焦帕金森病并发症中发生率高、药物疗效尚不确切的焦虑症这一现代医学治疗难点，在针刺应用有效却找不到数据证实其效用这一焦点上着力。以现代医学研究的规范模式，采用规范针刺刺激，以国际公认量表为疗效评定指标，以此肯定针刺治疗可降低帕金森病并发焦虑症患者的焦虑程度，证明针刺可以缓解升高的应激激素水平以减轻焦虑。研究线路清晰合理。研究遵循中医针刺诊疗规律，选穴处方依据传统中医理论和先前的临床实践。尤其值得称道的是该研究在细节上十分严谨，如所有患者均接受临床监测，特殊装置进针使研究操作者、两组受试者对组别和干预措施一无所知，所有患者的状态评估均由不了解研究设计且不知道患者分类的心理学家完成等；使研究结果可信，结论可靠，由此论文得以在SCI期刊发表，是针刺治疗临床研究的范例。

本研究也暴露出现行针刺研究中一些通病，如完全照搬西医模式研究使得中医个体化治疗难以展示，中医辨证在研究中难以体现等，类似问题尚需业界思考与重视。

何种情况下应单独使用，何种情况下应作为辅助增效手段的信息；③假电针未输出电流，理论上较难对患者实施盲法，尤其对于有针刺经验的中国患者而言。

2. 述评二

研究设计和过程实施方面，为达到评估电针治疗抑郁症患者失眠的疗效的研究目的，研究人员设计了一项多中心、患者-评估者双盲的1∶1∶1随机对照试验，样本量计算依据现有研究设定优效界值、一型错误与统计效能，并在干预试验结束后采用Bang盲法指数验证了盲法实施的有效性，从根本上确定了样本量满足要求与试验设计的有效性，减少潜在的偏倚，提高结果的可靠性，底层设计切实可行。

临床研究方法学及统计方法的选择及应用方面，本研究采用延续最后一次观察的原则对缺失数据进行替换处理，有效避免了样本量的流失。然而，为进一步增强结果的稳健性，建议补充采用更为普遍的多重插补法进行敏感性分析。值得肯定的是，研究严格遵循意向性分析原则构建统计分析数据库，有效应对了试验过程中可能出现的受试者脱落和违反方案等情况。由于试验采用多中心设计，且多次重复测量，数据层次结构特征明显，采用适用于独立性假设不满足情形的混合效应模型进行主要结果数据分析是科学合理的。此外，研究者针对多重比较采用Bonferroni校正，有效控制了一型错误，从统计学角度进一步保障了结果的真实性和可靠性。

第十九节 "Effectiveness of Acupuncture for Anxiety Among Patients With Parkinson Disease: A Randomized Clinical Trial" 相关介绍和述评

一 论文介绍

1. 中文题目：针刺治疗帕金森病患者焦虑症的有效性：一项随机临床试验
2. 作者：Jing-qi Fan, Wei-jing Lu, Wei-qiang Tan, Xin Liu, Yu-ting Wang, Nan-bu Wang, Li-xing Zhuang
3. 主要单位：广州中医药大学，广州中医药大学第一附属医院
4. 发表期刊：*JAMA Network Open*
5. 发布日期：2022年9月21日
6. SCI源文献：FAN J, LU W, TAN W, et al. Effectiveness of Acupuncture for Anxiety Among Patients With Parkinson Disease: A Randomized Clinical Trial [J]. JAMA Netw Open, 2022, 5 (9): e2232133.
7. 内容简介：本研究为单中心、随机、双盲、假对照临床试验。为了观察针刺对帕金森病患者焦虑症的干预效果，将70例帕金森病合并焦虑症患者随机分为真针

周）的匹兹堡睡眠质量指数的变化。得出结论：与假针刺联合标准护理组和仅标准护理组相比，电针组睡眠质量在第8周显著改善，并在第32周持续有效。

3组研究周期均为32周，包括8周的干预期和24周的观察性随访。治疗频率为每周3次，每次留针30 min，持续8周，共24次治疗。研究由6名针灸师（每个中心2名）执行，所有针灸师在试验前均接受了电针（electroacupuncture，EA）和假针刺（sham acupuncture，SA）干预方法的标准化培训。同时，所有患者均接受了由精神科医师指导的标准护理。

电针联合标准护理组常规针刺方法选穴百会（GV20）、神庭（GV24）、印堂（EX-HN3）、安眠（EX-HN22）、神门（HT7）、内关（PC6）和三阴交（SP6），使用0.25 mm×25 mm或0.30 mm×40 mm的真针进行针刺，患者进针后采用捻转或提插手法诱发得气感。随后，将电针仪的2个电极分别连接到百会、印堂处的针柄上，给予连续波，强度以患者耐受程度为准。

假针刺联合标准护理组使用钝头针模拟针刺过程，患者在钝头针接触皮肤时会感受到轻微的刺痛感，但实际上并未刺入皮肤。此外，虽然附近放置了电针仪，但所有参数均设置为0，仅保留指示灯闪烁。

研究人员建议接受标准护理的患者在试验期间进行定期锻炼、保持健康饮食，并控制压力水平。此外，还要求他们定期服用抗抑郁药、镇静剂或安眠药。精神科医师指导所有患者接受标准护理治疗，并在患者病情发生变化时提供专业建议。

二 专家述评（针灸学专家，临床研究方法学及卫生统计学专家）

1. 述评一

失眠是抑郁主症之一，常与抑郁共病，两者相互作用，严重影响患者的身心健康。目前，抗抑郁药、失眠的认知行为疗法及安眠药是指南推荐的有效手段，但面临药物不良反应、认知行为疗法可及性低、患者依从性和认可度有待提高等诸多问题。如何提高疗效、减少药物不良反应是医疗界面临的挑战。电针疗法在改善失眠和抑郁方面具有潜在疗效，但证据不足，尤其是针对失眠和抑郁共病的研究较少。该试验的目的是评价电针对失眠与抑郁共病患者睡眠障碍的改善效果，切入点明确，目标清晰。主要结局指标是国际公认的匹兹堡睡眠质量指数较基线的变化值，辅之以体动议记录的客观睡眠状况评价及抑郁焦虑程度评价，这能够有效反映电针对此类患者睡眠质量的改善效果。设置假电针对照是为了明确电针的净治疗效应，除外非特异性效应；标准护理对照可以显示电针疗法的临床价值。对试验结果的解读较为合理，表明为期8周的电针对失眠与抑郁共病的患者而言是较为有效和安全的。然而，该研究也存在一些不足之处：①基线未记录患者的抑郁程度及分类，亦缺乏抗抑郁药物使用情况的数据，因此无法判断患者的抑郁程度及药物使用是否对电针疗效产生影响；②未提供电针在

此人群仅占CD患者的1/3～2/3。加之大部分受试者不了解针灸，一周3次的针灸治疗时间也难以保证，这无疑增加了受试者的招募难度和研究的实施难度。

最后，投稿最初目标期刊为消化领域的顶刊 Gastroenterology。尽管投稿后编辑对本研究的创新性给予了肯定，并顺利送交外审，3位审稿专家提出了诸多宝贵意见。遗憾的是，由于期刊年发表量有限，最终综合考虑审稿专家的意见后，本研究被退稿了。随后，重新选定了综合性期刊柳叶刀子刊 eClinicalMedicine 作为投稿目标，并在2022年历经多轮修改后，最终顺利被录用。

回顾本研究整个过程，首先要在研究设计上潜心钻研，找准切入点。其次，要严格把控实施过程，注重细节。最后成果产出的过程中要细心慎重，反复推敲论证。总之，规范化研究是确保产出高质量的成果的重要因素之一。

吴焕淦
上海市针灸经络研究所

第十八节 "Effect of Electroacupuncture on Insomnia in Patients With Depression: A Randomized Clinical Trial" 相关介绍和述评

一、论文介绍

1. 中文题目：电针对抑郁症患者失眠的影响：一项随机临床试验

2. 作者：Xuan Yin, Wei Li, Tingting Liang, Bing Lu, Hongyu Yue, Shanshan Li, Victor W. Zhong, Wei Zhang, Xia Li, Shuang Zhou, Yiqun Mi, Huangan Wu, Shifen Xu

3. 主要单位：上海中医药大学附属市中医医院，复旦大学基础医学院，上海市第一人民医院嘉定分院

4. 发表期刊：JAMA Network Open

5. 发布日期：2022年7月7日

6. SCI源文献：YIN X, LI W, LIANG T, et al. Effect of electroacupuncture on insomnia in patients with depression: A randomized clinical trial [J]. JAMA Netw Open, 2022, 5 (7): e2220563.

7. 内容简介：本研究为双盲、随机、假对照临床试验，旨在探讨对于失眠与抑郁共病患者，电针疗法相较于假针刺和标准护理，在改善其睡眠质量和精神状态方面的有效性和安全性。研究纳入年龄为18～70岁、患有失眠症且符合《精神疾病诊断与统计手册》（第五版）中抑郁症分类标准的患者。将患者随机分为3组，即电针联合标准护理组、假针刺联合标准护理组及仅标准护理组，观察3组患者在干预结束时（第8

疗效评价和机制研究，为常规药物治疗反应不佳的轻中度活动性CD提供了一种安全、有效的治疗手段。

2. 述评二

（1）研究设计和过程实施

本研究评估了针刺治疗CD的疗效，并探讨其作用机制。研究团队采用多中心随机对照试验的方式开展研究，按照1∶1的比例将研究对象随机分为针灸组和假针灸组。两组受试者均接受每周3次的治疗，连续12周，随后进行36周的随访。在研究过程中，采用了盲法设计，不仅对研究对象设盲，还对针灸师、结局指标评估人员和统计学分析人员设盲。本研究的主要结局为治疗完成时的临床缓解率，次要结局为受试者在第24、36和48周的临床缓解率，C反应蛋白水平变化及CD内镜严重程度指数评分等。研究结果显示，针灸对活动性CD患者具有缓解和维持缓解的作用，其机制可能与促进肠道抗炎细菌的增多、增强肠道屏障功能等有关。研究思路清晰，设计合理，研究内容涉及疗效评价和机制探索，内容方面较为全面。

（2）临床研究方法学及统计方法的选择及应用

该临床研究为多中心的RCT研究，采用合理的样本量估算，确保了每组至少包含33例受试者。研究中对多个环节的研究者和研究对象设置盲法，并在研究结束时对研究对象开展了盲法猜测的调查，以评估本研究中盲法开展的可靠性。研究在统计分析上完全遵循意向性分析原则，将统计分析数据集分为意向性分析数据集和符合方案性数据集，两者相互验证。在本研究中，研究者对针刺的作用机制也做了大量的探索工作，开展生物信息学分析工作尝试探索相关细胞因子的调节作用。这些工作的开展不仅稳健地评估了针灸治疗的临床效果，还在一定程度上探索了针灸疗效产生的相关机制。

三 作者谈

本研究从构思到最终发表历经7年之久，在研究选题、临床实施及投稿等多个环节存在难点。首先，本设计与实施是基于团队先前发表的文章 *Randomized controlled trial: Moxibustion and acupuncture for the treatment of Crohn's disease*（*World J Gastroenterol*，2014）进行的。由于前期研究已评价了针灸治疗活动期CD患者的临床疗效与安全性，本研究势必要重新选题，力求从新的角度开展研究。

其次，在临床实施中，最困难的问题在于受试者的纳入速度。研究共纳入66例患者，但这一过程从首例患者入组至完成所有患者入组，持续了5年。审稿专家也指出了纳入周期较长的问题。这主要是因为CD发病率较低，近年来CD发病率和患病率在我国也急速攀升，但总患病率仍然较低。此外，本研究选择了CD药物响应不佳的人群，

床缓解的患者比例，定义为CD活动指数（CD activity index，CDAI）评分＜150分，且CDAI评分较基线下降≥70分。得出结论：与假针灸相比，针灸对活动期CD患者诱导和维持缓解有效，这一疗效可能与增加肠道抗炎细菌的丰度、增强肠道屏障功能以及调节循环Th1/Th17相关细胞因子的水平有关。

两组研究周期均为48周，包括12周的干预期和36周的观察性随访。治疗频率为每周3次，持续12周。

针灸组针刺选穴中脘（CV12），双侧上巨虚（ST37）、三阴交（SP6）、公孙（SP4）、太冲（LR3）、太溪（KI3）、合谷（LI4）、曲池（LI11）。在治疗过程中，采用一次性0.30 mm×40 mm或0.30 mm×25 mm针灸针，垂直刺入每个穴位20～30 mm，以得气为度（酸、胀、麻或沉重感）。艾灸选穴双侧足三里（ST36）和天枢（ST25），操作时将纯艾条点燃并固定在艾灸架上，使艾条距离穴位表面3～5 cm，确保穴位处皮肤表面的温度保持在43±1℃。针刺与艾灸治疗同步进行，每次持续30 min。

假针灸组使用平头假针（0.35 mm×40 mm）模拟真实针刺过程，刺入和针灸组相同的穴位，仅引起轻微疼痛，不刺入皮肤。假艾灸则是点燃与真艾灸同类型的艾条，但将艾条固定在距离穴位皮肤8～10 cm处，使穴位处皮肤表面温度维持在（37±1）℃。假针刺与假艾灸同样同步进行，每次持续30 min。

二　专家述评（针灸学专家，临床研究方法学及卫生统计学专家）

1. 述评一

药物疗法是多数疾病的常规治疗方案，而药物疗效不佳、药物耐受或者药物本身的副作用，都是针灸有可能发挥作用的切入点。必须结合针灸疗法本身特点，分析、验证针灸在药效替代、协同增效、协助减药、减少药物副作用等方面的作用或优势，提供高水平循证证据、阐明针灸作用机制，促进针灸融入现代医学体系。而本研究聚焦解决对常规药物治疗反应不佳的轻中度活动性CD患者，是一个很好的实践示范，明确12周针灸治疗可能通过调节肠道微生物组成和Th1/Th17细胞介导的炎症改善CD患者的疾病活动性。研究发现，针灸效应在治疗结束后可维持9个月，这也是针灸疗法作用优势的重要方面，即针灸是通过激活内源性保护机制发挥作用，因此即便治疗结束，依然可以看到效应的持续。

本研究的干预措施采用针刺与灸法联用。目前大多数高影响因子针灸临床评价研究均采用电针对比假电针。但在国内临床实践中，针与灸的联用非常普遍，因此这一干预措施设计对临床有更大的指导意义。同时，采用假针刺联合假艾灸实现有效对照，并充分报告了实施细节，这一模式值得借鉴推广。

综上所述，该研究针对药物疗法有短板的临床问题，开展了高质量的假对照针灸

（2）临床研究方法学及统计学方法的选择及应用

该临床研究为单中心的随机对照试验，研究对象在知情同意后被区组随机分为足三里电针疗法+标准护理组、天枢电针疗法+标准护理组和单独标准护理组（对照组），区组大小为6或9。研究团队通过随机分组平衡了不同干预组间研究对象的基线特征均衡性，确保在基线时接受不同干预的研究对象特征一致，便于评价干预措施的疗效。同时，研究采用区组随机分组，在一定程度上保障了不同组间研究对象样本量的一致性。由于本研究是3组设计的随机对照试验，该研究在样本量估算中将α调整为双侧0.025。在首要结局指标的评价上，研究团队采用生存分析的方法对结局指标进行评估，同时将 t 检验的分析结果作为敏感性分析结果。同时，本研究也采用了意向性分析原则，并对缺失数据进行了合理地填补，这些措施都保障了研究结果的可靠性和稳定性。

第十七节 "Acupuncture Improves the Symptoms, Intestinal Microbiota, and Inflammation of Patients With Mild to Moderate Crohn's Disease: A Randomized Controlled Trial" 相关介绍和述评

一 论文介绍

1. 中文题目：针灸可改善轻至中度克罗恩病患者的症状、肠道微生物群和炎症反应：一项随机对照试验

2. 作者：Chunhui Bao, Luyi Wu, Di Wang, Liming Chen, Xiaoming Jin, Yin Shi, Guona Li, Jingzhi Zhang, Xiaoqing Zeng, Jianhua Chen, Huirong Liu, Huangan Wu

3. 主要单位：上海中医药大学附属岳阳中西医结合医院；国家中医药管理局针灸免疫效应重点研究室；Department of Anatomy and Cell Biology, Stark Neurosciences Research Institute, Indiana University School of Medicine

4. 发表期刊：*eClinicalMedicine*

5. 发布日期：2022年2月12日

6. SCI源文献：BAO C, WU L, WANG D, et al. Acupuncture improves the symptoms, intestinal microbiota, and inflammation of patients with mild to moderate Crohn's disease: A randomized controlled trial [J]. EClinicalMedicine, 2022, 45: 101300.

7. 内容简介：本研究为随机、假对照、平行组临床试验，旨在探讨针灸对于药物反应不佳的轻度和中度活动性克罗恩病（Crohn's disease，CD）患者的有效性和安全性，并深入研究针灸对CD患者肠道微生物群和循环炎症标志物的影响。研究纳入66例患者，随机分配至针灸组或假针灸组分别进行干预，主要结局为完成治疗时达到临

单独标准护理组，即对照组，只采用标准化的术后管理。

二 专家述评（针灸学专家，临床研究方法学及卫生统计学专家）

1. 述评一

POI的管理是腹腔镜结直肠手术后常见且棘手的问题。POI会延长住院时间，增加医疗费用和再入院率，对患者的身心健康产生负面影响。既往有大量研究证实，电针可以促进胃肠道排空功能的恢复，但是缺乏对针刺在围手术期领域的应用。该研究探讨电针干预对POI的影响，旨在为腹腔镜结直肠手术快速康复管理中提供一种安全有效的非药物治疗手段。这将为针刺疗法在现代医学体系中的应用提供重要的支撑证据。

研究目的包括：①比较电针足三里和天枢这两个穴位在改善POI方面是否有疗效差别；②验证电针对于腹腔镜结直肠手术中能促进术后肠功能恢复这一假说。因此研究设足三里电针疗法+标准护理组、天枢电针疗法+标准护理组和单独标准护理组。电针组患者从术后第一天起，每日接受一次30 min电针治疗，持续4天或直至出院。标准护理组仅接受常规管理，以排除其他影响肠功能恢复的因素。结果显示，与单独标准护理组相比，足三里电针疗法+标准护理组在术后首次排气和排便时间显著缩短，而天枢电针疗法+标准护理组与单独标准护理组差异不显著，表明足三里在加速肠功能恢复方面更具优势。足三里电针疗法+标准护理组在液体和半流质饮食耐受时间上显示出优势。治疗过程中无严重不良事件。

本研究结果表明，足三里电针治疗可显著加速术后肠功能恢复，具有重要的临床应用潜力。本研究设计严谨，取穴少，针刺干预的实施细节明确。研究结果不仅证实了电针足三里的疗效，也为穴位的特异性提供了支撑证据。

2. 述评二

（1）研究设计和过程实施

本研究评估了针刺对腹腔镜下选择性结直肠手术后POI的治疗效果。该研究是一项单中心、三臂、前瞻性、随机对照试验，纳入了因结直肠癌接受选择性手术后POI的患者105例。患者被随机分为3组：足三里电针疗法+标准护理组、天枢电针疗法+标准护理组和仅接受标准治疗的对照组，并接受对应的干预措施干预。研究的主要结局是双结局指标（术后首次排气和排便时间），只有当这两个结局指标都有统计学意义时方可判定治疗有效。研究结果显示，在结直肠癌手术后的恢复期中，足三里穴位的电针疗法联合标准护理能够显著提高肠功能恢复效果。该研究思路清晰，设计合理，结局指标及其有效性的判定方法明确。

第十六节 "Effect of Acupuncture on Postoperative Ileus after Laparoscopic Elective Colorectal Surgery: A Prospective, Randomised, Controlled Trial" 相关介绍和述评

一 论文介绍

1. 中文题目：针刺对腹腔镜下择期结直肠手术后肠梗阻的影响：一项前瞻性、随机、对照试验

2. 作者：Jing-Wen Yang, Jia-Kai Shao, Yu Wang, Qian Liu, Jian-Wei Liang, Shi-Yan Yan, Si-Cheng Zhou, Na-Na Yang, Li-Qiong Wang, Guang-Xia Shi, Wei Pei, Cun-Zhi Liu

3. 主要单位：北京中医药大学针灸推拿学院国际针灸创新研究院，国家癌症中心/国家肿瘤临床研究中心/中国医学科学院北京协和医学院肿瘤医院结直肠外科

4. 发表期刊：*eClinicalMedicine*

5. 发布日期：2022年5月27日

6. SCI源文献：YANG J W, SHAO J K, WANG Y, et al. Effect of acupuncture on postoperative ileus after laparoscopic elective colorectal surgery: A prospective, randomised, controlled trial [J]. EClinicalMedicine, 2022, 49: 101472.

7. 内容简介：本研究为单中心、三臂、前瞻性的随机对照试验。为了探索在常规护理基础上，针刺不同单个穴位对术后肠梗阻（postoperative ileus，POI）的影响。将105例腹腔镜下择期结直肠手术后POI的患者随机（1∶1∶1）分为3组：足三里（ST36）电针疗法＋标准护理组；天枢（ST25）电针疗法＋标准护理组；单独标准护理组，观察3组受试者治疗前后首次排气时间和排便时间。得出结论：与仅接受常规护理相比，足三里电针疗法联合常规护理可显著促进腹腔镜下择期结直肠切除术后结直肠癌患者的肠功能恢复，天枢电针疗法联合常规护理则未显示出相同效果。

这三组患者从术后第一天开始接受标准化的术后管理，包括咀嚼口香糖或使用辅助药物。术后管理基于《加速康复外科中国专家共识暨路径管理指南（2018）》中的结直肠手术部分，包括多模式镇痛、患者控制镇痛加非甾体抗炎药、早期经口进食和早期活动。干预措施连续进行4天或直至出院。如果患者已停止静脉输液、已排便、使用口服镇痛药下地活动并且没有并发症的证据，则患者出院。

试验组，即两个电针疗法组患者除术后标准护理外，分别接受对足三里或天枢进行电针疗法。确定穴位刺入后，行30 s操作以获得得气，然后连接电针，电针刺激持续30 min，疏密波为2/100 Hz。两组的患者每天接受一次电针治疗，干预措施连续进行4天或直至出院。

长期预后。这一发现提示，耳针治疗在改善抑郁症症状方面可能具有潜在疗效，但还需进一步研究以确认其长期效果和稳定性。

在讨论部分，作者深入剖析了可能影响研究结果的因素，如样本量小、治疗周期短及随访丢失率高等，并据此提出了未来研究的改进方向。同时，作者还探讨了耳针治疗抑郁症的可能机制，包括迷走神经激活、下丘脑-垂体-肾上腺轴调节等，为深入理解耳针治疗抑郁症的生物学基础提供了思路。

综上所述，本文为耳针治疗抑郁症的疗效和安全性提供了初步证据。尽管主要结局未达到统计学上的显著差异，但次要结局的积极发现仍令人鼓舞。未来研究应进一步扩大样本量、延长治疗周期和随访时间，并采用更客观的评估工具来验证耳针治疗的长期效果和稳定性。同时，还应深入探讨耳针治疗抑郁症的具体机制，为临床提供更加科学、合理的治疗依据。

2. 述评二

这是一项多中心、随机对照、双盲的临床试验，于2023年3月至4月在巴西圣卡塔琳娜州的4所大学研究中心招募社区患者。研究目的是评价半永久针刺治疗抑郁症的有效性和安全性。试验组接受半永久针刺联合常规治疗，而对照组则接受假针刺联合常规治疗。研究采用PHQ-9问卷进行抑郁症状评估。主要结局为治疗后3个月PHQ-9评分改善50%或以上（即抑郁症康复）的参与者比例。样本量估计如下：假定两组间抑郁症状康复的差异为30%（SA组60%，NSA组30%）。在检验功效为80%、检验水准设为0.05的条件下，每组至少需要36例受试者。考虑到样本脱落，增加10%的样本量，因此每组需招募40例受试者，总计80例。随机化采用1∶1比例进行区组随机化，区组大小随机分配为4、6、8。数据分析采用意向性分析和改良意向性分析，并使用Fisher精确检验来比较两组间抑郁症恢复的比例。研究严格遵循CONSORT和STRICTA指南开展和报道结果，具有规范性。

从304名志愿者中筛选出74例患者进行随机化。意向性分析集中试验组37例、对照组37例。在3个月的主要结局评估时，累计27例患者（36%）失访。基于已搜集的数据，试验组24例患者的抑郁康复比例为58%，对照组23例患者的抑郁康复比例为43%。两组差异无统计学意义（$P=0.38$）所有的次要结局分析中，仅3个月时两组PHQ-9评分<5（抑郁缓解）的比例差异有统计学意义（试验组46%、对照组13%，$P=0.02$）。改良意向性分析和敏感性分析结果相似。两组不良反应与不良事件差异无统计学意义。该研究中，对照组的抑郁康复比例（43%）较样本量估计期望值（30%）高，提示存在安慰剂效应。样本估计时高估了两组间的差异，导致低估所需样本量。此外，实际失访率高于期望失访率。最终，整个研究有效样本量不足可能是未观察到有统计学差异结果的主要原因。

两组每周治疗2次，每次治疗15 min，共治疗6周，两耳交替进行，并指导受试者每天3次手动刺激每个穴位30 s。

SA组的治疗包括根据中医对抑郁症的诊断选择穴位。所有SA组参与者均使用耳郭上的6个预先设定的穴位：神门（TF4）、皮质下（AT4）、心（CO15）、肺（CO14）、肝（CO12）和肾（CO10）。采用EL11设备（NKL）确定穴位的准确位置，使用的半永久针的尺寸0.2 mm×2.5 mm，针刺深度为2.5 mm。

NSA组穴位包括外耳、面部区域及耳轮区域的4个非特异性穴位，这些穴位与精神健康症状无直接关联。使用EL11定位装置确认假针区域不是非神经反应点。对照组使用的针具尺寸为0.2 mm×1.0 mm，旨在实现更浅的针刺深度，针刺深度为1.0 mm。

二 专家述评（针灸学专家，临床研究方法学及卫生统计学专家）

1. 述评一

文章选题聚焦全球广泛关注的抑郁症问题，特别是针对巴西这一高患病率国家，深入探讨了耳针疗法在抑郁症治疗中的潜在价值。选题紧密围绕临床难点和热点问题，具有显著的现实意义和科研价值。抑郁症作为导致全球残疾的主要原因之一，其治疗依从性差、疗效不稳定等问题一直是临床关注的难点。本文旨在通过随机对照试验，科学评估耳针治疗抑郁症的疗效和安全性，为临床提供一种新的治疗选择。

本文在研究方法上严格遵循了科学规范，获得了伦理委员会的批准，并遵循临床试验报告统一标准（consolidated standards of reporting trials，CONSORT）和针刺临床试验干预措施报告标准（standards for reporting interventions in clinical trials of acupuncture，STRICTA），确保研究的科学性和透明度。通过随机化和盲法的应用，有效减少了偏倚，提高了研究结果的可靠性。

在耳针治疗的实施细节上，文章详尽描述了治疗过程，包括耳穴的选择、耳针规格、针刺深度和刺激方法等，充分展示了耳针治疗的合理性和可操作性。神门、皮质下、心、肺、肝、肾均为治疗抑郁症时常用的耳穴。尽管每周两次的治疗频率相较于国内标准较低，但考虑到国外患者的依从性和经济成本，有其一定的合理性。同时，通过设置对照组，采用浅刺非特异性穴位，并尽量避开神经反应点，以进一步验证耳针治疗的特异性疗效。此外，研究还特别强调了针灸师的专业背景，这些经验丰富的针灸师经过标准化培训，确保了耳针治疗的规范性和一致性。

研究结果显示，虽然SA组与NSA组在主要结局（抑郁症康复率）上无显著统计学差异，但SA组在次要结局（抑郁症缓解率）上却表现出明显优势。抑郁症的缓解对患者而言至关重要，其不仅有助于症状的改善，还能促进患者的社会心理功能恢复和

（2）临床研究方法学及统计学方法的选择及应用

采用意向性分析原则，尽可能保证数据分析人群与随机分组人群的一致性。使用线性混合模型对主要结局进行分析。线性混合模型允许数据中的相关性结构被明确建模，同时考虑固定效应和随机效应，从而较好地处理缺失数据，提供更准确的估计。在线性混合模型中，对不同组设置了相同的基线均值，称为约束纵向数据分析模型。与将基线作为协变量的传统模型相比，该模型能够为校正后的均值估计提供更合适的方差估计及可信区间估计。作为探索性分析目的，次要疗效指标的分析不需要考虑多重性问题。

第十五节 "Efficacy and Safety of Auricular Acupuncture for Depression: A Randomized Clinical Trial" 相关介绍和述评

一 论文介绍

1. 中文题目：耳针治疗抑郁症的疗效和安全性：一项随机临床试验

2. 作者：Daniel Maurício de Oliveira Rodrigues, Paulo Rossi Menezes, Ana Elise Machado Ribeiro Silotto, Artur Heps, Nathália Martins Pereira Sanches, Mariana Cabral Schveitzer, Alexandre Faisal-Cury

3. 主要单位：Department of Preventive Medicine, Faculdade de Medicina, Universidade de São PauloSão, Paulo, Brazil; Department of Biological and Health Sciences, University of Southern Santa Catarina, Palhoça, Brazil; Department of Health Sciences, Cruzeiro do Sul University, São Paulo, Brazil

4. 发表期刊：*JAMA Network Open*

5. 发布日期：2023年11月30日

6. SCI源文献：DE OLIVEIRA RODRIGUES D M, MENEZES P R, SILOTTO A E M R, et al. Efficacy and Safety of Auricular Acupuncture for Depression: A randomized clinical trial [J]. JAMA Netw Open, 2023, 6 (11): e2345138.

7. 内容简介：本研究为多中心随机临床试验，旨在评价耳针治疗抑郁症的疗效和安全性。将74例患者随机分配为针对抑郁症特异性耳针（specific auricular acupuncture，SA）组和非特异性耳针（nonspecific auricular acupuncture，NSA）组，观察两组受试者治疗3个月后抑郁症康复情况，即患者健康问卷（patient health questionnaire，PHQ-9）评分至少下降50%。得出结论：6周以上的耳针治疗是安全的。虽然两组之间在抑郁康复情况上没有显著统计学差异，但接受SA的患者在3个月后抑郁缓解（PHQ-9评分<5分）情况更好。

医疗设备的参与者，不采用电刺激。每次治疗总时间为30 min，留针20 min。

对照组：按摩治疗师首先进行5 min的治疗，包括引导式横膈膜呼吸练习、肋骨活动和枕骨放松，以增加副交感神经张力。根据主要疼痛部位，治疗师对该部位进行20 min按摩，然后向心脏方向进行推抚5 min。按摩时采用轻度至中度压力，包括按压、肌肉拉伸、主动/被动关节活动、等长收缩后放松、推抚、肌筋膜松解、体位松解和触发点松解，总治疗时间为30 min。

二、专家述评（针灸学专家，临床研究方法学及卫生统计学专家）

1. 述评一

晚期癌症患者的疼痛管理是临床治疗中的难点和热点问题。该试验针对这一问题，通过比较针刺和按摩两种非药物疗法，分析其在缓解晚期癌症患者疼痛方面的效果。该研究不仅关注疼痛本身，还涵盖了与疼痛相关的疲劳、失眠等症状，这些症状对患者的生活质量有着重大影响。研究的选题体现了对临床需求的深刻理解，以及对提高患者生活质量的追求，具有重要的临床价值和社会意义。

该研究中，由具有肿瘤诊治经验的针灸师或按摩治疗师实施治疗，他们接受了统一的培训，严格遵循治疗方案。治疗包括在患者身体疼痛最严重的区域进行针刺，并根据患者的合并症状选择配穴，但应进一步明确针刺深度、具体配穴等细节。该研究考虑到受试者间的个体差异，对干预方案进行个体化调整，确保了治疗的安全性和有效性。对照组的设置为按摩治疗，详细描述了其实施流程、部位及手法。由于治疗手段的特殊性，该研究未实施盲法。结果显示，针刺和按摩在减轻晚期癌症患者的疼痛及改善相关症状方面都具有积极效果，两种疗法之间未见显著差异。这一发现为晚期癌症患者的疼痛管理提供了新的视角和选择，强调了非药物疗法在综合治疗中的重要性。同时，研究也提示未来应整合这些非药物疗法进入临床治疗策略，以实现疾病综合管理。

2. 述评二

（1）研究设计和过程实施

该研究发表了试验方案，提高了研究的透明度。多途径招募患者，确保了受试者的多样性，有利于提高结论的外推性。患者基线卡氏评分不小于60分，预期寿命不少于6个月，确保患者能够顺利完成试验。患者基线疼痛程度为中重度，主要结局为过去1周内最严重而不是平均的疼痛程度，这些设计能够更客观地反映患者的疼痛改善程度。两组干预分别为针刺和按摩，无法对医师和患者设盲，但是，对主要研究者和统计师设盲，符合临床实际。采用分层区组随机化方法进行分组，避免了基线阿片类药物使用和中心因素对结果产生的影响。

性。对主要疗效指标的缺失进行了多重填补，避免缺失对结果的影响，并且使用4种敏感性分析评估结果的稳健性以提高可信度。

第十四节 "Acupuncture vs Massage for Pain in Patients Living With Advanced Cancer: The IMPACT Randomized Clinical Trial" 相关介绍和述评

一 论文介绍

1. 中文题目：针灸与按摩治疗晚期癌症患者的疼痛的效果对比：IMPACT随机临床试验

2. 作者：Andrew S. Epstein, Kevin T. Liou, Sally A. D. Romero, Raymond E. Baser, Greta Wong, Han Xiao, Zunli Mo, Desiree Walker, Jodi MacLeod, Qing Li, Margaret Barton-Burke, Gary E. Deng, Katherine S. Panageas, John T. Farrar, Jun J. Mao

3. 主要单位：Department of Medicine, Memorial Sloan Kettering Cancer Center; Department of Obstetrics, Gynecology, and Reproductive Sciences, University of California; Department of Epidemiology and Biostatistics, Memorial Sloan Kettering Cancer Center

4. 发表期刊：*JAMA Network Open*

5. 发布日期：2023年11月14日

6. SCI源文献：WANG W, LIU Y, YANG X, et al. Acupuncture vs Massage for Pain in Patients Living With Advanced Cancer: The IMPACT Randomized Clinical Trial [J]. JAMA Netw Open, 2023, 6 (2): e230310.

7. 内容简介：本研究为多中心随机临床试验。为了比较针刺与按摩对晚期癌症患者肌肉骨骼疼痛的影响，将298例受试者随机分为治疗组和对照组，分别给予干预，观察简明疼痛量表（brief pain inventory，BPI）评分从基线到第26周的变化，以及疲劳、失眠和生活质量。得出结论：在这项为期26周的随机临床试验中，针刺和按摩均有助于减轻晚期癌症患者的肌肉骨骼疼痛，改善疲劳、失眠，提高生活质量；然而，两种治疗方法之间没有显著差异。

治疗组和对照组治疗频次均为每周治疗1次，连续治疗10周，后每月进行1次加强治疗，总时长26周。

治疗组：针灸师在患者疼痛最严重的身体部位周围4个局部穴位针刺至少10~20根针，同时根据是否存在并发症在其他部位补充针刺。根据体型和穴位位置将针插入适当的深度。针灸师行针以达到得气，即有效针刺后出现的局部酸胀感。使用经皮电神经刺激装置以2 Hz频率对4个局部疼痛穴位处的针灸针进行电刺激。对于使用带电针刺操作；然后以0.1～0.2 mA的电流强度连接电极30 s。

二 专家述评（针灸学专家，临床研究方法学及卫生统计学专家）

1. 述评一

该研究选题聚焦解决癌症患者OIC，这一问题影响了绝大多数的癌症相关阿片类药物使用患者的生活质量，是亟待解决的临床难题。该研究探讨了电针对OIC的疗效，着眼点不仅在于为临床提供一种安全有效的治疗疗法，而且在于减轻阿片类药物的不良反应，具有重要的临床价值。

研究对针刺的细节进行详细的报告，包括电针的参数、针刺的深度等，这些细节对于实施的可重复性至关重要。研究采用了8周、24次的电针治疗方案，有助于评估电针治疗的长期效果和安全性。在试验实施期间，该研究不鼓励受试者接受其他的干预措施，但设置了应急用药，在保证客观评价电针疗效的同时保障了受试者的安全。研究中对针灸师资质的要求及统一培训，尽可能地做到针刺实施的标准化，降低了操作者效应。非穴浅刺的假电针对照设置、中央随机系统的随机方法及盲法评估，确保了研究的科学性和严谨性。

综上所述，该研究在选题上针对临床治疗中的重要问题，通过详细的治疗方案和科学的方法学应用，为OIC提供了一种安全有效的治疗手段，有助于改善癌症患者的生活质量。

2. 述评二

（1）研究设计和过程实施

该试验采用多中心设计，避免了从单个中心收集患者可能产生的选择偏倚，纳入的患者更具代表性。设置电针组和假电针组，避免了安慰剂效应对结果的影响。设置严格的纳入和排除标准，保证了患者特征的一致性，避免了潜在的混杂因素对结果的影响。纳入患者的预期寿命不少于6个月，避免因死亡而脱落，造成数据的缺失。针灸师不设盲，患者、结局测量者、数据管理员和统计师设盲，最大限度地保证了试验过程中的盲法，并且对盲法的成功率进行评估，既符合客观实际，又避免了信息偏倚。

（2）临床研究方法学及统计学方法的选择及应用

该试验使用中心随机化方法，提高了随机化分组的效率，降低了分组信息被泄露的风险。设置了一个主要结局，避免了多个主要结局引起的多重性问题，是将定量资料转化为定性资料的复合指标，标准严格，需要同时满足在8周治疗期间至少有6周每周排便至少3次，且每周排便次数比基线增加至少1次。样本量估计使用的指标也与主要结局一致。使用意向性分析原则，尽可能保证数据分析人群与随机分组人群的一致

第十三节 "Effects of Electroacupuncture for Opioid-Induced Constipation in Patients With Cancer in China: A Randomized Clinical Trial" 相关介绍和述评

一 论文介绍

1. 中文题目：电针疗法对中国癌症患者阿片相关便秘的疗效：一项随机临床试验

2. 作者：Weiming Wang, Yan Liu, Xiaofang Yang, Jianhua Sun, Zenghui Yue, Dianrong Lu, Kehua Zhou, Yuanjie Sun, Aihua Hou, Zhiwei Zang, Xiaoqing Jin, Chao Liu, Yuhang Wang, Jinna Yu, Lili Zhu, Zhishun Liu

3. 主要单位：中国中医科学院广安门医院针灸科，北京中医药大学东直门医院中医内科学教育部重点实验室，贵州中医药大学针灸推拿学院

4. 发表期刊：*JAMA Network Open*

5. 发布日期：2023年2月22日

6. SCI源文献：WANG W, LIU Y, YANG X, et al. Effects of Electroacupuncture for Opioid-Induced Constipation in Patients With Cancer in China: A Randomized Clinical Trial [J]. JAMA Netw Open, 2023, 6 (2): e230310.

7. 内容简介：本研究为多中心、假对照、随机临床试验，为了确定电针对癌症患者阿片相关便秘（opioid-induced constipation，OIC）的疗效，将100例受试者随机分为电针组和假电针组，观察总体反应者的比例，反应者定义为在8周治疗期间至少有6周每周排便至少3次，且每周排便量比基线增加至少1次者。得出结论：8周的电针治疗可以增加每周自发性排便（spontaneous bowel movements，SBM）的发生率，具有良好的安全性，并可以改善OIC患者的生活质量。

电针组和假电针组患者的疗程均为8周，每周3次（理想情况下每隔1天1次），每次30 min，之后进行8周的随访。在治疗前，需告知所有患者，其接受电针和假电针治疗的可能性分别为50%和50%，但可能疗效相似，并且由于刺激强度相对较低，其在治疗过程中可能会或不会感觉到刺激。为了避免交流，患者被分开治疗。为了评估盲法的成功性，在第8周治疗后5 min内，要求患者猜测其是否接受了常规电刺激。

电针组选取双侧天枢（ST25）、腹结（SP14）和上巨虚（ST37）。将电针仪（SDZ-V）连接在刺入双侧天枢、腹结、上巨虚等穴位的针柄上，设置频率为10 Hz，电流强度为0.5～4.0 mA的连续波，具体参数取决于患者的舒适度。

假电针组选取非穴位，即分别为双侧天枢、腹结水平向外2 cm处，以及双侧上巨虚外侧、位于胃经和胆经中间。将针垂直刺入非穴位，刺入深度为2～3 mm，但无须

质量。选题精准地捕捉到PD治疗中的难点和热点问题，通过探索电针治疗对PD患者运动功能和便秘的改善效果，为PD的综合治疗提供了新的视角，体现了中医针灸的潜在价值和应用前景。选题具有高度的临床实用性，对于改善PD患者的生活质量具有重要意义。

在针刺干预实施方面，整体设计科学合理，针刺操作由经验丰富的针灸师执行，要求他们至少有2年的工作经验，并遵循标准化流程，确保治疗的一致性和安全性，同时，针刺过程中注重"得气"感，并通过电针仪进行刺激，对这些细节的把握值得肯定。但该研究仍有可改进之处：首先，该研究观察了受试者接受12周电针治疗的效果，但对于电针治疗的长期效应（如超过半年的疗效）缺乏探讨，这限制了研究结论的普遍适用性和长期应用的指导价值。其次，设置等待治疗对照组在一定程度上控制了变量，但无法完全消除安慰剂效应的影响，未来研究可考虑加设假针刺组，以更准确地评估电针治疗的真实效果。最后，由于研究持续时间较长，不同研究中心可能在评价标准上有所差异，进而影响结果的一致性，同时，由于研究无法实现盲法，可能会产生一定的偏倚。

2. 述评二

该研究是一项多中心、随机对照、评估者单盲的临床试验，于2018年9月19日至2019年9月25日在中国4家三级医院进行。研究目的是评价电针联合常规药物治疗PD的安全性和有效性。试验组接受电针联合常规药物治疗，对照组接受常规药物治疗。主要结局是基线到治疗第12周UPDRS总分变化。根据预试验结果进行样本量估计，每组至少需要57例患者才能有90%的把握度在0.05的检验水准上识别到两组间UPDRS评分7.4的差异。考虑20%的退出率，总样本量增至144例。为了补偿中心效应和预先指定的亚组分析，样本量再次增至166例。患者按1∶1进行分层随机化，分层因素为研究中心和是否便秘。主要结局的缺失数据被假定为随机缺失，并采用多重填补法进行填补。采用广义线性模型，纳入基线UPDRS为协变量进行校正，评价两组间UPDRS变化值的差异。该研究方案获得4家医院伦理委员会批准，并在中国临床试验注册中心注册。该研究遵循临床试验报告统一标准（consolidated standards of reporting trials，CONSORT）和针刺临床试验干预措施报告标准（standards for reporting interventions in clinical trials of acupuncture，STRICTA），具有规范性。

两组基线资料均衡可比。在意向性分析中，试验组、对照组的基线UPDRS分别是（36.1±16.6）和（32.2±16.5）。治疗后12周，两组UPDRS分别是30.9（95%CI 27.3～34.4）和36.1（95%CI 32.2～39.9），两组UPDRS的变化值分别为−5.3（95%CI −6.9～−3.6）和3.9（95%CI 1.7～6.1），两组变化值差别为−9.1（95%CI −11.8～−6.4），组间差异有统计学意义（$P<0.001$）。在符合方案分析中，主要结局在两组间的结果基本相似，提示主要结局分析结果的稳健性。

5. 发布日期：2023年1月13日

6. SCI源文献：LI K, XU S, WANG R, et al. Electroacupuncture for motor dysfunction and constipation in patients with Parkinson's disease: a randomised controlled multi-centre trial [J]. EClinicalMedicine, 2023, 56: 101814.

7. 内容简介：本研究为多中心随机对照试验，为了调查电针联合常规药物治疗对帕金森病（Parkinson's disease，PD）运动功能障碍和便秘的疗效和安全性，将166例受试者随机分配至电针组和等待治疗对照组，并进行为期12周的治疗和12周的随访。研究以统一帕金森病评定量表（unified Parkinson's disease rating scale，UPDRS）从基线到第12周的变化为主要结局，次要结局包括评估运动症状和便秘严重程度，并记录依从性和不良事件。得出结论：与常规药物治疗相比，电针联合常规药物治疗可以显著增强PD患者的运动功能并增加排便次数，电针是治疗PD的一种安全有效的方法。

电针组在常规药物治疗基础上加用电针治疗，每周3次，每次30 min，共治疗12周。选取穴位包括前顶（GV21）透刺双侧悬颅（GB5）、前神聪（EX-HN1）透刺悬厘（GB6）、曲池（LI11）、合谷（LI4）、阳陵泉（GB34）、足三里（ST36）、三阴交（SP6）、太溪（KI3）、太冲（LR3）。便秘患者加天枢（ST25）、腹结（SP14）、上巨虚（ST37）。电针治疗持续30 min，疏密波为10/50 Hz，输出脉冲宽度为0.2 ms±30%。电流强度在1 mA至10 mA之间调整，直至穴位周围皮肤轻微颤动而不感到疼痛。

等待治疗对照组采用常规药物治疗。在本试验中，由于PD临床表现的复杂性及临床指南中的个性化治疗原则，其治疗受到严格限制。但是，如果参与者在入组前正在服药，则不能随意改变剂量。为了解决这一问题，不同药物的剂量将转换为左旋多巴每日等效剂量（levodopa equivalent dose，LED）。根据患者的便秘症状，提出以下用药建议。如果患者连续3天或3天以上没有排便，研究人员允许他们进行紧急治疗。患者有几种选择：①对于没有排便冲动的患者，建议按照以下方案服用口服乳果糖溶液，即每隔12 h服用15 ml口服乳果糖溶液；如果无效，第二天每隔12 h服用30 ml口服乳果糖溶液。②对于有排便冲动但无法排便的患者，建议通过直肠注射20 ml甘油灌肠剂。两天后对紧急治疗没有反应的患者建议联合采用上述两种治疗方法。指导患者不要使用任何其他紧急治疗。在排便日记中，记录每次紧急治疗的使用情况。如果使用了任何其他紧急治疗药物，也会记录在排便日记中。24周后，等待治疗对照组的所有患者均可接受与电针组相同的电针治疗。

二　专家述评（针灸学专家，临床研究方法学及卫生统计学专家）

1. 述评一

该论文聚焦PD患者的运动功能障碍和便秘问题，这两种症状严重影响患者的生活

持。研究的不足之处在于假电针没有电流输出，这可能会影响患者的盲法效果，但由于主要结局指标的客观性和盲法的成功实施，这种偏倚已被降至最低。

2. 述评二

本研究为一项多中心随机对照试验。干预措施为针刺治疗，文章清楚地描述了针刺操作者的要求，分别介绍了电针组和假电针组进行的针刺操作，以及穴位和非穴位设计。受试对象采用动态区组随机，对患者、手术操作者及观察员设盲。根据预试验的结果，估算了研究的样本含量，研究把握度设置为80%。结果部分按照随机对照试验的可比性分析、疗效比较和安全性评价的顺序进行报告。首先描述了两组的基线数据及其可比性。本研究疗效指标分析采用了意向性分析。在方法学部分，提到对主要指标的缺失值采用了最优和最差值填补的方法进行敏感性分析，但次要分析指标未进行填补。尽管前后描述存在一定差异（前面提到全部采用了意向性分析，但次要指标又未进行填补），但这对主要结论影响不大。统计学方法的描述部分概述了方法选择的原则、依据，但如果能够更具体地阐述会更为清晰明了，例如说明对正态分布的数据使用独立样本t检验，而对偏态数据使用Mann-Whitney U检验，并具体指出哪些指标使用t检验，哪些使用非参数检验。本研究为多中心随机对照试验，但未报告各中心的数据构成及是否存在中心效应。

整体而言，本研究采用多中心随机对照试验，设计合理，报告规范，统计学描述及推断简单、清晰、直观。

第十二节 "Electroacupuncture for Motor Dysfunction and Constipation in Patients with Parkinson's Disease: A Randomised Controlled Multi-centre Trial" 相关介绍和述评

一 论文介绍

1. 中文题目：电针治疗帕金森病患者运动功能障碍和便秘：一项随机对照多中心试验

2. 作者：Kunshan Li, Shifen Xu, Ruiping Wang, Xuan Zou, Huirong Liu, Chunhai Fan, Jing Li, Guona Li, Yiwen Wu, Xiaopeng Ma, Yiyi Chen, Chenfang Hu, Xiru Liu, Canxing Yuan, Qing Ye, Ming Dai, Luyi Wu, Zhaoqin Wang, Huangan Wu

3. 主要单位：上海中医药大学附属岳阳中西医结合医院，上海中医药大学附属上海市中医医院，同济大学附属皮肤病医院

4. 发表期刊：*eClinicalMedicine*

Electroacupuncture in the Treatment of Postoperative Ileus After Laparoscopic Surgery for Colorectal Cancer: A Multicenter, Randomized Clinical Trial [J]. JAMA Surg, 2023, 158 (1): 20-27.

7. 内容简介：本研究为多中心、随机、假对照临床试验。在采用加速术后康复（enhanced recovery after surgery，ERAS）方案的医学实践中，评估电针在缩短术后肠梗阻（postoperative ileus，POI）持续时间上的疗效。研究纳入249例患者，随机分为电针组和假电针组，排除1例诊断为肠结核的患者，主要结局指标为首次排便的时间，次要结局指标则包括其他患者报告的结局指标、术后住院时间、30天内的再入院率，以及术后并发症和不良事件的发生率。得出结论：在使用ERAS方案并接受腹腔镜手术的结直肠癌患者中，与假电针相比，电针可以显著缩短POI持续时间，并降低POI延长的风险。

电针组及假电针组患者均在术后接受连续4天的治疗，每次治疗30 min。

电针组穴位为中脘（CV12），双侧天枢（ST25）、足三里（ST36）和上巨虚（ST37）。针刺得气后，两侧足三里交叉连接神经穴位电刺激仪，刺激频率为2/100 Hz，刺激强度调整至可触发针柄轻微振动。

假电针组患者在4个非穴位点接受假电针刺激，针刺刺入深度为2～3 mm，无得气，未给予针刺手法操作。电极虽以与电针组相似方式连接到双侧非穴位，但神经穴位电刺激仪的内部线被切断，确保无电流输出。

二 专家述评（针灸学专家，临床研究方法学及卫生统计学专家）

1. 述评一

ERAS方案在结直肠癌手术中已广泛应用，但是POI仍是不可避免的并发症，目前尚无特效治疗手段。手术创伤和肠道操作引发的炎症反应是导致POI相关胃肠道运动障碍的关键病理机制。电针通过激活迷走神经-肾上腺通路减轻炎症，并可能通过减少POI中的局部肠道肌肉炎症保护平滑肌细胞，从而改善胃肠道的蠕动功能。这些机制可能是电针作为治疗POI和胃肠功能障碍的潜在选择的重要原因。研究者的前期试验显示，电针治疗较假电针缩短腹腔镜结直肠癌手术患者术后首次排便时间达12 h，并减轻了相关的胃肠功能障碍症状。基于前期研究、电针促进术后胃肠功能恢复的科学机制和预试验结果，提出电针可有效治疗POI的假设是合理且具有临床意义的。干预方案采用胃肠合穴与募穴的配合，这是在针灸经典理论指导下的优化设计。主要结局指标具有客观性，次要结局指标能够支持主要结果的有效性。假电针对照能够明确电针对胃肠功能的特异性促进效应。研究结果表明，电针作为ERAS方案的有力辅助手段，能够有效促进腹腔镜结直肠癌术后患者的胃肠功能恢复，这一结论具有较强的证据支

此外，该研究还使用严格的纳入与排除标准，如年龄、孕周、体质量减轻等，确保了研究对象的同质性，从而减少潜在的混杂因素，有助于提高研究结果的内部效度，即研究结果与干预之间的因果关系。研究通过使用PUQE评分对NVP的严重程度进行标准化评估，使得结果的比较更加客观和一致。

（2）临床研究方法学及统计学方法选择与应用

该研究采用意向性治疗分析原则，可有效减少由于试验退出或违反试验方案导致的偏倚。使用链式多重填补法来处理缺失数据也在一定程度上减少了由于数据缺失带来的偏倚。

该研究采用因子方差分析方法有效处理了多种干预措施之间的相互作用，提供了不同治疗组合的独立效应的详细分析。此外，重复测量线性混合模型用于评估时间序列数据中的治疗效果，这种方法充分利用纵向数据的优势，提高了统计效率。

对于二元变量的处理，该研究应用了改进的泊松（Poisson）回归模型。这种方法能够有效应对二项分布数据中方差异常的情况，并提供准确的估计值。

综上所述，本文在研究设计、方法学选择、统计分析应用方面展示出较高的科学性和严谨性。然而，未来研究可以进一步加强对复杂交互效应的样本量计算，并考虑多重比较的校正方法，以提高结果的稳健性和解读的可靠性。在未来的研究中，为减少Ⅰ类错误的影响，可以考虑采用多重检验校正方法来增强次要结果的稳健性。

第十一节 "Electroacupuncture vs Sham Electroacupuncture in the Treatment of Postoperative Ileus After Laparoscopic Surgery for Colorectal Cancer: A Multicenter, Randomized Clinical Trial" 相关介绍和述评

一 论文介绍

1. 中文题目：比较电针与假电针治疗腹腔镜结直肠癌术后肠麻痹：一项多中心随机临床试验

2. 作者：Yu Wang, Jing-Wen Yang, Shi-Yan Yan, Yun Lu, Jia-Gang Han, Wei Pei, Jing-Jie Zhao, Zhi-Kai Li, Hang Zhou, Na-Na Yang, Li-Qiong Wang, Ying-Chi Yang, Cun-Zhi Liu

3. 主要单位：北京中医药大学针灸推拿学院，国际针灸创新研究院；青岛大学附属医院；首都医科大学附属北京朝阳医院

4. 发表期刊：*JAMA Surgery*

5. 发布日期：2023年1月1日

6. SCI源文献：WANG Y, YANG JW, YAN SY, et al. Electroacupuncture vs Sham

接受假针刺者进行指压刺激内关。

多西拉敏-吡哆醇和安慰剂药物具有相同的外观、大小、气味和味道。受试者在睡前服用2片多西拉敏-吡哆醇或安慰剂，共服用14天。如果用药2天后PUQE评分评估的症状未改善，则增加1片。每日最大剂量为4片。

二 专家述评（针灸学专家，临床研究方法学及卫生统计学专家）

1. 述评一

中重度NVP不仅影响孕妇生活质量，严重者会因无法忍受而终止妊娠。针刺在我国被广泛应用于妊娠期呕吐治疗，但中重度NVP存在治疗方法不足、缺乏有效性证据及治疗个体化需求的临床问题。该研究为针刺对中重度NVP的有效性和安全性提供了高质量的临床依据，可为NVP提供个体化治疗方案。该研究在全国范围内13家三级医院开展针刺多中心、随机、2×2析因设计、大样本的临床研究，探究针刺联合缓释抗组胺药物多西拉敏-吡哆醇治疗中重度NVP的有效性及安全性。通过为期2周的干预，各组受试者分别执行真针刺+多西拉敏-吡哆醇、假针刺+多西拉敏-吡哆醇、真针刺+安慰剂、假针刺+安慰剂治疗。选取了和胃止呕经典选穴内关、足三里，结合患者脾胃虚弱、肝火旺盛、痰湿中阻等证型个体化的合理配穴，选择安慰剂或假针刺进行合理对照，试验设计科学严谨，最终284例受试者完成干预。结果显示，无论单纯针刺、止吐药多西拉敏-吡哆醇，还是两者联合治疗，孕吐严重程度评分降幅均大于其各自的对照组，联合治疗效果更佳，可减少止吐药用量。该研究在选题、临床问题提炼、治疗方案设计及针刺干预实施等方面都体现了高度的专业性和创新性，形成高级别循证医学证据，为今后综合治疗及妊娠呕吐指南制定提供新的见解和方法。

2. 述评二

（1）研究设计和过程实施

该研究为一项多中心、双盲、安慰剂对照试验，分析针刺对中重度NVP孕妇的疗效和安全性。文章在研究设计和过程实施方面展示出良好的结构和执行质量，值得肯定。

首先，该研究采用多中心设计，涵盖全国13家医院，这种大型多中心设计可增加结果的普适性，减少个别医院的偏倚，同时增强对目标人群的代表性，有助于提高研究结论的外部效度。

其次，研究采用双盲设计，这一设计能够有效减少观察者偏倚和期望效应的影响，确保试验结果的客观性和准确性。随机分组通过计算机生成和统计分析系统（SAS）的PLAN程序执行，随机化方案的预先打印和分发进一步确保了盲法的有效性。

第十节 "Acupuncture and Doxylamine-Pyridoxine for Nausea and Vomiting in Pregnancy: A Randomized, Controlled, 2×2 Factorial Trial" 相关介绍和述评

一 论文介绍

1. 中文题目：针刺联合多西拉敏-吡哆醇治疗妊娠期恶心呕吐：一项随机、对照、2×2析因设计试验

2. 作者：Xiao-Ke Wu, Jing-Shu Gao, Hong-Li Ma, Yu Wang, Bei Zhang, Zhao-Lan Liu, Jian Li, Jing Cong, Hui-Chao Qin, Xin-Ming Yang, Qi Wu, Xiao-Yong Chen, Zong-Lin Lu, Ya-Hong Feng, Xue Qi, Yan-Xiang Wang, Lan Yu, Ying-Mei Cui, Chun-Mei An, Li-Li Zhou, Yu-Hong Hu, Lu Li, Yi-Juan Cao, Ying Yan, Li Liu, Yu-Xiu Liu, Zhi-Shun Liu, Rebecca C. Painter, Ernest H.Y. Ng, Jian-Ping Liu, Ben Willem J. Mol, Chi Chiu Wang

3. 主要单位：黑龙江中医药大学第一附属医院，杭州师范大学药学院，徐州市中心医院妇产科

4. 发表期刊：*Annals of Internal Medicine*

5. 发布日期：2023年6月20日

6. SCI源文献：WU X K, GAO J S, MA H L, et al. Acupuncture and Doxylamine-Pyridoxine for Nausea and Vomiting in Pregnancy: A Randomized, Controlled, 2×2 Factorial Trial [J]. Ann Intern Med, 2023, 176 (7): 922-933.

7. 内容简介：本研究为多中心、随机、双盲、安慰剂对照、2×2析因试验。为了评估针刺、多西拉敏-吡哆醇及两者联合对中重度妊娠恶心呕吐（nausea and vomiting of pregnancy，NVP）的疗效和安全性，将352例妊娠早期存在中重度NVP的女性随机分为4组：真针刺+多西拉敏-吡哆醇组、假针刺+多西拉敏-吡哆醇组、真针刺+安慰剂组、假针刺+安慰剂组，评估受试者治疗前后妊娠恶心呕吐专用量化（pregnancy-unique quantification of emesis and nausea，PUQE）评分。得出结论：针刺、多西拉敏-吡哆醇治疗中重度NVP均有较好的疗效，二者联合可能比单独治疗产生更大的潜在益处。然而，这种疗效的临床意义尚不确定。

各组针刺频次相同，均每天1次，每次30 min，连续2周。受试者在一个舒适的环境中单独接受针刺或假针刺，且不与其他受试者交流。

接受真针刺者根据脾胃虚弱、肝火旺盛、痰湿中阻3种中医证型进行取穴。主穴为内关（PC6）、足三里（ST36）。辅穴：脾胃虚弱证，加中脘（CV12）；肝火旺盛证，加太冲（LR3）；痰湿中阻证，加丰隆（ST40）。

短的不足；④针对CSU的病证特点，采用国际认可的UAS7量表为主要疗效指标，以评估针刺治疗CSU的疗效；⑤在辅助干预措施方面，仅允许在紧急状况下按需服用规定剂量的抗组胺药；⑥针刺组及假针刺组的实施者为接受培训且通过考核的针灸师；⑦研究过程规范，研究结果的可信度高。

2. 述评二

（1）研究设计和过程实施

这项针对针刺治疗CSU的多中心、随机、假对照试验，在试验设计上展现出严格的临床研究标准和细致的过程控制。

首先，该研究选择了3个不同城市的三级医院作为研究中心，确保了患者样本的多样性和结果的普遍性，增强了研究结果的外部效度，使其更广泛适用于不同地区和人群。

其次，该研究采用了1∶1∶1的随机分配方法，确保了针刺组、假针刺组和等待治疗组的组间平衡。研究中使用的在线响应系统生成随机序列，并通过手机短信分配组别，有效防止了随机化过程中的人为干预和偏倚，展现了研究团队在随机化和分配隐藏过程中的严谨性。

该研究的盲法实施也比较严谨。患者、结果评估者和统计员均不知分配情况，且研究团队在干预结束时进行了盲法可信度评估，确保了盲法有效性。

（2）临床研究方法学及统计学方法的选择及应用

这项研究在统计分析中选用了多种适合的统计学方法，为结果的可靠性和科学性提供了强有力的支持。

对于主要结局和部分次要结局使用线性回归模型，为主要结果提供了清晰的量化评估。此外，研究团队在分析中进行了 *Bonferroni* 调整，减少了多重比较带来的Ⅰ型错误风险。同时该研究将UAS7的最小临床重要差异设定为10，从而能够清晰地评估不同治疗组之间的临床效果差异，而不仅仅是统计学上的显著性。

在处理缺失数据方面，本研究使用链式方程多重填补法。这种方法能够有效地处理数据缺失问题，并最大限度地减少因缺失数据而导致的偏倚。

值得注意的是，研究还进行了两次亚组分析，以探讨不同患者群体中的治疗效果。这种分层分析为不同患者亚群提供了更详细的效果评估，有助于个性化治疗的制定。

总之，该研究在临床研究方法的应用和统计学方法的选择上表现出十分严谨的态度。合理的研究设计与严谨的统计学方法确保了结果的科学性和可靠的临床应用价值。然而，尽管该研究已考虑到多种潜在的偏倚来源并进行调整，未来的研究仍可以通过增加样本量和延长针刺干预时间，进一步验证结果的可靠性和长期效果。

Chronic Spontaneous Urticaria: A Randomized Controlled Trial [J]. Ann Intern Med, 2023, 176 (12): 1617-1624.

7. 内容简介：本研究为多中心、随机、假对照试验。为了探究针刺对慢性自发性荨麻疹（chronic spontaneous urticaria，CSU）的疗效是否优于假针或等待治疗，将330例CSU患者以1∶1∶1的比例随机分配为3组，即针刺组、假针刺组和等待治疗组，观察3组患者治疗4周后7日荨麻疹活动度评分（weekly urticaria activity score，UAS7）与基线的平均变化。得出结论：与假针刺和等待治疗相比，针刺对UAS7的改善更优，但干预与对照的差异无统计学意义。

针刺组、假针刺组和等待治疗组均接受标准短期（按需）H1抗组胺药治疗，即在紧急情况下，每天服用10 mg氯雷他定，若氯雷他定无效每天服用10 mg依巴斯汀。另外，所有患者都被要求每天记荨麻疹日记，记录CSU症状和伴随用药情况。

针刺组患者在前两周接受10次针刺治疗，在随后的两周再接受6次针刺治疗（共16次）。针刺穴位包括曲池（LI11）、血海（SP10）、足三里（ST36）、天枢（ST25）、三阴交（SP6）、神门（HT7）和中脘（CV12），直到产生得气感。每次治疗留针30 min。

假针刺组患者接受的针刺次数、频率与针刺组相同，但是治疗为假穴非穿透性针刺干预。

等待治疗组患者除了标准的抗组胺药治疗外，不接受任何其他治疗。

二 专家述评（针灸学专家，临床研究方法学及卫生统计学专家）

1. 述评一

（1）选题分析

慢性荨麻疹是临床常见过敏性疾病，针灸治疗效果明显，但缺少高质量临床研究证据。该研究以CSU为研究对象，通过三家中心的随机对照试验，证实了针刺治疗本病具有良好的效果，研究有助于拓展针灸临床应用范围，选题具有较重要的学术价值和临床意义。

（2）针刺干预的实施

该研究与针灸临床结合密切，研究方案在中国临床试验注册中心注册（ChiCTR1900022994）。研究有如下特点：①研究分为针刺组、假针刺组和等待治疗组，其中假针刺组的假针刺实施采用非穴非刺入方式；②选用的曲池、血海、足三里、天枢、三阴交、神门、中脘是治疗本病共识性较强的腧穴；③在治疗频率与疗程方面，慢性荨麻疹的抗组胺药治疗一般规律性应用3～6个月，药物控制病情2～4周，在临床中针刺治疗一般也需较长疗程以更好地改善症状、控制病情，本研究为期4周的疗程虽然偏短，但会明显提高研究的可行性，而且4周共16次的高频治疗也可能具有弥补疗程偏

2. 述评二

（1）研究设计和过程实施

该研究在附件中提供了完整试验方案，增强了研究的透明度。通过招募较大样本受试者，提升了研究人群的代表性。受试者至少有3个月膝关节疼痛史且NRS评分达到3级或以上，有效避免了因自愈因素导致的疗效夸大，同时提高了结局指标的灵敏度。通过排除多种既往治疗史，减少了其他干预对疗效评估的潜在影响。研究采用4或6长度的混合区组随机序列，并结合密封不透明信封进行隐蔽分组。由于无法对受试者和干预提供者施盲，混合区组随机可避免每个区组的最后1例受试者分组被预测。通过对评估人员实施盲法，降低了主观因素带来的测量偏倚。

（2）临床研究方法学及统计学方法的选择及应用

主要分析遵循意向性治疗原则，提供了更为保守的治疗效应估计，使评价结果更为严格。采用线性混合模型比较组间效应差，可降低混杂因素对结果的影响，但研究未具体报告所调整的固定或随机效应协变量，影响了统计分析的透明性。研究失访率较高，而缺失数据的处理方式报告不明确，故不能排除缺失数据对结果的影响。缺乏主要结局多个测量点的多重性校正说明，统计推断可能受到多重性影响。疗效分析未进行基于符合方案集的敏感性分析，使得主分析结果的稳健性缺乏额外验证。但在成本效益分析中进行了5000次bootstrap抽样，提高了分析结果的稳健性。

第九节 "Efficacy of Acupuncture for Chronic Spontaneous Urticaria: A Randomized Controlled Trial" 相关介绍和述评

一 论文介绍

1. 中文题目：针刺治疗慢性自发性荨麻疹的疗效：一项随机对照试验

2. 作者：Hui Zheng, Xian-Jun Xiao, Yun-Zhou Shi, Lei-Xiao Zhang, Wei Cao, Qian-Hua Zheng, Feng Zhong, Ping-Sheng Hao, Ying Huang, Ming-Ling Chen, Wei Zhang, Si-Yuan Zhou, Yan-Jun Wang, Chuan Wang, Li Zhou, Xiao-Qin Chen, Zuo-Qin Yang, Zi-Hao Zou, Ling Zhao, Fan-Rong Liang, Ying Li

3. 主要单位：成都中医药大学针灸推拿学院，成都中医药大学养生康复学院，四川大学华西医院中西医结合科

4. 发表期刊：*Annals of Internal Medicine*

5. 发布日期：2023年11月14日

6. SCI源文献：ZHENG H, XIAO X J, SHI Y Z, et al. Efficacy of Acupuncture for

（ST35）、足三里（ST36）、阴陵泉（SP9）、血海（SP10）、阳陵泉（GB34）、鹤顶（EX-LE2）及内膝眼（EX-LE4）。SAA组干预分为两个疗程，第一个疗程为第一周，受试者需每日进行穴位按压练习30 min，随后揉搓穴位及活动膝关节；第二个疗程在第一个疗程结束后进行，受试者继续进行穴位按压练习（30 min）并接受KHE培训（30 min），每天训练2次，每次2 h，两个疗程共计12周。

KHE组受试者按照相同的时间表和持续时间接受KEH培训，每天训练2次，每次2 h，共12周。在12周研究结束后，KHE组受试者接受与SAA组相同干预的补偿治疗。KHE是基于香港特别行政区政府卫生署长者健康服务网站的资料修改而来的。KHE讲师为接受过物理治疗师培训的注册护士。

二 专家述评（针灸学专家，临床研究方法学及卫生统计学专家）

1. 述评一

（1）选题分析

本研究选题精准地聚焦临床中广泛存在且难以根治的膝骨关节炎，特别针对50岁以上的中老年人群。该文将SAA作为一种潜在的解决方案进行探讨，旨在避免药物副作用的同时，提升患者的治疗依从性。这种疗法不仅贴近临床实际需求，还补充了现有研究的空白，尤其体现在其研究设计的严谨性、穴位选择的精准性、临床应用的广泛性及疗效评估的科学性等方面。通过构建关键临床问题，系统评估了SAA的短期与中期效果，并进行卫生经济学分析，从多个维度验证这一治疗方法的可行性及经济性。这些研究成果不仅为临床治疗膝骨关节炎提供了新的证据支持，也为后续相关研究奠定了坚实基础，具有较高的临床价值。

（2）干预措施的实施

该文的干预措施设计合理，充分考虑了中老年膝关节骨关节炎患者的病程长、恢复难的临床特点。治疗组的干预方案包括热身、穴位按压、揉膝及移动膝盖等多层次操作；穴位选择均基于传统中医经络理论，涵盖了与膝关节功能密切相关的胃经、脾经和胆经等经络；各穴位的按压手法也经过精心设计，融合了手指与鱼际的不同力度和技巧；在充分体现了中医治疗特色的同时，也对操作的方法及时长进行了严格地把控。该研究对指导患者治疗的人员资质进行了严格筛选和专业培训，确保了干预措施的专业性与准确性。治疗组采用SAA联合KHE培训，对照组仅接受KHE培训，这样的设计保证了研究的科学性与对比性，有效评估了SAA在膝骨关节炎治疗中的独立效果。此外，若研究能进一步设计成SAA联合KHE与假SAA联合KHE对照，将能更深入地排除安慰剂效应，评估SAA的特异性治疗效果。

尚不清晰，应明确何谓"重大方案偏差"。对于缺失值，通过多重插补法进行多次插补，取每个插补后数据集分析结果的平均值作为最终估算结果，可降低插补中的偶然因素对结果的影响。通过设定一个指标在一个时间点的测量结果作为主要结局，避免了多重性问题对结论的影响。

第八节 "Self-Administered Acupressure for Probable Knee Osteoarthritis in Middle-Aged and Older Adults: A Randomized Clinical Trial" 相关介绍和述评

一 论文介绍

1. 中文题目：自我穴位按压法治疗中老年疑似膝骨关节炎：一项随机临床试验

2. 作者：Wing-Fai Yeung, Shu-Cheng Chen, Denise Shuk Ting Cheung, Carlos King-Ho Wong, Tsz Chung Chong, Yuen Shan Ho, Lorna Kwai Ping Suen, Lai Ming Ho, Lixing Lao

3. 主要单位：香港理工大学护理学院，香港理工大学中医药创新研究中心，香港理工大学智能老龄化研究院

4. 发表期刊：*JAMA Network Open*

5. 发布日期：2024年4月19日

6. SCI源文献：YEUNG WF, CHEN SC, CHEUNG DST, et al. Self-Administered Acupressure for Probable Knee Osteoarthritis in Middle-Aged and Older Adults: A Randomized Clinical Trial [J]. JAMA Netw Open, 2024, 7 (4): e245830.

7. 内容简介：本研究为随机、对照、临床试验。为了评估自我按压穴位（self-administered acupressure，SAA）在减轻中老年人膝关节疼痛方面的有效性。研究纳入314例疑似膝骨关节炎的中老年人受试者，随机分为SAA组（干预组）与膝关节健康教育（knee health education，KHE）组（对照组）。主要结局指标为两组受试者在12周时的数值评级量表（numerical rrating scale，NRS）疼痛评分。次要结局指标包括西部安大略和麦克马斯特大学骨关节炎量表（Western Ontario and Mcmaster University osteoarthritis index，WOMAC）、六维健康调查短表（short form 6 dimensions，SF-6D）、起坐行走测试（timed up and go，TUG）和快速步态速度（fast gait speed，FGS）测试。得出结论：SAA联合简短的KHE在改善疑似膝骨关节炎的疼痛和关节活动方面有效且具有成本效益。

SAA组接受SAA干预及KHE课程。穴位按压选穴包括梁丘（ST34）、犊鼻

二 专家述评（针灸学专家，临床研究方法学及卫生统计学专家）

1. 述评一

TMD是常见且治疗难度较大的疾病，本文针对TMD探索了针刺疗法在减轻疼痛、改善关节功能方面的作用，是一项具有重要临床意义的随机对照试验。

本研究的选题聚焦TMD的治疗难点和热点问题，提出了关键临床问题：如何通过非药物治疗减轻TMD患者的疼痛和改善其关节功能。当前，尽管已有多种治疗TMD的方法，但许多疗法在效果和安全性方面尚存在争议，且缺乏高质量的随机对照试验。

60例TMD患者随机分为针刺组和假针刺组，每组30例，每周治疗3次，持续4周，选取的穴位包括双侧合谷、阳陵泉及患侧听宫、颊车和下关，操作过程中注重得气反应。这些穴位和手法的选择基于经典文献和现代研究，确保了治疗的合理性和科学性。假针刺组则采用无创针刺，通过特制的假针装置模拟针刺操作，保证了受试者的盲法效果。

研究结果显示，针刺组在第4、8周的疼痛强度显著低于假针刺组，且在下颌开口和运动、下颌功能限制、抑郁-焦虑-压力等方面均有显著改善。针刺组的反应率和患者满意度也明显高于假针刺组，两组之间的安全性差异无统计学意义。研究强调了针刺作为一种有效的非药物治疗方法在TMD中的应用价值。

2. 述评二

（1）研究设计和过程实施

该研究试验方案在国际平台上前瞻性注册，提高了方案的透明度。纳入标准中要求TMD疼痛至少持续3个月，可降低疾病自愈对结果的影响。排除了筛选前1个月接受过其他治疗者，以避免延滞效应的影响。采用基于网络的交互系统进行区组化随机分组，可提高随机化、分配隐藏和盲法执行的可靠性。基于Park假针装置对患者施盲，可有效降低实施过程的破盲率，从而保障假针刺组患者的依从性和消除安慰剂效应的影响。主要结局为视觉模拟评分（visual analogue score，VAS）量表，该量表可有效评估TMD的疼痛强度，但未描述该量表最小临床重要差异，使得分析结果缺少一个重要参照。

（2）临床研究方法学及统计学方法的选择及应用

样本量计算中未明确组间共同标准差，导致无法重复计算过程。统计分析基于意向性分析原则，该原则下的效应估算结果相对保守，即更严格标准验证针刺的疗效。采用符合方案集进行敏感性分析，可检验主分析结果的稳定性，但符合方案集的定义

第七节 "Effect of Acupuncture for Temporomandibular Disorders: A randomized Clinical Trial" 相关介绍和述评

一 论文介绍

1. 中文题目：针刺对颞下颌关节紊乱病的影响：一项随机临床试验
2. 作者：Lu Liu, Qiuyi Chen, Tianli Lyu, Luopeng Zhao, Quan Miao, Yuhan Liu, Limin Nie, Feiyu Fu, Shuting Li, Chenxi Zeng, Yixin Zhang, Peiyue Peng, Woyu Wang, Ying Lin, Bin Li
3. 主要单位：首都医科大学附属北京中医医院针灸科，针灸神经调控北京市重点实验室
4. 发表期刊：QJM: An International Journal of Medicine
5. 发布日期：2024年5月6日
6. SCI源文献：LIU L, CHEN Q, LYU T, et al. Effect of acupuncture for temporomandibular disorders: A randomized clinical trial [J]. QJM, 2024, 117(9): 647-656.
7. 内容简介：本研究为单中心、单盲、随机对照试验。为了探讨针刺是否能减轻颞下颌关节紊乱病（temporomandibular disorders，TMD）患者的疼痛强度，将60例TMD患者随机（1:1）分为针刺组和假针刺组分别进行干预，观察两组受试者从基线到第4周的每周疼痛强度变化（主要结局）。次要结局和探索性指标包括第4周和第8周时疼痛强度降低≥30%或≥50%的受试者比例、下颌开口和运动的变化值、慢性疼痛分级量表（graded chronic pain scale，GCPS）、下颌功能限制量表20（jaw functional limitations scale-20-item，JFLS-20）、抑郁-焦虑-压力量表21（depression, anxiety and stress scales-21，DASS-21）、匹兹堡睡眠质量指数（Pittsburgh sleep quality index，PSQI）、压力痛阈值（pressure pain threshold，PPT）及表面肌电图。得出结论：与假针刺相比，针刺可显著缓解TMD患者的疼痛，改善身心功能。

针刺组和假针刺组治疗频次均为每周3次，每次30 min，共4周。两组穴位均为双侧合谷（LI4）、阳陵泉（GB34），患侧听宫（SI19）、颊车（ST6）和下关（ST7）。受试者采用仰卧位，穴位处皮肤消毒。

针刺组采用一次性不锈钢针刺针（直径0.35 mm、长70 mm），通过引导装置刺入皮肤，并使用自粘贴垫固定在皮肤上。通过提插捻转手法使患者得气。

假针刺组采用假针刺方法，假针与真针规格相同，但针尖钝且能在针柄内滑动，通过Park假针装置插入，并使用自粘贴垫固定在皮肤上。操作流程与针刺组相同，但没有刺入皮肤，无得气。

深度及角度等。假针刺组采用相同穴位浅刺的方式，相对于针刺组的刺入深度及刺激方式而言，给予受试者较为微弱的刺激，有利于保持受试者的盲法。但刺入型假针通常比非刺入型假针有更大的效应（除安慰剂效应之外，具有更大的生理性效应），进而缩小与针刺组之间的差别。该研究的结果也验证了这一点，作者也对该问题进行了相应讨论。

（2）临床研究方法学及统计学方法的选择及应用

从整体上来看，本研究的统计学方法较为规范。①样本量计算：样本量计算基于事先确定的两次比较进行了检验水准α的调整，并考虑了不依从的比例、脱落率及可能发生沾染的比例，但并未给出基于上述考虑后，最终确定的样本量是多少例。②统计分析：统计分析以多因素分析方法为主，充分考虑了研究过程中可能的影响因素，并较为全面地对分析细节做了报告，给出具体的纳入模型的协变量及相关参数的设置。缺失数据处理是统计分析中的关键内容，研究采用了混合效应模型进行分析，该模型可处理缺失数据，因此，无须专门进行缺失数据的填补。但为了评估该结果的稳健性，研究采用多重填补进行敏感性分析，值得借鉴。

三 作者谈

DLSS是老年人高发病，间歇性跛行是其致残的主症。药物治疗疗效有限，证据不足；10%～40%接受手术的患者出现并发症和背部手术失败综合征，指南建议非药物干预如个体化训练和综合手法作为初始治疗，但其疗效很有限。针刺治疗下腰痛有效，并且得到指南推荐，但是对DLSS引起的神经缺血性疼痛和间歇性跛行疗效证据不足。研究者预试验和长期临床经验表明，深刺大肠俞方案有较好疗效。基于此，我们提出针刺可有效缓解DLSS患者疼痛性间歇性跛行的假说，设置假针刺对照的多中心随机试验以评价针刺的有效性，主要指标为改良RMDQ较基线变化值，以及与假针刺的差异（基于MCID），并且治疗后随访半年以评价针刺疗法的临床价值和优势。

实施过程的难点主要是针刺方案的依从性和数据的可靠性保障，每家分中心都进行了2～3次现场监察，所有患者数据都进行了溯源核查。

论文总结的难点主要是结果解读和阐释，主要指标有统计学意义，但未达到MCID，仍谨慎地下结论针刺可以缓解神经源性间歇性跛行；组间差值虽未达到MCID，但两组自身与基线比较均超过MCID；为保障对患者设盲成功，假针刺组采用穴位微针刺，但其有较强的非特异性效应和一定的特异性效应，从而降低了针刺的特异性效应值；其他次要指标如臀腿痛评分、腰椎管狭窄症状和躯体功能评分等都支持针刺疗效优于假针刺；腰椎管狭窄间歇性跛行没有特效疗法。

刘志顺
中国中医科学院广安门医院

异未达到最小临床重要差异（minimal clinically important difference，MCID）；治疗6周的效果可能会持续24周。

针刺组和假针刺组治疗频次均为每周3次，共6周18次治疗。两组选用相同穴位，包括双侧肾俞（BL23）、大肠俞（BL25）、委中（BL40）、承山（BL57）、太溪（KI3）。

针刺组操作：将75 mm的针直刺刺入大肠俞，进针深度50～70 mm，并在受试者感到电击样针感向下放射至膝盖和后小腿时立即提起1～2 mm。将40 mm的针直刺刺入肾俞、委中和承山。以45°的角度向下斜刺刺入太溪，进针深度15～30 mm。除大肠俞外，所有穴位在进针后立即进行提插捻转，平补平泻操作30 s，留针30 min，每10 min行针1次，以达到得气效果。

对照组选用假针刺疗法。将针刺入上述所有穴位，深度为2～3 mm，但不进行任何行针操作，留针30 min。

二　专家述评（针灸学专家，临床研究方法学及卫生统计学专家）

1. 述评一

本论文在研究背景中提到，虽然指南推荐腰椎管狭窄患者接受非药物疗法，但是缺乏高质量的循证证据支持，因此，该研究的选题着眼于DLSS患者中的间歇性跛行问题，主要评价指标是个体主观感受的报告结局。尽管从优效性检验的角度，针刺改善水平未达到MCID，不具备临床意义，但综合主、次要评价指标和随访记录来看，依然可以发现针刺对以神经源性跛行性疼痛症状为主的DLSS患者的疼痛特异性残疾有缓解效果，本研究对于该领域的针刺试验具有十分重大的启发和指导意义，值得针刺临床试验的研究者们学习。

本研究有严格的标准化针刺方案，从针刺的进针角度、深度及行针手法到得气都有清晰的描述。而假针刺组采用相同穴位浅刺，不可避免地引入穴位的安慰剂效应。尤其是在痛症的研究中，基于患者对于疼痛感受的阈值不同，穿透的假针带来的安慰剂效应可能会较其他疾病更甚，正如本文在改进部分提到，在后续的研究中建议采取不破皮的假针刺对照，降低安慰剂效应的影响。因此，在不同的研究中，对照组干预方式的选择显得尤为重要。根据研究病种和针刺穴位，考虑不同的对照组干预方式，对结果和结论都有至关重要的影响。

2. 述评二

（1）研究设计和过程实施

该项研究采用多中心、随机、对照设计，主要有以下几方面特点：本研究采用假针刺设计和区组随机的方式进行随机化，更好地减少随机化过程中的可预见性，做到了随机隐藏。对干预措施部分的描述非常详细，尤其是针刺，详细地描述了每个穴位的针刺位置、

压力等一系列混杂因素的干扰。

另外，关于我们在投稿时面临过的问题，因为成瘾性疾病的特殊性，不同国家地区对于阿片类药物的管控程度不同，因此我们的研究结论在不同地区期刊看来所具有的临床指导意义、公共卫生也就不同，甚至会对不同地区相关的卫生政策产生影响，这一点在以往临床研究投稿时并不常见。

许能贵
广州中医药大学

第六节 "Effect of Acupuncture on Neurogenic Claudication Among Patients With Degenerative Lumbar Spinal Stenosis: A Randomized Clinical Trial" 相关介绍和述评

一 论文介绍

1. 中文题目：针刺对退行性腰椎管狭窄症患者神经源性跛行的影响：一项随机临床试验

2. 作者：Lili Zhu, Yuanjie Sun, Jing Kang, Jun Liang, Tongsheng Su, Wenbin Fu, Wei Zhang, Rongshui Dai, Yan Hou, Hong Zhao, Weina Peng, Weiming Wang, Jing Zhou, Ruimin Jiao, Biyun Sun, Yan Yan, Yan Liu, Zhishun Liu

3. 主要单位：中国中医科学院广安门医院针灸科，北京中医药大学东直门医院中医内科学教育部重点实验室，陕西省中医院针灸科

4. 发表期刊：*Annals of Internal Medicine*

5. 发布日期：2024年7月2日

6. SCI源文献：ZHU L L, SUN Y J, KANG J, et al. Effect of Acupuncture on Neurogenic Claudication Among Patients With Degenerative Lumbar Spinal Stenosis: A Randomized Clinical Trial [J]. Ann Intern Med, 2024, 177 (8): 1048-1057.

7. 内容简介：本研究为多中心随机临床试验。为了探讨针刺治疗退行性腰椎管狭窄症（degenerative lumbar spinal stenosis，DLSS）的疗效，将以神经源性间歇性跛行疼痛症状为主的196例DLSS患者随机分配为针刺组和假针刺组，分别进行干预，观察两组受试者治疗前后改良罗兰-莫里斯残疾问卷（Roland-Morris disability questionnaire，RMDQ）相对于基线的分数变化，以及改良RMDQ达到最小（较基线减少30%）和显著临床意义改善（较基线减少50%）的受试者比例。得出结论：针刺可能缓解DLSS患者以神经源性间歇性跛行疼痛症状为主的疼痛特异性残疾，尽管与假针刺组比较，差

盲态的方法，如结果评估者、研究中心的医师和护士、数据收集者和统计学家等对分组情况不知情；在实施过程中，每天都观察到医师给予患者美沙酮治疗剂量的记录，持续8周，这种严格的操作确保了数据的准确性。

另外在固定干预措施的情况下，对针刺医师的资质要求和统一培训是保证质量的重要因素，值得提倡。①关于样本量的描述问题的考虑：样本量估算需要两组84例，因为新型冠状病毒肺炎疫情，预计脱落率将从最初估计的15%增加至30%，这在疫情期间是可以理解的，因此，将实际受试者招募目标提高至120例，实际入组了116例，完成8周治疗和第20周随访的样本量为105例，脱落率是12.5%。这个案例表明，样本量的估计是一个范围，小的调整没有影响到实际研究结果。②关于主要观察指标的精确性测量和质量控制：该试验的一项主要结局被定义为干预8周后与基线相比美沙酮剂量减少20%或更多的受试者比例，这个指标至关重要。因此，要求入组的所有受试者每天去诊所，每日摄取一次由诊所医师管理的美沙酮。之后，独立观察员会从医师那里获得美沙酮的每日消耗量，进而记录美沙酮的剂量。研究结果证明，针刺组美沙酮剂量减少20%或更多的患者比例达到62%，远高于对照组的29%。

（2）临床研究方法学及统计学方法的选择及应用问题讨论

该研究的统计分析和图表的表达规范且先进，是一个较好表达纵向研究和连续测量与报告的案例，统计分析方法描述细致，可供同道参考学习。

关于讨论中深入分析的问题，例如文中提到，根据美国和加拿大美沙酮维持治疗的标准和临床指南，每2周减少美沙酮剂量5%被认为是有效的，本研究正文结果和讨论中没有提供针刺组每2周减少美沙酮的实际剂量和患者比例，无法与美国和加拿大美沙酮维持治疗的标准和临床指南做对比，是小小的遗憾。

三 作者谈

从我国开始大力打击吸毒贩毒之后，在国家对阿片类药物的严格管控下，国内已经极少出现新的阿片类药物成瘾患者，但社区美沙酮门诊依然在为自愿戒毒的人群提供美沙酮药物替代治疗，可见阿片类药物依赖并没有得到根本的解决。我们的初衷是希望能通过针刺实现对阿片类药物的完全戒断，让美沙酮维持治疗患者能够彻底摆脱药物依赖，回归社会。

在针刺试验进行的过程中，对照组干预方式的选择一直是团队反复讨论的重点。针刺的特殊性决定了其只能对患者施盲，在以往的针刺临床研究中，对照组可以选择"非经非穴"或"穴位浅刺"，但我们的研究对象是长期服用美沙酮的人群，具有多疑、安全感缺失等特点，因此我们研发了外观完全一致的针刺盲法辅助装置，通过底部开口区分，分别用在针刺组与假针刺组。这样不仅可以保证盲法的顺利实施，同时受试者不会产生抵抗情绪，能够充分信任研究人员、配合治疗，减少心理作用带来的精神

adone Reduction: A Randomized Clinical Trial [J]. Ann Intern Med, 2024, 177 (8): 1039-1047.

7. 内容简介：本研究为多中心、双臂、随机、假针刺对照试验。为了评估针刺与假针刺对美沙酮减量的疗效，将每天到门诊就诊且已使用美沙酮至少6周、患有阿片类药物使用障碍的65岁及以下成年人随机分为针刺组和假针刺组，观察美沙酮剂量较基线水平减少20%及以上的患者比例和患者对阿片类药物的渴求程度。得出结论：8周针刺治疗在减少美沙酮剂量和降低阿片类药物渴望方面优于假针刺。

针刺组和假针刺组治疗频率为每周3次，共8周，进行24次治疗，每次留针30 min，每个穴位行针操作10 s，每10 min行针1次，共行针3次。两组均使用安慰装置，将装置放置在穴位上，将尖头/钝头的针插入导管，快速敲击管的顶部使针向下，然后取出导管，将装置和针留在原位，穴位为"定神针""四神针""手智针"。

针刺组使用尖头的针。

对照组选用假针刺疗法。将尖头的针更换为钝头的针，钝头的针不会刺入皮肤，但患者会感到模拟实际针刺的刺痛感。

二 专家述评（针灸学专家，临床研究方法学及卫生统计学专家）

1. 述评一

阿片类药物成瘾属全球严峻的公共卫生问题。阿片类药物成瘾致死率高，易加速传染病传播，并诱发各种犯罪活动，严重影响社会稳定，并造成严重的经济负担。尽管美沙酮维持治疗能短暂改善阿片类药物成瘾症状，但不良反应多，显然非药物疗法对减少美沙酮用量、降低阿片类药物成瘾的意义重大。

广州中医药大学许能贵教授团队以针刺为切入点，开展多中心的随机对照试验，采用针灸名家靳瑞创制的特色疗法"靳三针"，选取"定神针""四神针""手智针"作为针刺干预位点，观察比较为期8周、每周3次的针刺与假针刺对118例美沙酮维持治疗受试者的疗效，并在干预结束后进行12周随访。研究结果证实针刺对减少美沙酮剂量和降低阿片类药物渴望方面优于假针刺，并在一定程度上提高睡眠质量。"靳三针"重在"调神治神"，对于精神类疾病疗效确切。本研究采用"靳三针"作为针刺疗法思路确切，有章可循。此外，研究中设置了一名独立研究人员监督受试者与医师之间的对话，以避免他们沟通有关分组的问题。这一设置有益于数据管理和质控效率的提升。由于针刺干预的复杂性，假针刺通常难以实施，该团队采用自创的非刺入性假针刺装置对118例受试者成功施盲，为完成本次高质量的临床试验"保驾护航"。

2. 述评二

（1）研究设计和过程实施

这是一项规范设计的RCT研究，随机法和盲法的实施较为严谨，设计了多种保持

量方差分析比较两组主要指标的差异性。从临床角度考虑，失语症持续时间可能是影响疗效评价的混杂因素，文中采用亚组分析（分层策略）进行评价，并在重复测量方差分析时，将基线时失语症持续时间作为协变量纳入方差分析模型，调整了该混杂因素的影响，使得结论更客观、可信。此外，统计分析遵循了意向性原则（intention to treat，ITT），对于脱落者的缺失数据，研究采用了随机缺失假设下的多重插补方法进行敏感性分析。

（3）小结

这是一篇质量较高的临床试验研究，属于首次开展的多中心、假针刺对照、随机临床试验，评估针刺治疗对中风后运动性失语症患者的临床疗效。

但从统计学设计角度，仍有几个问题值得探讨。①多重性问题：文中统计学方法中提到不同时间点比较时采用Bonferroni校正来调整P值，解决多重比较问题。但值得注意的是，该研究的主要疗效指标有2个，即治疗第6周时WAB的AQ和CFCP评分。那么，在假设检验时，无论针对AQ还是CFCP评分，检验水准应该为0.025，而非0.050，以避免假阳性结果的出现。②ITT分析时缺失值填补问题：文中采用了随机缺失假设下的多重插补方法。该法近年来在临床研究中越来越多地被使用。但考虑到研究中较多的时间窗（6个），测量指标的量表特性，传统的处理方法如LOCF（临近值填补）、BOCF（基线值填补）、WOCF（最差值填补）仍不失为一种备选，可在敏感性分析时考虑使用，避免假阳性结果。

第五节 "Effect of Acupuncture for Methadone Reduction: A Randomized Clinical Trial" 相关介绍和述评

一 论文介绍

1. 中文题目：针刺干预美沙酮减量的疗效：一项随机临床试验

2. 作者：Liming Lu, Chen Chen, Yiming Chen, Yu Dong, Rouhao Chen, Xiaojing Wei, Chenyang Tao, Cui Li, Yuting Wang, Baochao Fan, Xiaorong Tang, Shichao Xu, Zhiqiu He, Guodong Mo, Yiliang Liu, Hong Gu, Xiang Li, Fang Cao, Hongxia Xu, Yuqing Zhang, Guowei Li, Xinxia Liu, Jingchun Zeng, Chunzhi Tang, Nenggui Xu

3. 主要单位：广州中医药大学针灸康复临床医学院，华南针灸研究中心临床研究与大数据实验室；江苏医药职业学院中医系；广东省中医院审计科

4. 发表期刊：*Annals of Internal Medicine*

5. 发布日期：2024年7月9日

6. SCI源文献：LU L M, CHEN C, CHEN Y M, et al. Effect of Acupuncture for Meth-

而言，疗效的持续性具有重要意义。实际上，本研究结果之所以具有说服力，不仅在于第6周的即时效果，更在于部分患者疗效显著改善持续至第6个月。

主要结局是分析干预措施有效性的关键。假设结果仅在第6周显示临床意义，而后期组间差异不显著，是应该肯定针刺在治疗中风后运动性失语症的即时有效性，还是应该因其缺乏长期作用否定针刺干预的临床意义呢？显然，此时，以第6周作为主要结局的随访时间缺乏一定的合理性。

慢性疾病的症状改善可能存在一定的波动，因此，更为合理的主要结局的随访时间应该由患者通过权衡针刺治疗的受益、风险、治疗负担等之后决定。这样既能避免因在某类慢性疾病中缺乏"时间持续性"而全盘否定针刺效果，也能避免因针刺仅在某时段内有效而草率得出针刺有效的结论，确保研究结论更加严谨。从患者角度出发设计临床试验，将得到更加符合临床实践和患者需求的试验结果，从而更好地支持试验结果推广、临床指南制定及临床循证决策。倾听患者的声音，应该成为未来临床研究的一项重要原则。

2. 述评二

（1）研究设计和实施过程

该研究为多中心、随机化、单盲设计的临床试验。临床研究中PICOST六要素在文中的方法部分都有较为准确的描述。从受试对象的纳入和排除标准、对照组的定义和划分、干预方案的解析、结局指标的定义，到研究设计中关键环节（如随机化、样本量、盲法）的应对，本文均进行了较为详实的介绍，尤其是干预方法，其中针刺角度和深度、手法方向和频率、留针时间等细节均在附录中给出，效应指标的定义也非常细致地给出。此外，文中对于中央随机化处理器、单盲实施过程等也有简略但精准的描述，提升了对研究过程和研究结果的可信度。

关于试验的实施过程，文章做了简略但清晰的描述，即在正文Figure 1中报告了受试者从入组到完成试验的流程。

文章构思和撰写很好地遵循了临床试验报告统一标准（consolidated standards of reporting trials，CONSORT），较为完整准确地报告了设计、实施、分析及结果解读全过程，可读性较强。

（2）临床研究方法学及统计学方法的选择及应用

作为一项随机对照试验（randomized controlled trial，RCT）研究，该文对于干预措施、受试对象、试验效应三要素，以及需要遵循的随机化、对照、重复三原则都有简洁准确的叙述。对于设计中的关键环节，比如中央随机化处理器完成随机入组、如何实施单盲法、样本量的确定及其依据，面面俱到。尤其是对干预措施的描述非常详实，一套标准化的操作指南增加了读者和评审者的好感和信心。

针对前瞻性研究设计、重复测量的疗效指标属于定量资料，研究采用了重复测

天津中医药大学

4．发表期刊：*JAMA Network Open*

5．发布日期：2024年1月22日

6．SCI源文献：LI B, DENG S, ZHUO B, et al. Effect of Acupuncture vs Sham Acupuncture on Patients With Poststroke Motor Aphasia: A Randomized Clinical Trial [J]. JAMA Netw Open, 2024, 7 (1): e2352580.

7．内容简介：本研究为多中心、假对照随机临床试验。为了研究针刺对中风后运动性失语症患者的语言功能、神经功能和生活质量的影响，将首次中风后运动性失语症的成年患者随机分为手针组和假针刺组，两组均接受语言培训和常规治疗。主要结局是治疗第6周时西方失语症成套测验（Western aphasia battery，WAB）的失语商（aphasia quotient，AQ）和中国式功能性语言沟通能力检测法（Chinese functional communication profile，CFCP）评分。次要结局包括WAB子项目、波士顿诊断性失语症检查法（Boston diagnostic aphasia examination，BDAE）、美国国立卫生研究院卒中量表（National Institutes of Health stroke scale，NIHSS）、脑卒中专用生活质量量表（stroke-specific quality of life scale，SS-QOL）、脑卒中失语症生活质量量表39（stroke and aphasia quality of life scale-39，SAQOL-39）及根据中医理论体系揭示综合健康状况的中医健康量表。次要结局的统计学分析在发病后2周、4周、6周、12周及6个月进行。得出结论：在语言训练的基础上，与假针刺相比，针刺治疗能够有效改善中风后运动性失语症患者的语言功能，提高患者的生活质量。

手针组和假针刺组分别进行手针治疗和假针刺治疗，均为每周5次，每次30 min，共30个疗程。同时，两组均需进行30次语言训练，连续6周（每周5次，每次60 min）。

手针组按照标准的醒脑开窍针刺方案进行手针治疗，包括固定的进针角度和深度、操作方向和频率、留针时间。手针组患者针刺8个固定穴位，包括内关（PC6，双侧）、水沟（GV26）、三阴交（SP6，双侧）、极泉（HT1，患侧）、尺泽（LU5，患侧）、委中（BL40，患侧）、廉泉（CV23）及旁廉泉（CV23旁边，双侧）。通过针刺刺激诱发得气感觉，留针30 min。

假针刺组选用假针刺疗法，在手针组选定的穴位水平方向上选择8个假穴位，包括非经络点和非经络位置，并且间隔为1寸（1寸≈25毫米，定义为患者大拇指指间关节宽度），不引起得气感觉，留针30 min。

二 专家述评（针灸学专家，临床研究方法学及卫生统计学专家）

1. 述评一

本研究探讨了针刺对中风后运动性失语症的疗效。研究者选取治疗后的WAB的AQ和CFCP评分（第6周）作为主要结局，这种设计颇为常见。但对于慢性疾病患者

第二章 SCI源期刊高质量针灸临床研究述评

针对前瞻性研究设计、重复测量的疗效指标属于定量资料，研究采用了混合效应模型（无结构协方差矩阵）评价3组主要指标的差异性；对于临床反应、不良事件等定性指标采用了卡方检验。统计分析遵循了意向性分析原则，对于不可避免的脱落造成的疗效指标缺失，采用了基于单调回归的多重填补方法进行处理，并对主要结果做了敏感性分析，发现结果依然保持稳定。

（3）小结

这是一篇质量较高的临床试验研究，证实了针刺治疗放射性口干症的临床疗效和安全性。除作者提到的几点不足之处，仍有一些问题值得警惕和思考。①统计学意义和临床意义：文中计算样本含量时明确提到"每组之间XQ评分（0~100分尺度）差异为10个点，被认为具有临床意义"，然而，文中主要结果（Table 2）中的XQ评分的修正均数（调整了基线XQ评分后），包括附录Supplementary Online Content中etable1、2提供的真实均数，针刺与假针刺、标准口腔卫生两个对照组XQ评分的均差都未达到10分，比如第4周的XQ评分的修正均值，针刺组为50.59，假针刺组为54.99，标准口腔卫生组为57.26，在附录etable1的真实值也是如此。大约7分的分差是否有临床意义？针对这个问题，可以从年龄、种族、职业、基线XQ评分等入手，进行亚组分析，探索针灸治疗潜在的更佳获益人群。当然，考虑安全性、经济性等综合评价后，针刺仍不失为一个好的选择。②脱落的影响：文中结果部分详述了三组的脱落率，针刺组为2.4%，假针刺组为10.6%，标准口腔卫生组为23.8%，为什么标准口腔卫生组脱落如此之高？能从一定程度上反映TA的依从性更好吗？还需要从脱落者特征入手，评价脱落对结果外推造成的影响。比如，伤残/无法工作者、非洲裔美国人、美洲印第安人或阿拉斯加原住民占50%，土著美国人或太平洋岛民退出率都很高。

由此延伸，研究持续了8年，多家中心参与，有没有中心效应存在（某家或某些中心的质控不佳导致脱落率更高）？

第四节 "Effect of Acupuncture vs Sham Acupuncture on Patients With Poststroke Motor Aphasia: A Randomized Clinical Trial" 相关介绍和述评

一 论文介绍

1. 中文题目：针刺与假针刺对中风后运动性失语症患者的疗效：一项随机临床试验

2. 作者：Boxuan Li, Shizhe Deng, Bifang Zhuo, Bomo Sang, Junjie Chen, Menglong Zhang, Guang Tian, Lili Zhang, Yuzheng Du, Peng Zheng, Gonglei Yue, Zhihong Meng

3. 主要单位：国家中医针灸临床医学研究中心，天津中医药大学第一附属医院，

究发现针刺干预可以促进患者唾液分泌并改善。然而，由于盲法缺失、无假针刺对照或样本量小等因素，针刺治疗头颈癌放疗后口干的疗效仍缺乏高质量证据。鉴于此，作者设计了该项多中心、随机、盲法、三臂、安慰剂对照的3期临床试验。研究将接受放疗的头颈癌患者随机分为针刺组、假针刺组和标准口腔卫生组，针刺周期4周，每周2次，每次20 min，选取14个穴位进行干预。假针刺以非穿透性、伸缩式针头装置刺激穴位旁开部位。所有患者均接受标准口腔护理。主要结局指标是第4周时患者的口干问卷（xerostomia questionnaire，XQ）评分。这项纳入258例头颈部癌症患者的随机临床试验结果显示，与标准口腔护理相比，针刺在改善头颈癌患者的口干症症状和总体生活质量方面是有效的。尽管存在安慰针效应的可能性，但假针刺治疗的疗效甚微，且与总体生活质量的改善无关。本研究涉及的机制虽然尚不明确，但已有研究报道这种针刺机制可能与筋膜介导的中枢神经系统效应、针刺刺激后某些神经肽增加而导致的血管舒张和微循环改善有关。

2. 述评二

（1）研究设计和过程实施

该研究很好地报告和诠释了临床研究中PICOST六要素，包括Participants/Patients（研究对象/患者）、Intervention（干预措施）、Control/Comparison（对照或比较措施）、Outcome（研究结局）、Study design（研究设计）和Time（时间）。受试对象的入选和排除标准、对照组的定义和划分、3组干预方案的解释说明、结局指标的定义，以及研究设计中的关键环节（如随机化、样本量、盲法）的详细解析、试验周期都在文章中得以体现，从而增强了研究过程与结果的可信度。

关于试验的实施过程，文章做了清晰的描述，从2013年7月开始到2015年4月试验基地转移，直至2021年6月结束，这一过程在正文及补充材料中均有详细介绍。这样一项持续8年的随机、盲法、三臂、多中心的临床试验并不多见，其可持续性、受试者脱落、质量控制等方面均面临诸多挑战。然而，作者在正文Figure 1. 中很明智地报告了受试者从入组到完成实验的流程图（Patient Flowchart），以详实的数据在一定程度上减少了质疑。

文章的行文过程很好地遵循了临床试验报告统一标准（consolidated standards of reporting trials，CONSORT）准则，将研究的设计、实施、分析及结果解读全过程较为完整准确地报告出来，可读性较强。

（2）临床研究方法学及统计学方法的选择及应用

作为一项随机对照试验（randomized controlled trial，RCT）研究，该文对干预措施、受试对象、试验效应三要素，以及需要遵循的随机化、对照、重复三原则做了详细描述。尤其是决定试验成败的关键环节部分，如采用自适应最小化法进行动态随机化，盲法设置中假针刺组穴位点的选取，避免盲法失败的应对措施，样本量的确定及其依据，甚至研究所用的针，作者在文中均做了叙述或详述，很大程度上增强了读者对研究质量的信心。

University of TexasMD Anderson Cancer Center, Houston; Department of Social Sciences & Health Policy, Wake Forest University School of Medicine, Winston-Salem, North Carolina; Department of Biostatistics &Data Science, Wake Forest University School of Medicine, Winston-Salem, North Carolina

4. 发表期刊：*JAMA Network Open*

5. 发布日期：2024年5月13日

6. SCI源文献：COHEN L, DANHAUER S C, GARCIA M K, et al. Acupuncture for Chronic Radiation-Induced Xerostomia in Head and Neck Cancer: A Multicenter Randomized Clinical Trial [J]. JAMA Netw Open, 2024, 7 (5): e2410421.

7. 内容简介：本研究为随机、盲法、三臂、安慰剂对照试验，旨在比较针刺、假针刺及标准口腔卫生在治疗放射性口干症（由头颈部癌症放疗引起）方面的效果，将258例患者随机分配至针刺组、假针刺组或标准口腔卫生组，所有患者均接受标准口腔卫生，观察3组患者在基线、第4周（主要评估时间点）、第8周、第12周及第26周的口干症症状和生活质量的差异。得出结论：放疗结束后1年或更长时间内，针刺在治疗慢性放射引起的口干症方面比假针刺或标准口腔卫生更有效。

针刺组和假针刺组治疗频次均为每周2次，每次持续20 min，共进行4周。对于治疗反应轻微的患者，再给予4周治疗。

针刺组共针刺14个部位，包括双侧耳穴：神门（TF4）、零点、唾液腺2；承浆（CV24），双侧列缺（LU7），双侧商阳（LI1-prime），双侧照海（KI6）；于中渎（GB32）放置1处安慰针。

对照组选用假针刺疗法，其时间安排与针刺组相同。假针刺疗法采用经过验证的非穿透性的、伸缩式针头，该针头配备可分离装置，能够安全地附着在皮肤上而不穿透皮肤。在耳轮上，选择3个非阳性穴位点，分别位于耳郭中央，标记为helix2、helix3和helix4。对于体穴的操作，假针刺点则选择在以下非活动穴位上，假针刺点1：位于下颏上神庭（GV24）下方0.5寸及侧面各0.5寸的非活性点；假针刺点2：位于手少阳三焦经和手阳明大肠经之间的支沟（SJ6）径向0.5寸和近端0.5寸的非活性点；假针刺点3：位于手少阳三焦经和手阳明大肠经之间，温溜（LI7）与下廉（LI8）之间的上方2寸处的非活性点；假针刺点4：位于足阳明胃经和足少阳胆经之间，足三里（ST36）下方1.0寸及侧面0.5寸的非活性点。

二　专家述评（针灸学专家，临床研究方法学及卫生统计学专家）

1. 述评一

头颈癌放疗后，超过50%的患者会出现唾液分泌不足（口干症），严重影响其生活质量。尽管目前尚无可靠方法彻底治疗急性和慢性放疗引起的口干症状，但一些随机观察研

者，然而，在结果中却未报告患者对针刺治疗的依从情况，从而可能低估针刺疗效。

总之，本研究选题精准，针对PD患者临床治疗难点及关键点，针刺干预报告较为详细，但关于针刺治疗方案的合理性、针刺操作、针灸师资质及患者依从性等方面的阐述仍有待进一步加强。

2. 述评二

本研究为单中心、随机对照试验研究。干预措施为针刺治疗，论文严格按照临床试验报告统一标准（consolidated standards of reporting trials，CONSORT）撰写，清晰阐述了受试对象的纳入标准，针刺组、假针刺组分别进行的针刺操作，以及穴位和非穴位设计。受试对象采用简单随机、单盲设计，即患者不知道分组情况。此外文章还强调了统计分析人员盲法。根据预试验的结果，估算了研究的样本量，研究把握度设置为90%，脱落率按照20%预估。结果部分按照随机对照试验的可比性分析、疗效比较和安全性评价的顺序进行报告。首先描述了两组的基线数据，进行可比性分析，在描述的基础上也报告了统计学结果（P值）。本研究疗效指标分析采用全数据集分析，而根据针刺组40例和假针刺组38例均为全部完整的病例，因此事实上亦满足符合方案集。但文中又阐述了采用随机填补的方式获得全数据集数据进行分析，但报告的数据例数显示是40例和38例，这部分陈述使读者感到费解。统计学方法的描述部分陈述了方法选择的原则和依据，结合研究中在3个时间点获取效果数据，按照重复测量的设计，选择了线性混合效应模型分析组别效应、时间效应和组别-时间交互效应，并结合折线图展示结果。

整体而言，本研究采用单中心、随机对照试验，设计合理，报告规范，统计描述与推断方法合理，逻辑清晰，推论合理。

第三节 "Acupuncture for Chronic Radiation-Induced Xerostomia in Head and Neck Cancer: A Multicenter Randomized Clinical Trial" 相关介绍和述评

一 论文介绍

1. 中文题目：针刺治疗头颈癌慢性放射性口干症：一项多中心随机临床试验

2. 作者：Lorenzo Cohen, Suzanne C. Danhauer, M. Kay Garcia, Emily V. Dressler, David I. Rosenthal, Mark S. Chambers, Andrew Cusimano, W. Mark Brown, Jewel M.Ochoa, Peiying Yang, Joseph S. Chiang, Ora Gordon, Rhonda Crutcher, Jung K. Kim, Michael P. Russin, Joshua Lukenbill, Mercedes Porosnicu, Kathleen J. Yost, Kathryn E. Weaver, Glenn J. Lesser

3. 主要单位：Department of Palliative, Rehabilitation, and Integrative Medicine, The

4. 发表期刊：*JAMA Network Open*

5. 发布日期：2024年6月26日

6. SCI源文献：YAN M, FAN J, LIU X, et al. Acupuncture and Sleep Quality Among Patients With Parkinson Disease: A Randomized Clinical Trial [J]. JAMA Netw Open, 2024, 7 (6): e2417862.

7. 内容简介：本研究为单中心、随机、双盲、假对照临床试验。为了探讨针刺辅助治疗睡眠质量差的帕金森病（Parkinson's disease，PD）患者的有效性和安全性，将78例受试者随机分为针刺组和假针刺组，分别进行干预，观察两组受试者在基线、治疗4周结束时和随访8周时帕金森病睡眠量表（Parkinson's disease sleep scale，PDSS）评分的变化，以及治疗完成率、不良事件等。得出结论：针刺有助于改善PD患者的睡眠质量和生活质量。

针刺组和假针刺组治疗频次均为每周3次，每次30 min，持续4周。两组均使用研究团队自主研发的针刺装置，患者均采取仰卧位并佩戴不透明眼罩。两组选用相同穴位，包括：四神针（Si Shenzhen）、神庭（GV24）、印堂（EX-HN3）、合谷（LI4）、太冲（LR3）、三阴交（SP6）、神门（HT7）、足三里（ST36）、申脉（BL62）、照海（KI6）。穴位定位和常规消毒后，医师将针刺装置紧贴穴位皮肤，然后进行针刺。

针刺组将一次性无菌不锈钢针放入针刺装置上相应的针管，将针插入持针器上相应的15°/90°进针口，快速、无痛进针。

假针刺组使用相同规格钝头针（不刺穿皮肤进入皮下组织），针刺方法同针刺组。

二 专家述评（针灸学专家，临床研究方法学及卫生统计学专家）

1. 述评一

睡眠障碍是PD常见的非运动症状，也是PD治疗药物常见的副作用。睡眠障碍不仅严重影响PD患者的生活质量，而且会加速患者运动症状和非运动症状恶化，成为影响PD患者转归的主要原因。然而，目前PD患者睡眠障碍的治疗药物虽然在一定程度上可以改善睡眠，但经常伴随副作用，亟需寻找新的安全有效的疗法。既往研究显示，针刺可用于治疗失眠，改善PD患者睡眠障碍，但是研究和证据质量相对较低。因此，本研究聚焦影响PD患者转归的关键点及治疗难点，在分析针刺治疗PD睡眠障碍临床研究现状的基础上，设计高质量临床试验，以提供高质量的研究证据。

参考既往研究，本研究中针刺治疗方案选择常用的安神定志及脾、胃经穴位，腧穴定位依据国家标准《经穴名称与定位》（GB/T 12346—2021），报告了针具选择、治疗频次及疗程，尤其是详细描述了针刺辅助装置的操作方法以实现患者盲法。然而，本研究仍有待改进之处，治疗方案中穴位选择不同于既往研究而未给出解释，未介绍各穴位操作细节及针灸师资质要求。文中虽然指出数据分析针对至少接受1周治疗患

并通过适应性随机化和双盲法来减少偏倚，从而增强研究结果的内部效度。总体而言，研究设计在控制变量和减少干扰因素方面呈现出较高的严谨性，尤其是多层次的评估体系，包括临床症状（如CAPS-5评分）和生理反应（如恐惧增强惊吓反应）的评估，使研究结果更为全面和有力。然而，该设计仍有改进空间。首先，研究仅在单一地点进行，可能限制了结果的外部有效性。其次，虽然采用了适应性随机化以确保分组平衡，但由于研究样本的特殊性（即仅限于战斗退伍军人），结果的普适性可能受到限制。此外，研究在对受试者进行长期随访方面存在不足，无法全面评估针刺的长期疗效。

（2）临床研究方法及统计学方法的选择及应用

在临床研究方法上，本研究选择验证性RCT设计，结合盲法，将假针刺作为对照组，为评估针刺的特异性效果提供了科学依据。主要分析方法采用意向性治疗（intention to treat，ITT）分析和完成治疗模型，确保了结果的稳健性。统计分析采用了广义线性模型和重复测量方差分析，有效控制了数据的相关性，并在处理组间差异时显示了适当的效力。研究通过使用Cohen d效应量评估了治疗效果的大小，进一步验证了结果的临床意义。

尽管如此，统计学方法上仍存在一些需要注意的问题。首先，虽然研究对针刺干预PTSD症状的减少效果进行了评估，但未能对多重假设检验进行充分调整，这可能增加第一类错误的风险。其次，在处理中途退出的受试者数据时，尽管采用了ITT分析，但由于退出原因的复杂性，可能导致结果的偏倚。最后，研究中对假针刺组的有效性讨论较少，而假针刺本身可能产生一定的生理效应，这在解释结果时应更为谨慎。

综上所述，该研究在设计和方法学应用上具有明显的优点，尤其是在随机化、盲法及多维度结果评估方面。然而，在外部效度、统计学方法的细化处理及假针刺组的讨论方面仍有改进空间。总体而言，该研究为针刺在PTSD治疗中的应用提供了有价值的证据，但在结论的普遍性和严谨性方面应持谨慎态度。未来的研究应进一步探索针刺疗效的长期性及其与其他治疗方法的相对效力。

第二节 "Acupuncture and Sleep Quality Among Patients With Parkinson Disease: A Randomized Clinical Trial" 相关介绍和述评

一 论文介绍

1. 中文题目：针刺对帕金森病患者睡眠质量的影响：一项随机临床试验
2. 作者：Mingyue Yan, Jingqi Fan, Xin Liu, Yingjia Li, Yuting Wang, Weiqiang Tan, Yuanyuan Chen, Jun He, Lixing Zhuang
3. 主要单位：广州中医药大学第一临床医学院，广州中医药大学，广州市番禺中医院

肾俞（BL23）及风池（GB20）。除标准穴位外，还会根据中医诊断模式选择另外3个穴位，以针对受试者的症状加减穴位。所有针刺组受试者接受2/100 Hz疏密波治疗。

对照组选用假针疗法。本研究中的假针（微针）疗法有3个要素定义。第一是针刺位置，假针刺位置位于实际参考点外侧或内侧2 cm处，预计不会影响PTSD症状。第二是与标准针刺相比，刺入深度较浅（＜0.25英寸）。第三是由于刺入深度和不起作用的假电刺激器来完成假效果而导致相对无刺激。标准针刺位点和假针刺位置之间的实际距离是相近的，设置将考虑：①附近的针灸经络分布；②浅表或深层的解剖特征；③每例受试者的身体比例（同身寸）。研究者将假针刺部位列为前部或后部，并注意保持在经络外。针灸师不会进行任何获得"得气"的操作，假针只会调整至更浅的深度，以尽量减少报告的刺痛或刺激等感觉。该方案还交替使用11个仰卧位穴位和14个俯卧位穴位，并对成对穴位连接假电针。

二 专家述评（针灸学专家，临床研究方法学及卫生统计学专家）

1. 述评一

药物疗法和心理疗法对创伤后应激障碍有效，但患者依从性差。该试验以PTSD退伍军人为研究对象，选题新颖，进一步扩大了针刺的临床适应范围。

针刺组治疗频次为每周2次，疗程为15周（24次），每次留针30 min，基本满足临床疗效产生所需的强度要求。针刺方案采用半标准化选穴，结合教材、专家共识及对受试者的评估，归纳出四大证型，确定治疗必选的主穴，针灸师每次治疗前进行四诊，并选择仰卧位和俯卧位交替治疗以避免穴位疲劳。双侧分布的穴位连接电针，频率为2/100 Hz。针刺治疗方案的制定和实施能够反映中医特色。针刺深度及电流频率在既往临床研究方案及试验结果报告中未见报道。

为兼顾盲法实施，试验采用微针疗法作为假针刺对照组，从针刺部位、深度和刺激强度出发进行设置，尽可能减小生物学治疗效应。以非经、非穴作为施术部位（针刺组经穴旁2 cm左右），同时须兼顾不同患者体型，并避开关键解剖标志。对穴位进行浅刺，深度不超过0.25英寸。拟破皮感，不行手法、不得气，电针仪指示灯亮但无电流输出。为确保盲法实施，选穴数量、治疗频次与针刺组完全相同，诊疗环境布置、物品准备、操作流程及同患者沟通方法均按照标准流程进行。对照组选择及实施得当。

2. 述评二

（1）研究设计和过程实施

该研究采用随机对照试验（randomized controlled trial，RCT）设计，旨在评估针刺对战斗相关PTSD的临床和生物学效应。研究采用两组平行对照的方法，假设标准针刺在减少PTSD症状和改善恐惧消退反应方面优于假针刺。研究的实施严格遵循伦理规范，

第二章
SCI 源期刊高质量针灸临床研究述评

第一节 "Acupuncture for Combat-Related Posttraumatic Stress Disorder: A Randomized Clinical Trial" 相关介绍和述评

一 论文介绍

1. 中文题目：针刺治疗战斗相关创伤后应激障碍：一项随机临床试验

2. 作者：Michael Hollifield, An-Fu Hsiao, Tyler Smith, Teresa Calloway, Tanja Jovanovic, Besa Smith, Kala Carrick, Seth D. Norrholm, Andrea Munoz, Ruth Alpert, Brianna Caicedo, Nikki Frousakis, Karen Cocozza

3. 主要单位：Tibor Rubin VA Medical Center, Long Beach, California; Department of Psychiatry and Behavioral Sciences, GeorgeWashington School of Medicine & Health Sciences, Washington, DC; Department of Medicine, Health Policy Research Institute and General Internal Medicine, University of California, Irvine

4. 发表期刊：*JAMA Psychiatry*

5. 发布日期：2024年2月21日

6. SCI 源文献：HOLLIFIELD M, HAIAO A F, SMITH T, et al. Acupuncture for Combat-Related Posttraumatic Stress Disorder: A Randomized Clinical Trial [J]. JAMA Psychiatry, 2024, 81 (6): 545-554.

7. 内容简介：本研究为双臂、双盲、前瞻性、假对照随机临床试验。为了探讨对于创伤后应激障碍（posttraumatic stress disorder，PTSD）患者，针刺在减少PTSD症状或恐惧增强惊吓反应方面是否比假针刺的治疗效果更佳，将93例患者（退伍军人）随机分为针刺组和假针刺组，并分别进行干预，观察两组受试者治疗前后PTSD量表评分和恐惧增强惊吓反应。得出结论：与假针刺相比，针刺治疗PTSD效果显著。

针刺组和假针刺组治疗频次均为每周2次，每次1 h，疗程为15周。每次治疗包括问诊（10 min）、脉诊舌诊（5 min）、标准针刺得气（10 min）、留针（30 min）、拔针和观察（5 min）。

针刺组仰卧位共针刺11个穴位，包括双侧太冲（LR3）、内关（PC6）、神门（HT7）、足三里（ST36）、三阴交（SP6），以及印堂穴（EX-HN3）；俯卧位共针刺14个穴位，包括双侧厥阴俞（BL14）、心俞（BL15）、肝俞（BL18）、脾俞（BL20）、胃俞（BL21）、

(3): 291-294.

［5］ 洪寿海, 张盈盈, 徐福. 近7年高影响因子SCI期刊针灸RCT研究分析与探讨 [J]. 浙江中医药大学学报, 2021, 45 (7): 718-725.

［6］ 丁楠. 针灸临床实践指南共识过程的方法学研究 [D]. 北京: 中国中医科学院, 2023.

［7］ 邱瑞瑾, 魏旭煦, 关之玥, 等. 中医药领域核心指标集研究现状及展望 [J]. 中国循证医学杂志, 2023, 23 (2): 211-220.

［8］ 林静怡, 申屠慰, 季昭臣, 等. 近5年国内针灸随机对照临床试验文献质量分析 [J/OL]. 上海针灸杂志, 2024: 1-9[2024-09-26]. https://doi.org/10.13460/j.issn.1005-0957.2024.11.0004.

［9］ 石云舟, 周思远, 郑倩华, 等. 国际高质量针灸随机对照试验特征分析[J]. 世界中医药, 2018, 13 (7): 1580-1583.

［10］ 岗卫娟, 巩昌镇, 景向红. 中西方针刺随机对照试验的比较研究 [J]. 中国针灸, 2022, 42 (1): 3-7, 22.

［11］ 樊伟铭, 孙驰雲, 张晶潾, 等. 针刺临床随机对照试验改进方法的探究 [J]. 上海针灸杂志, 2024, 43 (1): 104-110.

［12］ 张子星. 基于国外高质量针灸临床试验评价安慰针刺设置因素及合理性研究 [D]. 天津: 天津中医药大学, 2023.

［13］ 郭秋蕾, 刘清国, 战河, 等. 安慰针刺对照在临床研究中的应用与思考 [J]. 针灸临床杂志, 2017, 33 (11): 1-3.

［14］ 刘佳惠, 马宁, 董旭, 等. 安慰针刺对照设计的研究现状及应用分析 [J]. 上海针灸杂志, 2022, 41 (3): 318-322.

［15］ 刘晓玉, 马培宏, 刘保延, 等. 针刺临床试验中假针刺对照报告指南与清单 (SHARE) 解读 [J]. 中国循证医学杂志, 2024, 24 (7): 838-844.

［16］ FAN J Q, LU W J, TAN W Q, et al. Effectiveness of Acupuncture for Anxiety Among Patients With Parkinson Disease: A Randomized Clinical Trial [J]. JAMA Netw Open, 2022, 5 (9): e2232133.

［17］ YAN M, FAN J, LIU X, et al. Acupuncture and Sleep Quality Among Patients With Parkinson Disease: A Randomized Clinical Trial [J]. JAMA Netw Open, 2024, 7 (6): e2417862.

［18］ 王毓婷, 刘鑫, 徐子乔, 等. 一种用于双盲安慰针刺研究的辅助装置 [J]. 中国针灸, 2022, 42 (3): 351-354.

三 小结与展望

中国在针灸领域的卓越成果推动了全球针灸临床研究的进步，取得了显著成就。高质量的针灸临床研究广泛涵盖了疼痛、消化系统疾病、神经系统疾病等多个领域，展示出针灸疗法的多元应用潜力。这些研究采用了包括电针、手针和激光针在内的多种针刺方法，以满足不同疾病的治疗需求。值得注意的是，假针刺的设置在针灸临床研究中占据了重要地位，它通过科学严谨的对照设计，提升了针灸治疗效果评估的证据质量，从而确保了研究结果的准确性和可靠性。然而，临床研究内容重复和质量不高等问题依然存在，这在一定程度上造成了科研资源的浪费。

在2023年举办的中国·天津第十六届国际针灸学术研讨会上，在世界针灸学会联合会刘保延主席的召集下，30位中医药及临床研究专家围绕"研究者发起的中医药临床研究体系建设"召开闭门会议，形成了《研究者发起的中医药临床研究天津共识》。该共识旨在团结和组织中医药界人士，探索并推动符合中医药特色的临床研究，促进中医药在全球范围内的广泛应用及其价值的充分体现。

展望未来，应加强不同国家和地区之间的交流与合作，构建跨学科的针灸临床研究团队，将多领域的新技术和新方法应用于针灸临床研究，以促进其多元化发展，这是提升针灸临床研究质量的重要途径。在传统医学理论的基础上，结合现代科学技术，构建符合针灸临床研究特点的实验范式和评价方案，以形成高质量的针灸临床证据，完善针灸疾病谱，优化针灸治疗方案，为提升全人类的健康水平贡献针灸力量。

执笔人：石江伟、沈燕、樊官伟、王金贵、张艳军（均来自天津中医药大学第一附属医院，国家中医针灸临床医学研究中心）；刘保延、刘志顺、何丽云（中国中医科学院）

参 考 文 献

[1] 闫世艳, 熊芝怡, 刘晓玉, 等. 2010—2020年针灸临床研究现状及展望 [J]. 中国针灸, 2022, 42 (1): 116-118, 120.

[2] KASPER S, BANCHER C, ECKERT A, et al. Management of mild cognitive impairment (MCI): The need for national and international guidelines [J]. World J Biol Psychiatry, 2020, 21(8): 579-594.

[3] 李少源, 荣培晶, 张悦, 等. 基于耳穴迷走神经电刺激技术的"脑病耳治"思路与临床应用 [J]. 中医杂志, 2020, 61 (24): 2154-2158.

[4] 洪寿海, 吴菲, 丁沙沙, 等. 近5年SCI高影响因子期刊针灸相关文献分析 [J]. 中国针灸, 2015, 35

别在于后者具有正确的穴位名称和明确的主治作用。二者通过利用人体部位效应的差异来降低针刺的作用,但与不刺入相比,浅刺更容易导致阴性结果[12]。在设置假针刺时,需要在保障盲法的基础上,实现"盲法最大化、效应最小化"的目标。因此,基于上述假针刺的特性,建议参考假针刺报告的SHARE指南,以提高假针刺报告的透明度[15]。

在针灸随机对照试验中,所选用的安慰针刺装置主要以Streitberger和Park的设计为主(图11)。这两种装置均不刺破皮肤,但能够产生类似于针刺的痛觉。研究[11]表明,这两种装置能够有效实现患者的盲法设定。在纳入的52篇研究中,有12篇文献(占23.08%)提及安慰针刺装置的应用。此外,国内学者也在积极研发新型安慰针刺装置,相关成果已在国际高质量期刊上发表(图12)[16-18]。

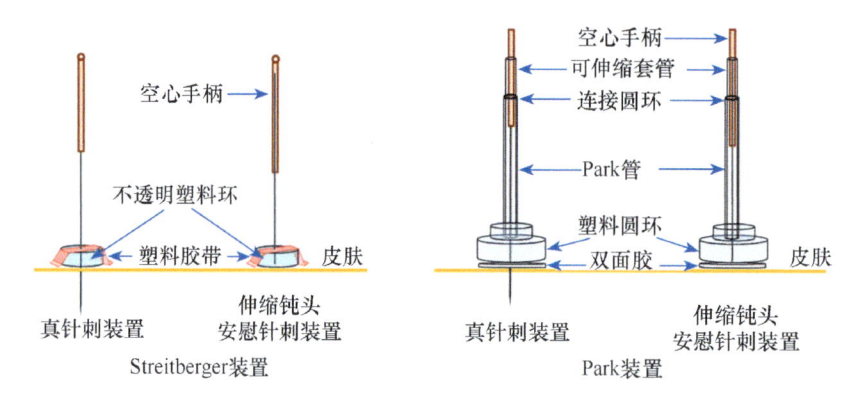

图11 Streitberger和Park安慰针刺装置示意图

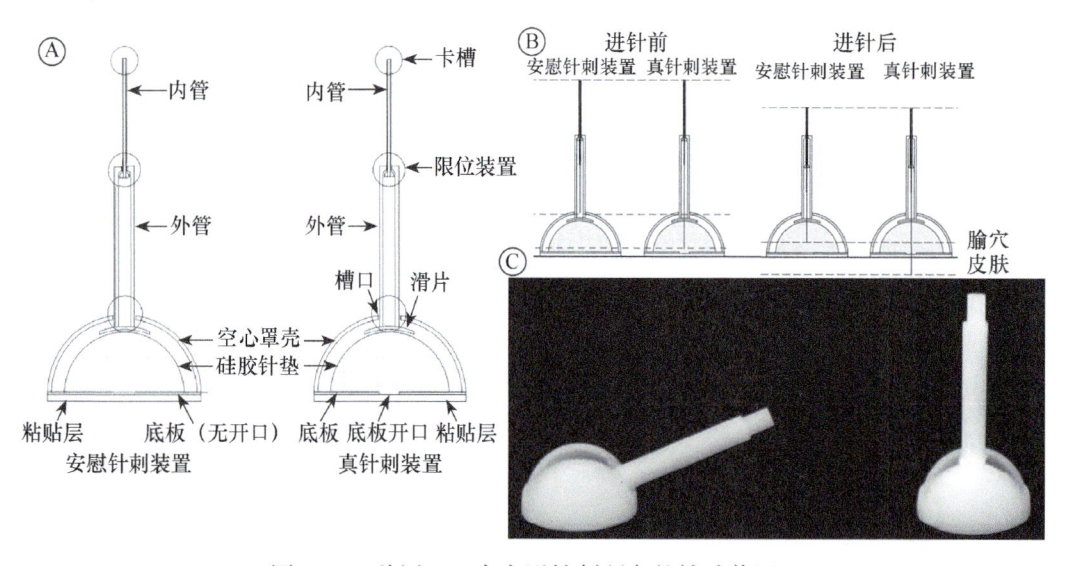

图12 一种用于双盲安慰针刺研究的辅助装置

注:A.安慰针刺与真针刺装置结构示意图;B.安慰针刺与真针刺操作示意图;C.新型辅助针刺装置实物图。

3. 从解释性随机对照试验到真实世界研究：针灸临床试验的发展趋势与范式思考

纳入的文献中共有17篇（32.69%，17/52）涉及验证性检验及优效性检验/非劣效性检验，其中组别设置为针刺组、假针刺组和对照组（包括西药组或常规护理组）。针刺组与假针刺组的比较能够揭示针灸特异性效应及其有效性；而针刺组与西药组或常规护理组的比较则可用于评估针灸的优效性和安全性。有研究[10]表明，由于中国和西方国家在针刺随机对照试验研究的需求、起点、目的、设计、预试验、研究者、针刺治疗方案、针刺方案来源、方法学质量、研究结果、结论、数量、发表偏倚及研究不足等方面存在显著差异，使得中国学者的针灸临床研究阳性结果率为71.43%，而国外学者的则为59.18%。中西学者对针灸结果的不同报告推动了对针灸特异性效应的验证（71.15%，37/52；图10），成为针灸临床研究的重要焦点。真实世界研究强调在真实临床环境中评估干预措施的临床结局，从而获得高质量且具有广泛外推性的循证依据[11]。结合针灸的特性，从解释性随机对照试验、实用性随机对照试验到以临床疗效为导向的真实世界研究，建立遵循针灸自身规律的科研新范式，以促进针灸临床证据的积累与完善，已成为当前针灸学科亟待解决的重要任务。

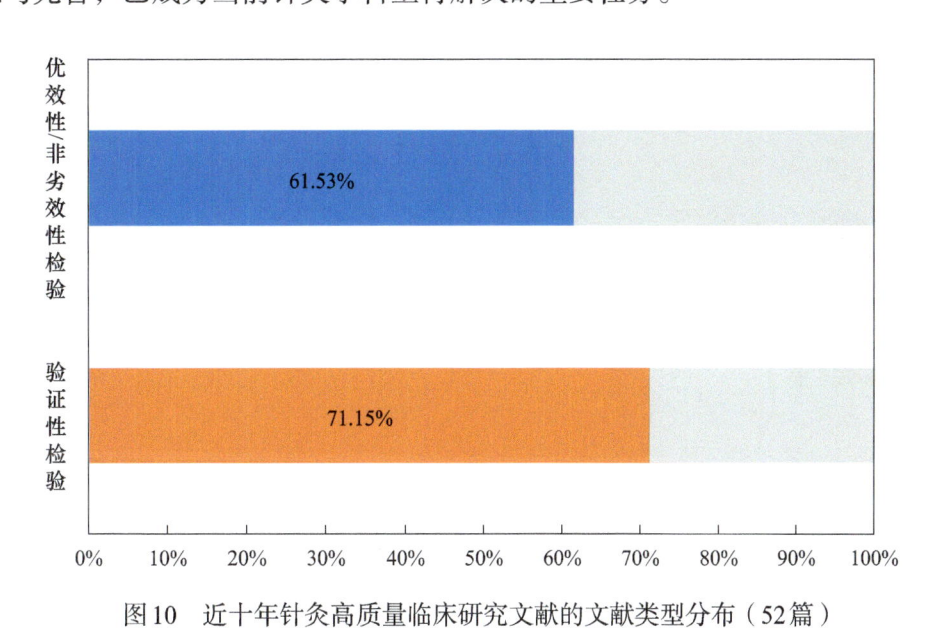

图10 近十年针灸高质量临床研究文献的文献类型分布（52篇）

4. 针灸特异性效应验证：安慰针刺设计的争议与进展

安慰针刺是国际公认的验证针灸特异性效应的重要对照方法，对确保高质量随机对照试验至关重要[12]。然而，目前安慰针刺的设计仍然存在较大争议[13]。安慰针刺的设计方案主要包括：真穴假刺（不破皮）、假穴浅刺及非治疗相关穴位浅刺等。真穴假刺的盲法效果较差，破盲风险较大，但其优点在于不刺破皮肤，激活人体感受器的程度有限，从而不产生特异性治疗效果[14]。假穴浅刺与非治疗相关穴位浅刺的主要区

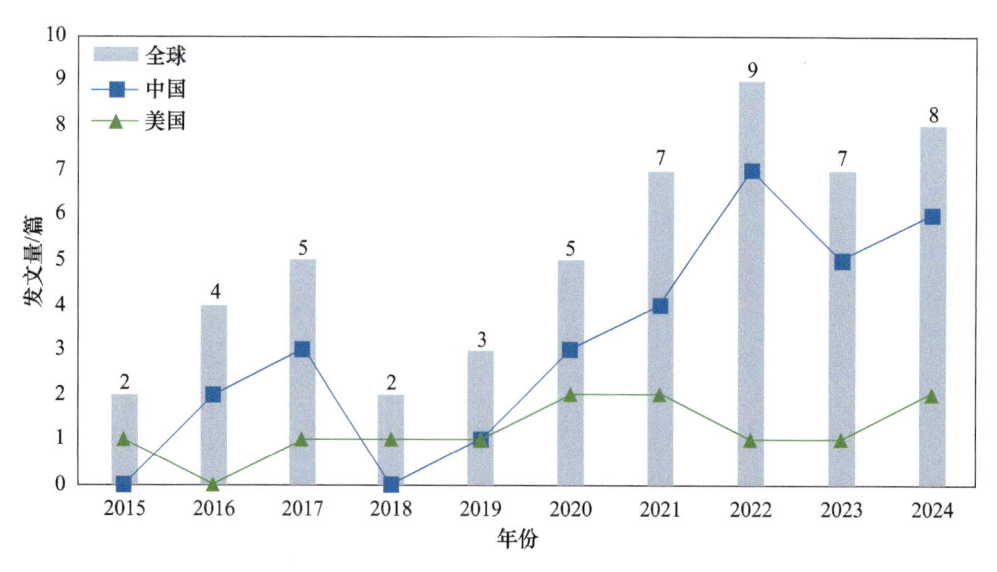

图8　近十年针灸高质量临床研究文献发表国家趋势（52篇）

注：2024年数据截至7月31日。

2. 针灸治疗的疾病种类不断扩展

疼痛仍是高质量针灸临床试验的主要研究焦点之一。有研究通过检索PubMed数据库中2010—2018年影响因子（impact factor，IF）>5的针灸随机对照试验发现，肿瘤及疼痛是研究热点[9]。近年来，针灸治疗的疾病种类逐步从癌症及其并发症扩展至消化系统疾病。同时，针灸在治疗精神障碍、心血管疾病、盆底疾病及皮肤病等多个领域均取得了一定成效，表明针灸在多种疾病的治疗中展现出广阔的前景。然而，仍需更多高质量的循证医学证据予以支持（图9）。

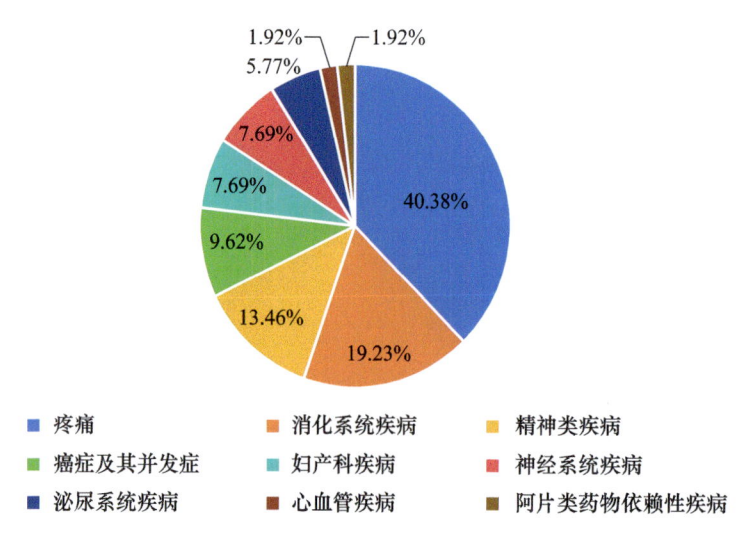

图9　近十年针灸高质量临床研究文献的病种分布（52篇）

注：部分文献的病种为共病，本文将这类文献同时放入多个病种。

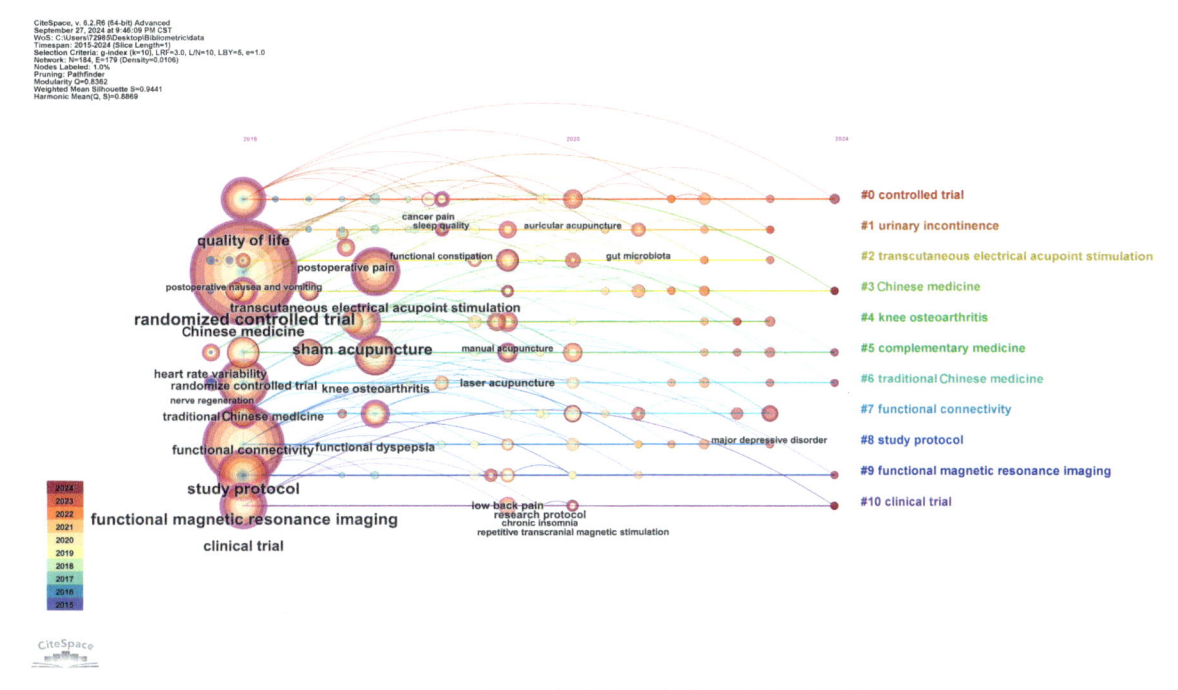

图7　中国SCI源期刊针灸临床试验关键词时间线趋势图

甲是体表唯一有迷走神经分布的区域，且存在直接向孤束核投射的神经纤维，从而能够快速诱发耳-脑反射以发挥调控作用，已研制出耳迷走神经刺激仪[3]。耳穴不仅是中医经典理论与现代科学交流与融合的典范，更成为连接中医针灸学与脑科学的桥梁。此外，针灸临床应用的多样化也得到充分体现，如原发性痛经（primary dysmenorrhea，频次10）、功能性便秘（functional constipation，频次6）及结直肠癌（colorectal cancer，频次7）等疾病的治疗均展现出针灸的独特疗效。

二　近十年针灸临床试验高影响因子SCI源期刊文献分析

本研究对近十年来高影响因子SCI源期刊上发表的针灸临床试验文献进行系统检索，共纳入52篇文献。从文献的发表趋势、疾病种类分布、样本量、干预措施及假针刺设置等方面，总结了全球学者在针灸临床试验设计上的特点，以期为今后开展高质量的针灸临床试验提供参考依据。

1. 中国高质量研究数量稳步提升

检索获得的52篇文献涉及9个国家。其中，中国团队发表了31篇（59.62%，31/52），美国团队发表了12篇（23.08%，12/52），如图8所示。与既往研究[4-5]相比，中国在高质量针灸临床研究方面的数量持续增长，已然跃升至领先地位。这一成就得益于中国学者的积极探索与努力，他们不断利用高质量的随机对照试验证据来构建科学的针灸临床决策体系[6-8]。

· 8 ·

第一章 近十年针灸临床研究进展

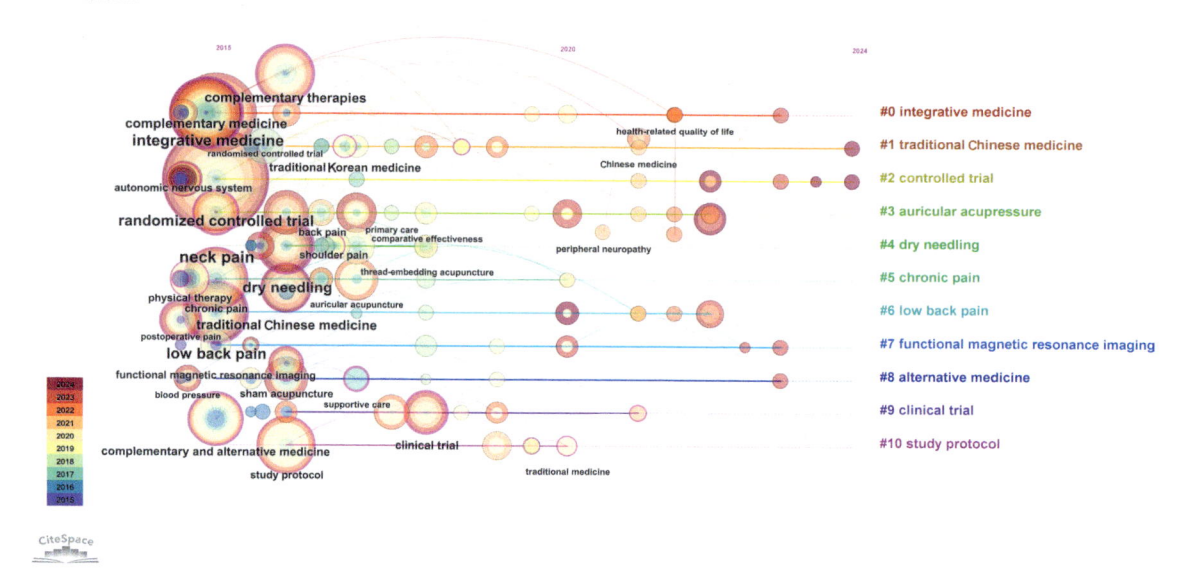

图6 国外SCI源期刊针灸临床试验关键词时间线趋势图

对照试验是探索针灸特异性和有效性的关键研究方法，而生存质量则反映出针灸在综合调节人体状态方面的独特优势，展现了其疗效。②在2017年至2018年间，耳针（auricular acupuncture，频次16）和耳穴贴压（auricular acupressure，频次14）逐渐成为新的研究热点。③在2019年至2024年间，轻度认知障碍（mild cognitive impairment，频次7）和功能性磁共振成像（functional magnetic resonance imaging，频次8）成为主要研究焦点。考虑到目前轻度认知障碍尚无"金标准"药物，且西医治疗面临着价格昂贵与长期使用副作用大等问题，这些因素严重影响了患者的生活质量[2]。针灸能够刺激神经活动，调整大脑区域的神经网络，从而改善认知功能受损的状况。

（2）中国针灸临床试验关键词时间线趋势分析

在回顾中国针灸临床研究的时间线趋势图（图7）时，发现中西方针灸临床研究的关键词呈现出交替发展的趋势，反映了双方在研究方向上的交流与融合。①在2015年至2016年间，研究方案（study protocol，频次180）和功能性磁共振成像（functional magnetic resonance imaging，频次70）在中国针灸临床研究中占据了显著的地位。这表明中国研究者高度重视研究设计与方法的严谨性，致力于推动临床研究的标准化进程。值得注意的是，与西方相比，中国更早引入功能性磁共振成像技术来阐释针刺机制，体现了中国在这一领域的领先地位。②在2017年至2019年间，经皮穴位电刺激（transcutaneous electrical acupoint stimulation，频次59）这一新型针灸技术因其非侵入性刺激腧穴的特点而备受关注。同时，膝骨关节炎（knee osteoarthritis，频次48）和术后疼痛（postoperative pain，频次10）展示了针灸在疼痛管理领域的广泛应用。③在2020年至2024年间，耳穴（auricular acupuncture，频次11）成为中国研究的热点。基于耳

· 7 ·

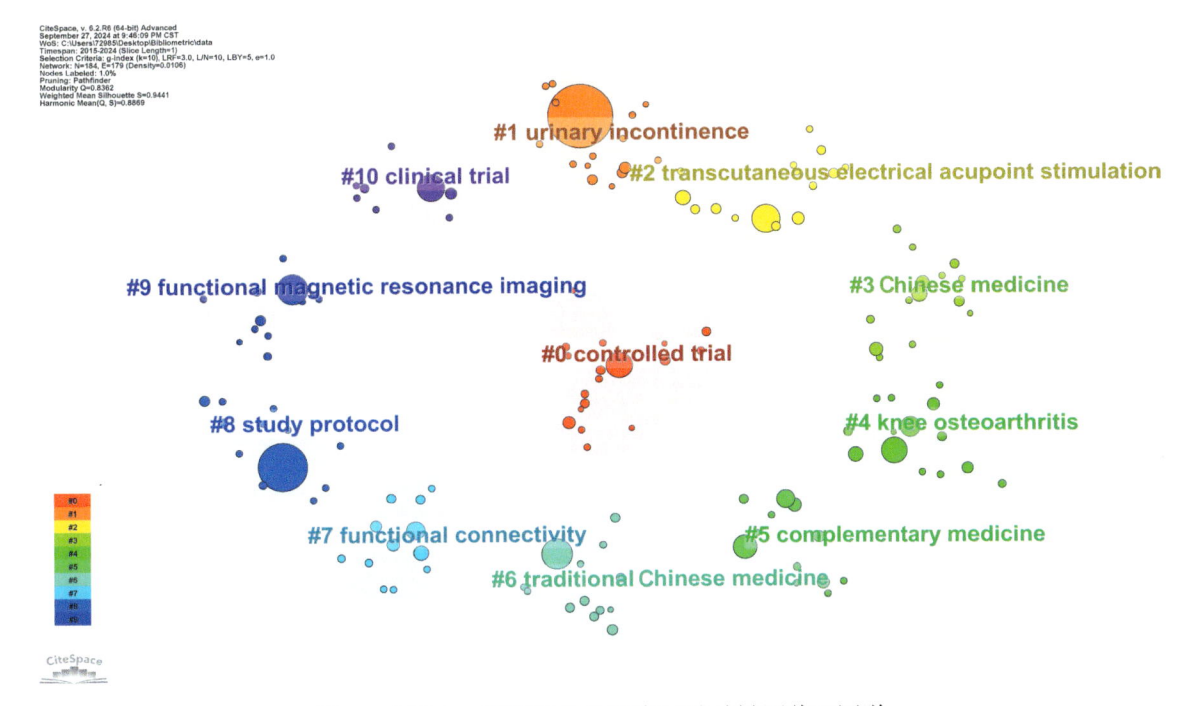

图5 中国SCI源期刊针灸临床试验关键词共现图谱

表2 中国SCI源期刊针灸临床试验关键词聚类标签

分组	聚类号	标签名	关键词数量	轮廓值	年份	主要标签词
Ⅰ	#0	对照试验	18	0.939	2019	对照试验；辅助化疗；癌痛；阿片类药物相关性便秘；非药物治疗
	#5	队列研究	13	0.963	2019	队列研究；补充医学；肌肉骨骼失调症；神经根型颈椎病；雷火灸
Ⅱ	#2	经皮穴位电刺激	15	0.978	2018	经皮穴位电刺激；乳腺癌；术后镇痛；癌症相关疲劳；乳癌根治术
	#3	耳穴贴压	14	0.988	2020	耳穴贴压；中药；缺血性中风；慢性紧张性头痛；术后肠梗阻
Ⅲ	#1	尿失禁	17	1.000	2019	尿失禁；巨刺；针灸；假针刺；慢性失眠
	#4	膝骨关节炎	14	0.991	2019	膝骨关节炎；临床疗效；青龙摆尾针刺法；全膝置换术；假针刺
	#6	心律失常	13	0.937	2018	心律失常；中药；迷走神经激活；自主神经系统；针感
	#8	功能性肛门直肠痛	12	1.000	2020	功能性肛门直肠痛；八髎穴；老年患者；研究方案；穴位注射
	#10	退行性脊柱病	9	0.839	2020	退行性脊柱病；术后疼痛；浮针；对照试验；失眠
Ⅳ	#7	功能连接	12	0.849	2019	功能连接；机器学习；多元模式分析；餐后不适综合征；重度抑郁
	#9	功能性磁共振成像	12	0.986	2019	功能性磁共振成像；特异性疗效；非特异性疗效；腰痛；慢性疼痛

表 1　国外 SCI 源期刊针灸临床试验关键词聚类标签

分组	聚类号	标签名	关键词数量	轮廓值	年份	主要标签词
Ⅰ	#5	慢性疼痛	10	0.955	2017	慢性疼痛；肌筋膜疼痛综合征；穴位埋线；耳针；麻醉并发症
	#6	腰痛	10	0.956	2019	腰痛；激光针灸；临床试验方案；对照试验；术后疼痛
	#9	膝骨关节炎	8	0.889	2017	膝骨关节炎；手针；激光针灸；耳针；物理治疗
Ⅱ	#2	蜂针	14	1.000	2017	蜂针；对照试验；慢性颈痛；心律失常；自主神经
	#3	耳穴贴压	11	0.871	2018	耳穴贴压；补充疗法；干针；激光针刺；传统针灸
	#4	干针	11	0.982	2016	干针；激痛点；慢性疼痛；慢性颈痛；肱骨外上髁炎
Ⅲ	#0	整合医学	17	0.920	2019	整合医学；妇科肿瘤；化疗后失眠；化疗后恶心；替代疗法
	#1	中药	17	1.000	2018	中药；耳穴；揿针；舌诊；定性研究
	#8	替代医学	9	0.928	2017	替代医学；小儿肿瘤；结合医学；支持疗法；药物相关性抑郁
	#10	补充疗法	6	0.963	2019	补充疗法；轻度认知障碍；研究方案；对照试验；传统医学
Ⅳ	#7	功能性磁共振成像	9	1.000	2018	功能性磁共振成像；多元模式分析；腧穴特异性；假针刺治疗效果；针灸期望

（2）中国针灸临床试验关键词聚类分析

11 个聚类可大致分为 4 类（图 5，表 2）。Ⅰ针灸研究方法学（#0、#10）：从范围来看，目前的针灸临床研究仍以对照试验为主，其次为队列研究。Ⅱ常见的针刺干预方法（#2、#3）：中国学者对经皮穴位电刺激、穴位贴压、浮针等多种针灸技术进行了深入研究。而国外学者对青龙摆尾针法、巨刺法、雷火灸等传统针灸方法表现出浓厚的兴趣。Ⅲ针灸适应证（#1、#4、#6、#8、#10）：近年来，针灸试验涵盖了多种病症的临床应用，包括尿失禁、膝骨关节炎、心律失常、功能性肛门直肠痛及退行性脊柱病。Ⅳ针灸效应机制（#7、#9）：神经影像学的发展，尤其是功能性磁共振成像技术的广泛应用，为直观揭示针灸的效应机制提供了可能，这一趋势在国内外均保持一致。

5. 针灸临床研究关键词时间线趋势分析

（1）国外针灸临床试验关键词时间线趋势分析

国外针灸临床试验关键词时间线趋势图（图 6）揭示了国外针灸临床研究在不同年份的研究热点与话题。①在 2015 年至 2016 年间，随机对照试验（randomized controlled trial，频次 103）和生存质量（quality of life，频次 59）这两个关键词显著突出。随机

系统（autonomic nervous system，频次14）的功能显著改善患者的心理状态。

此外，在癌症（cancer，频次37）治疗领域，针灸展现出其独特的价值，能够有效缓解化疗所引发的副作用［如化疗诱导的周围神经病变（chemotherapy-induced peripheral neuropathy，频次11）］，并显示出改善癌症相关疲劳（cancer-related fatigue，频次11）的潜力。

这些研究成果丰富了针灸在现代医学体系中的应用场景，为广大患者提供了更加多元、有效的治疗选择。

4. 针灸临床研究关键词聚类分析

（1）国外针灸临床试验关键词聚类分析

11个聚类可大致分为4个方向（图4，表1）。Ⅰ针灸适应证（#5、#6、#9）：痛症（肌筋膜疼痛综合征、腰痛、膝骨关节炎、术后疼痛）作为针灸的优势病种，在国外受到广泛关注。Ⅱ针灸技术（#2、#3、#4）：主要涉及蜂针、耳穴贴压、干针等多样化的针灸方法。同时，在其他分类中，激光针灸、手针、耳针、穴位埋线、揿针等也为临床应用提供了丰富的选择。Ⅲ针灸在疾病治疗中的角色（#0、#1、#8、#10）：国外常将针灸作为补充替代疗法，应用于癌症及其并发症（如妇科肿瘤、小儿肿瘤）、轻度认知障碍等疾病。Ⅳ针刺机制研究：功能性磁共振成像为探索腧穴特异性及真假针刺疗效对比的机制提供了新的视角。

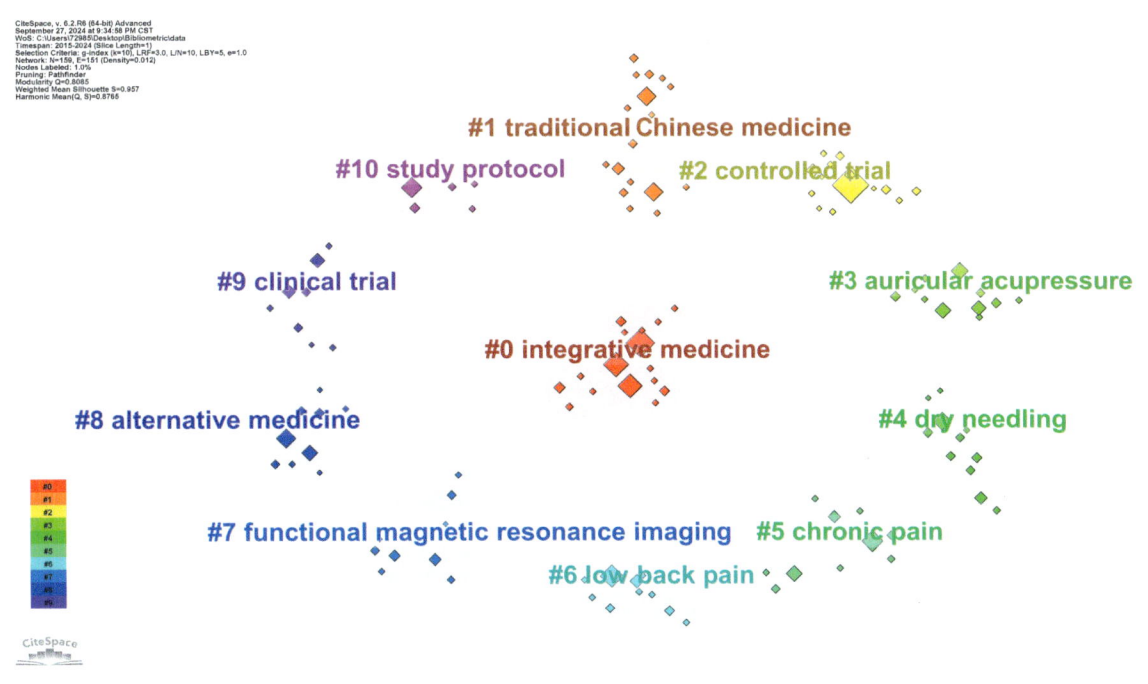

图4　国外SCI源期刊针灸临床试验关键词共现图谱

跃的科研态势，形成了一个多元化、国际化的针灸研究生态。

3. 针灸临床研究关键词共现分析

在研究方法方面，随机对照试验（randomized controlled trial，频次417）是探索和验证针刺疗效的主要手段，其次为队列研究（cohort study，频次10）和个案报道（case report，频次8）。

针灸形式多样，除常见的针刺（acupuncture，频次1167）和电针（electroacupuncture，频次245）外，新型针刺技术如经皮穴位电刺激（transcutaneous electrical acupoint stimulation，频次77）、激光针灸（laser acupuncture，频次38）、耳针（auricular acupuncture，频次35）和干针（dry needling，频次30）也逐渐引起关注。这些频次的差异直观地反映了不同针刺方法在研究中的被重视程度。

在综合医学（integrative medicine，频次47）与传统中医（traditional Chinese medicine，频次96）的广泛框架下，针灸的研究范畴不再局限于疼痛管理，而是深入拓展至心理健康领域［包括抑郁症（depression，频次61）；焦虑症（anxiety，频次59）］，以及多种慢性疾病的干预中。针对焦虑症与抑郁症，针灸疗法能够通过调节自主神经

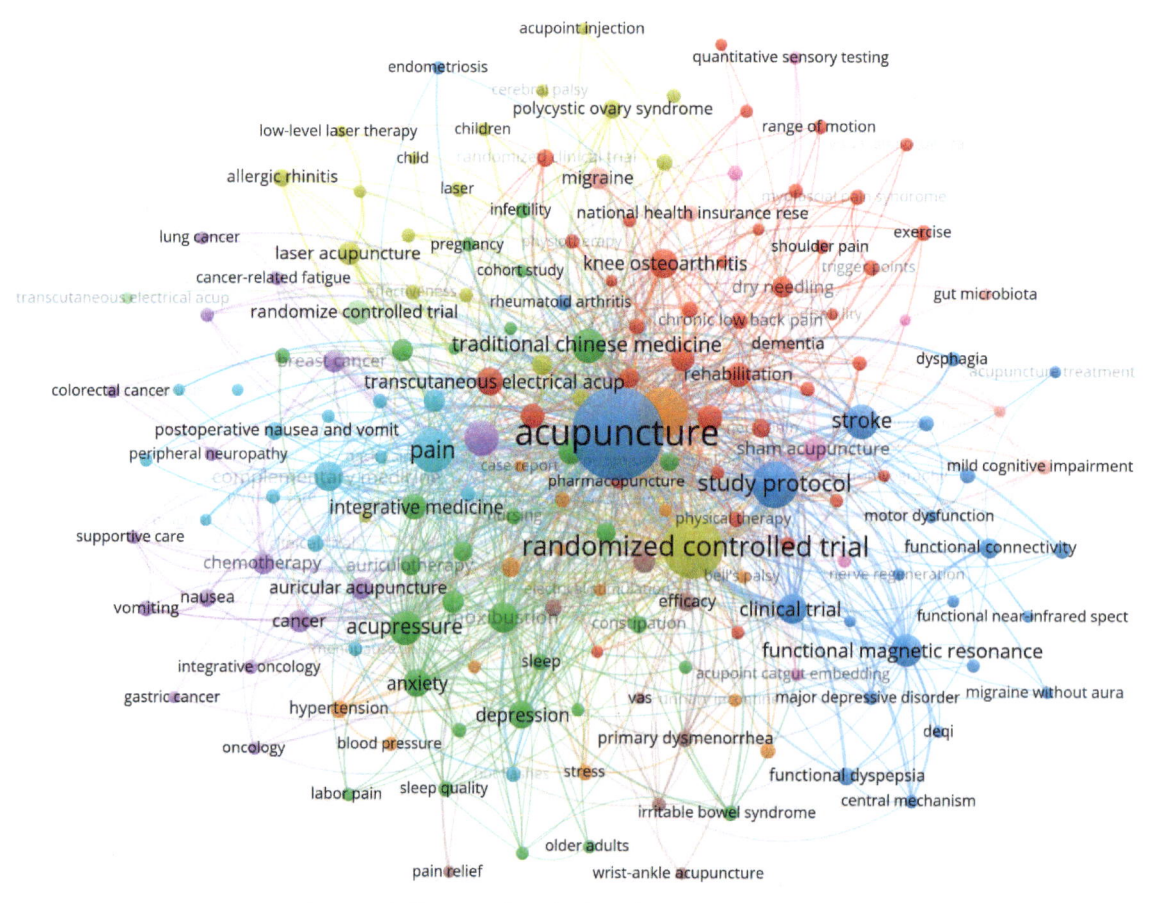

图3　国内外SCI源期刊针灸临床研究关键词共现图

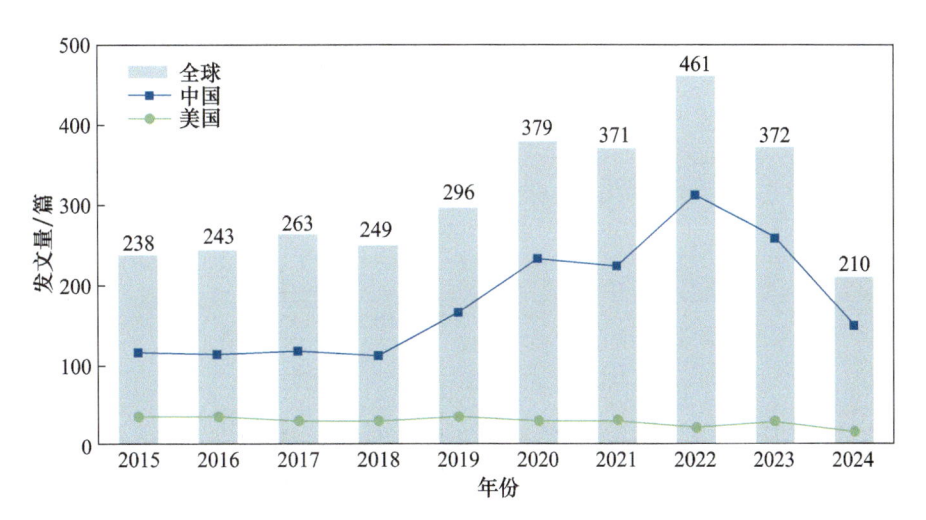

图 1　SCI源期刊针灸临床试验年度发文量趋势

注：2024年数据截至7月31日。

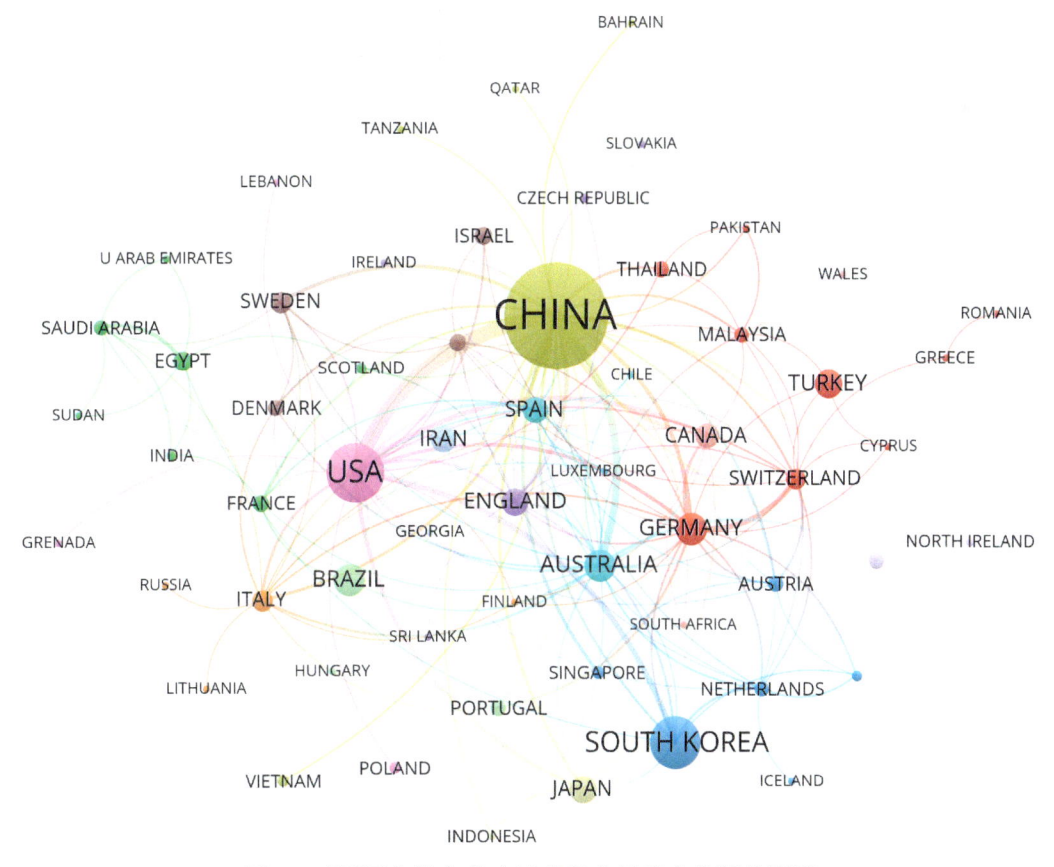

图 2　不同国家针灸临床试验发文量及合作网络图谱

特别是在疼痛管理、心理健康及综合医疗的应用方面，促进了针灸与其他疗法的综合应用，为针灸的国际推广创造了有利条件。此外，韩国的研究更侧重于针灸治疗月经不调和更年期症状等妇科疾病的效果验证，而澳大利亚的研究则重点关注针灸在慢性疼痛和运动损伤等领域的疗效。此外，土耳其、英国和日本在针灸研究中也展现出活

第一章
近十年针灸临床研究进展

针灸是中医药学的重要组成部分。目前，针灸已在全球196个国家和地区得到广泛传播和应用，能够治疗的病种多达461种，涉及病症972种[1]。近年来，针灸临床研究取得显著进展，其研究成果相继发表于 JAMA（《美国医学会杂志》）、Annals of Internal Medicine（《内科学年鉴》）、The BMJ（《英国医学杂志》）等国际临床研究权威期刊，表明国际学术界对针灸临床研究的关注不断加深。为进一步提升国际针灸临床研究的水平，特对近十年来针灸临床试验的研究进展进行梳理，归纳出国际针灸临床研究的趋势和特征如下。

一 近十年SCI源期刊针灸临床试验的可视化分析

本文以Web of Science数据库为数据来源，检索2015年1月至2024年7月被科学引文索引（Science Citation Index™，SCI）收录的针灸临床试验相关文献。采用CiteSpace 6.2.R6和VOSviewer 1.6.20软件对国内外针灸临床试验的发表时间、地域分布、关键词共现及聚类等进行可视化分析。

1. 年度发文量趋势

总体来看，在过去的十年中，针灸临床试验文献的数量虽有波动，但整体呈上升趋势。其中，2022年发表文献数量最多，2020年和2022年显示出显著增长。中国在针灸临床试验文献方面的发文量在2021年与2023年间略有波动，但整体呈现出显著上升的态势，近年来更是展现出强劲的增长势头，如图1所示。

2. 不同国家发文量及合作网络图谱

全球针灸临床试验的分布主要集中于中国和美国。在过去的十年中，中国的总发文量为1823篇（占总发文量的59.15%，即1823/3082），美国423篇（占14.02%，即423/3082），韩国（排名第三，发文量311篇）、澳大利亚（排名第四，发文量98篇）、德国（排名第五，发文量94篇）和巴西（排名第六，发文量92篇）在针灸研究中也发挥了重要作用。中国的研究领域广泛且成果丰硕，涵盖了针灸的临床应用、现代医学技术与针灸的各个方面，尤其在疼痛管理、肿瘤辅助治疗及康复等领域表现突出。从图2可见，中国作为针灸疗法的发源地，在全球范围内与众多国家和地区开展合作，极大地提升了全球对针灸研究的兴趣。美国在针灸临床研究领域同样展现出卓越的成就，

第四十节 "Effect of Acupuncture vs Sham Acupuncture or Waitlist Control on Joint Pain Related to Aromatase Inhibitors Among Women With Early-Stage Breast Cancer: A Randomized Clinical Trial" 相关介绍和述评 ……110

第四十一节 "Effect of Acupuncture vs Sham Acupuncture on Live Births Among Women Undergoing in Vitro Fertilization: A Randomized Clinical Trial" 相关介绍和述评 ……113

第四十二节 "Effect of Electroacupuncture on Urinary Leakage Among Women With Stress Urinary Incontinence: A Randomized Clinical Trial" 相关介绍和述评 ……116

第四十三节 "Effect of Acupuncture and Clomiphene in Chinese Women With Polycystic Ovary Syndrome: A Randomized Clinical Trial" 相关介绍和述评 ……118

第四十四节 "The Long-Term Effect of Acupuncture for Migraine Prophylaxis: A Randomized Clinical Trial" 相关介绍和述评 ……120

第四十五节 "Rewiring the Primary Somatosensory Cortex in Carpal Tunnel Syndrome With Acupuncture" 相关介绍和述评 ……122

第四十六节 "A Randomised Controlled Trial Examining the Effect of Acupuncture at the EX-HN3 (Yintang) Point on Pre-operative Anxiety Levels in Neurosurgical Patients" 相关介绍和述评 ……125

第四十七节 "Acupuncture as an Integrative Approach for the Treatment of Hot Flashes in Women With Breast Cancer: A Prospective Multicenter Randomized Controlled Trial (AcCliMaT)" 相关介绍和述评 ……127

第四十八节 "Acupuncture for Chronic Severe Functional Constipation: A Randomized Trial" 相关介绍和述评 ……129

第四十九节 "Acupuncture for Menopausal Hot Flashes: A Randomized Trial" 相关介绍和述评 ……132

第五十节 "Transcutaneous Acupoint Electrical Stimulation Pain Management After Surgical Abortion: A Cohort Study" 相关介绍和述评 ……134

第五十一节 "Electroacupuncture Versus Gabapentin for Hot Flashes Among Breast Cancer Survivors: A Randomized Placebo-Controlled Trial" 相关介绍和述评 ……136

第五十二节 "Alexander Technique Lessons or Acupuncture Sessions for Persons With Chronic Neck Pain: A Randomized Trial" 相关介绍和述评 ……139

第三章 《研究者发起的中医药临床研究天津共识》内容与解读 ……142

第一节 研究者发起的中医药临床研究天津共识 ……142

第二节 《研究者发起的中医药临床研究天津共识》解读 ……143

疾病索引（ICD-11） ……146

第二十七节	"Effect of Briefing on Acupuncture Treatment Outcome Expectations, Pain, and Adverse Side Effects Among Patients With Chronic Low Back Pain: A Randomized Clinical Trial" 相关介绍和述评	77
第二十八节	"Effect of Acupuncture on Atrial Fibrillation Stratified by CHA_2DS_2-VASc Score— A Nationwide Cohort Investigation" 相关介绍和述评	79
第二十九节	"Greater Somatosensory Afference With Acupuncture Increases Primary Somatosensory Connectivity and Alleviates Fibromyalgia Pain via Insular γ-Aminobutyric Acid: A Randomized Neuroimaging Trial" 相关介绍和述评	81
第三十节	"Efficacy of Intensive Acupuncture Versus Sham Acupuncture in Knee Osteoarthritis: A Randomized Controlled Trial" 相关介绍和述评	83
第三十一节	"Electroacupuncture vs Prucalopride for Severe Chronic Constipation: A Multicenter, Randomized, Controlled, Noninferiority Trial" 相关介绍和述评	86
第三十二节	"Manual Acupuncture Versus Sham Acupuncture and Usual Care for Prophylaxis of Episodic Migraine Without Aura: Multicentre, Randomised Clinical Trial" 相关介绍和述评	88
第三十三节	"Effect of Acupuncture for Postprandial Distress Syndrome: A Randomized Clinical Trial" 相关介绍和述评	92
第三十四节	"Electroacupuncture Trigeminal Nerve Stimulation Plus Body Acupuncture for Chemotherapy-Induced Cognitive Impairment in Breast Cancer Patients: An Assessor-participant Blinded, Randomized Controlled Trial" 相关介绍和述评	94
第三十五节	"Effect of Acupuncture vs Sham Procedure on Chemotherapy-Induced Peripheral Neuropathy Symptoms: A Randomized Clinical Trial" 相关介绍和述评	97
第三十六节	"Effect of Electroacupuncture vs Sham Treatment on Change in Pain Severity Among Adults With Chronic Low Back Pain: A Randomized Clinical Trial" 相关介绍和述评	99
第三十七节	"Acupuncture as Adjunctive Therapy for Chronic Stable Angina: A Randomized Clinical Trial" 相关介绍和述评	102
第三十八节	"Effect of True and Sham Acupuncture on Radiation-Induced Xerostomia Among Patients With Head and Neck Cancer: A Randomized Clinical Trial" 相关介绍和述评	105
第三十九节	"Acupuncture Versus Cognitive Behavioral Therapy for Insomnia in Cancer Survivors: A Randomized Clinical Trial" 相关介绍和述评	107

第十三节	"Effects of Electroacupuncture for Opioid-Induced Constipation in Patients With Cancer in China: A Randomized Clinical Trial" 相关介绍和述评	44
第十四节	"Acupuncture vs Massage for Pain in Patients Living With Advanced Cancer: The IMPACT Randomized Clinical Trial" 相关介绍和述评	46
第十五节	"Efficacy and Safety of Auricular Acupuncture for Depression: A Randomized Clinical Trial" 相关介绍和述评	48
第十六节	"Effect of Acupuncture on Postoperative Ileus after Laparoscopic Elective Colorectal Surgery: A Prospective, Randomised, Controlled Trial" 相关介绍和述评	51
第十七节	"Acupuncture Improves the Symptoms, Intestinal Microbiota, and Inflammation of Patients With Mild to Moderate Crohn's Disease: A Randomized Controlled Trial" 相关介绍和述评	53
第十八节	"Effect of Electroacupuncture on Insomnia in Patients With Depression: A Randomized Clinical Trial" 相关介绍和述评	56
第十九节	"Effectiveness of Acupuncture for Anxiety Among Patients With Parkinson Disease: A Randomized Clinical Trial" 相关介绍和述评	58
第二十节	"Effectiveness of Acupuncture for Pain Control After Cesarean Delivery: A Randomized Clinical Trial" 相关介绍和述评	60
第二十一节	"Acupuncture for the Treatment of Diarrhea-Predominant Irritable Bowel Syndrome: A Pilot Randomized Clinical Trial" 相关介绍和述评	63
第二十二节	"Comparison of Acupuncture vs Sham Acupuncture or Waiting List Control in the Treatment of Aromatase Inhibitor-Related Joint Pain: A Randomized Clinical Trial" 相关介绍和述评	65
第二十三节	"Effect of Adjunctive Acupuncture on Pain Relief Among Emergency Department Patients With Acute Renal Colic Due to Urolithiasis: A Randomized Clinical Trial" 相关介绍和述评	68
第二十四节	"Effect of Acupoint Hot Compress on Postpartum Urinary Retention After Vaginal Delivery: A Randomized Clinical Trial" 相关介绍和述评	70
第二十五节	"Effectiveness of Electroacupuncture or Auricular Acupuncture vs Usual Care for Chronic Musculoskeletal Pain Among Cancer Survivors: The PEACE Randomized Clinical Trial" 相关介绍和述评	72
第二十六节	"Efficacy of Acupuncture for Chronic Prostatitis/Chronic Pelvic Pain Syndrome: A Randomized Trial" 相关介绍和述评	75

目 录

第一章 近十年针灸临床研究进展……………………………………………………………1

第二章 SCI源期刊高质量针灸临床研究述评……………………………………………14

第一节 "Acupuncture for Combat-Related Posttraumatic Stress Disorder: A Randomized Clinical Trial" 相关介绍和述评……………………………14

第二节 "Acupuncture and Sleep Quality Among Patients With Parkinson Disease: A Randomized Clinical Trial" 相关介绍和述评………………16

第三节 "Acupuncture for Chronic Radiation-Induced Xerostomia in Head and Neck Cancer: A Multicenter Randomized Clinical Trial" 相关介绍和述评……18

第四节 "Effect of Acupuncture vs Sham Acupuncture on Patients With Poststroke Motor Aphasia: A Randomized Clinical Trial" 相关介绍和述评……………21

第五节 "Effect of Acupuncture for Methadone Reduction: A Randomized Clinical Trial" 相关介绍和述评……………………………………………………24

第六节 "Effect of Acupuncture on Neurogenic Claudication Among Patients With Degenerative Lumbar Spinal Stenosis: A Randomized Clinical Trial" 相关介绍和述评……………………………………………………………27

第七节 "Effect of Acupuncture for Temporomandibular Disorders: A randomized Clinical Trial" 相关介绍和述评……………………………………………30

第八节 "Self-Administered Acupressure for Probable Knee Osteoarthritis in Middle-Aged and Older Adults: A Randomized Clinical Trial" 相关介绍和述评………32

第九节 "Efficacy of Acupuncture for Chronic Spontaneous Urticaria: A Randomized Controlled Trial" 相关介绍和述评………………………………………34

第十节 "Acupuncture and Doxylamine-Pyridoxine for Nausea and Vomiting in Pregnancy: A Randomized, Controlled, 2×2 Factorial Trial" 相关介绍和述评………37

第十一节 "Electroacupuncture vs Sham Electroacupuncture in the Treatment of Postoperative Ileus After Laparoscopic Surgery for Colorectal Cancer: A Multicenter, Randomized Clinical Trial" 相关介绍和述评…………………………39

第十二节 "Electroacupuncture for Motor Dysfunction and Constipation in Patients with Parkinson's Disease: A Randomised Controlled Multi-centre Trial" 相关介绍和述评……………………………………………………………41

前　言

针灸起源于中国，拥有悠久的历史和深厚的文化底蕴，现已在196个国家和地区得到传播和应用，逐步融入主流医学体系。然而，目前在国际范围内针灸相关立法仍显不足，许多国家和地区的针灸从业人员尚未获得合法地位。因此，提供和推广高质量的针灸临床及基础研究成果，制定并宣传针灸相关标准与规范，已成为推动针灸国际化发展的当务之急。

世界针灸学会联合会（简称"世界针联"）与中国国家中医针灸临床医学研究中心携手，依托世界针联科技工作委员会及《中华针灸电子杂志》，对近十年针灸临床研究进行了系统总结。从SCI数据库中遴选出发表于2015年1月至2024年7月的52篇高影响因子的针灸临床研究文献，并邀请60位来自针灸学、临床方法学及统计学领域的专家学者对这些文章进行深入学习，围绕临床价值、设计方法及特点、对针灸发展的影响，以及存在的问题与建议等方面进行评述。基于此，形成了《针灸临床研究证据蓝皮书（2015—2024）》（简称"蓝皮书"），并于在英国伦敦召开的第七届国际针灸学术研讨会上进行宣讲与发布。蓝皮书同时刊载了《研究者发起的中医药临床研究天津共识》及其重点解读，旨在提升针灸学科的临床研究水平，产生更多高质量的证据，以真实可靠的科学数据推动针灸的传播与应用。

世界针联计划每年发布一次蓝皮书，为广大针灸从业人员提供针灸临床研究的最新动态和进展，同时为公众健康干预、针灸相关立法及其进入医保与主流医学体系等提供全面、准确、有科学数据支撑的高质量研究证据。循证医学的创始人、世界针联科技工作委员会主任委员 Gordon H. Guyatt 教授为此蓝皮书撰写了序言，期待针灸界能够借助循证医学的思路与方法，开辟出自己独特的临床研究之路。感谢所有为蓝皮书付出努力的同事与同行们。

刘保延
世界针灸学会联合会主席
国际欧亚科学院院士
中国中医科学院学部委员

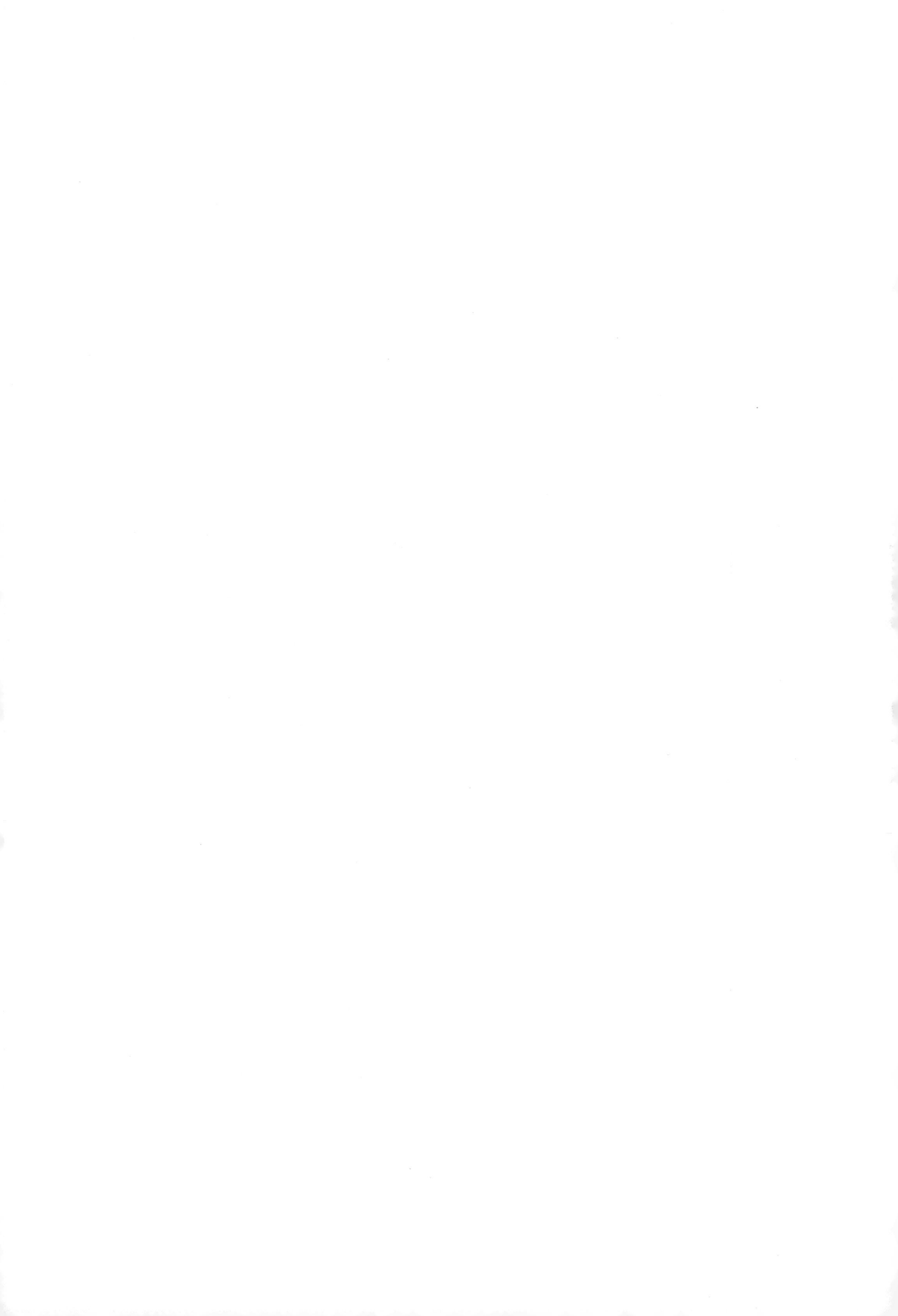

序 言

自古以来，针刺疗法便如同一条绵延不绝的丝线，将东西方医学的智慧与实践紧密相连。在二十一世纪的今天，这门古老的医术与科学，正以崭新的面貌展现出前所未有的活力与深度。我，Gordon H. Guyatt，作为循证医学的创始人和长期致力于循证医学研究的学者，有幸见证了这一领域的巨大变迁，更荣幸能为这本《针灸临床研究证据蓝皮书（2015—2024）》撰写序言。

过去十年，中国和其他国家的学者在针刺领域发表的高影响力临床研究，不仅为全球医学界提供了丰富的数据与洞见，更推动了针刺疗法从传统经验走向现代科学的进程。这些研究如同一盏盏明灯，照亮了针刺疗法的科学之路，让其在循证医学的框架下，展现出更为坚实的基础与广阔的应用前景。

本书精心挑选了近十年国内外学者在针刺领域最具代表性和影响力的临床研究，通过行业专家深入浅出的点评，展现了针刺疗法在痛症、神经系统疾病、消化系统疾病等多个领域的应用与成效。这些研究探索了针刺疗法的有效性和安全性，为针刺疗法的进一步发展提供了坚实的科学依据。

能够通过本书与广大读者分享这些研究的精华，我深感荣幸。我相信，无论您是患者、医疗从业者、科研人员，还是对传统医学充满好奇的探索者，都能从这些研究中获得新的启示和思考。让我们一同踏上这趟"探索之旅"，感受针刺疗法与现代科学碰撞出的火花，见证古老智慧与现代医学的完美融合。

愿《针灸临床研究证据蓝皮书（2015—2024）》能成为连接东西方医学的桥梁，为推动全球医疗健康事业的进步贡献一份力量。

Gordon H. Guyatt
循证医学创始人
加拿大皇家科学院院士
麦克马斯特大学教授

在全球医疗体系日益重视循证医学的背景下，《针灸临床研究证据蓝皮书（2015—2024）》的发布标志着针灸研究迈上一个更高的台阶。我们将以疗效为导向，深入探讨针灸的机制与原理，力求为患者提供更具科学依据的治疗方案。

——韩济生院士

《针灸临床研究证据蓝皮书（2015—2024）》的发布是对针灸科学化、标准化的又一重要推动。我们将继续挖掘针灸学科的潜力，将丰富的临床经验转化为临床疗效证据，以科学的力量为传统医学赋能，让针灸为人类健康作出更大的贡献！

——石学敏院士

《针灸临床研究证据蓝皮书（2015—2024）》一书不仅是对过去十年针灸临床研究成果的总结，更是为未来针灸学科发展夯实了科学基础。希望将这些高质量循证证据转化和推广应用，推动针灸学术与现代医学融合创新发展，丰富新时代健康医学研究内容，施惠人类的健康福祉！

——张伯礼院士

中国工程院院士1名，国医大师1名，全国名中医1名，享受国务院政府特殊津贴专家5名。有博士后合作导师4名，博士研究生导师10名，硕士研究生导师47名，二级学会会长/主任委员5名、副会长/副主任委员10名。构建了全国最大的协同创新网络，拥有网络协作单位218家，覆盖全国31个省、自治区、直辖市。"世界针灸看中国、中国针灸看天津"，医院针灸学科在国内外针灸领域一直居于领军地位，在中华中医药学会、中国中医科学院组织的2021—2023年度中医医院学科（专科）学术影响力评选中蝉联针灸学科全国第一，引领针灸学科的发展。

权单位，拥有国家级教学团队1个，是国家中医药管理局中医药高层次人才培养综合基地、首批国家中医住院/全科医生规范化培训基地、国家住院医师规范化培训中医与中医全科重点专业基地、国家中医临床教学培训示范中心。

医院始终坚持走"科技兴院，院兴科技"之路，拥有国家中医针灸临床医学研究中心、国家中医临床研究基地、国家药物临床试验机构等一批国家级科技平台和国家中医药管理局脑病针刺疗法重点研究室等16个省部级科技平台，成立中医药临床研究中心。近5年承担国家"重大新药创制"科技重大专项、国家重点研发计划"中医药现代化"重点专项、国家自然科学基金重点项目等重大科研任务31项，牵头承担中药新药临床试验项目63项，获得国家科技进步奖5项、省部级科技进步一等奖16项。2023年度中医医院学科（专科）学术影响力评价——综合排名第8名，针灸学排名第1名，中医推拿学、中医儿科学均排名第2名，中医心病学排名第3名。2022年度中国医院科技量值（STEM）排名第75位。

医院先后与美国、俄罗斯、德国、日本、韩国等40余个国家建立合作关系，已连续举办16届国际针灸学术研讨会，主办首届中国·东盟传统医药国际论坛，建设海外中心3个。

医院坚持以习近平新时代中国特色社会主义思想为指导，秉承"心存乎仁、行止于善"的院训，坚持"发展事业，服务社会，维护健康，造福人类"的办院宗旨，以学科建设为统领，以改革创新为动力，以人才队伍和现代化管理为支撑，努力建设更高水平教学研究型中医医院，奋力开创医院高质量发展新局面。

针灸部为医院龙头科室，由15个病区、南北院门诊、针灸研究所、《中华针灸电子杂志》编辑部组成。在中国工程院院士、国医大师石学敏教授的带领下，历经70年的建设、发展与创新，已成为国内最大的针灸临床、科研、教学基地和国际交流中心。开放床位1000张，年门诊量60万余人次，年出院患者2万余人次，累计治疗中风病患者3300万余人次。针灸临床服务能力全国第一。

针灸部是国家重点学科（2002年）、国家中医药管理局重点学科（2001年）和高水平中医药重点学科（2023年）、天津市"重中之重"学科（2005年），并先后被确立为全国针灸临床研究中心（1988年）、国家中医临床研究基地（2008年）、国家临床重点专科建设单位（2011年）、国家中医药管理局区域针灸诊疗中心（2018年）、国家中医药管理局优势专科建设单位（2021年、2024年）。

针灸部目前有4个稳定的研究方向：醒脑开窍理论科学内涵及其创新研究；优势病种临床评价及作用机制研究；针灸规范化；针灸交叉创新。近年来，共承担各级科研课题432项，其中在针刺治疗中风病、高血压病、认知障碍等优势病种方面承担国家级课题69项，省部级课题105项，获国家科技进步奖1项，省部级一等奖3项、二等奖24项、三等奖27项。

针灸部人才团队为国家教育部"长江学者和创新团队发展计划"创新团队。拥有

国家中医针灸临床医学研究中心

2019年5月，中国科学技术部、国家卫生健康委员会、中央军事委员会后勤保障部、国家药品监督管理局联合发布《关于认定第四批国家临床医学研究中心的通知》，10个疾病领域的18家医院被认定为"国家临床医学研究中心"。天津中医药大学第一附属医院被认定为"国家中医针灸临床医学研究中心"。

天津中医药大学第一附属医院始建于1954年，是天津市历史最悠久、建设规模最大的中医医疗机构，是国家医学中心创建单位、国家中医针灸临床医学研究中心、国家区域医疗中心建设输出医院、国家中医药传承创新工程重点中医医院、国家中医临床教学培训示范中心、国家中医药服务出口基地，是国家中医临床研究基地、国家区域中医（专科）诊疗中心、国家中医优势专科建设单位、首批国家中医住院医师规范化培训基地、国家中医药高层次人才综合培养基地、国家中医疫病防治及紧急医学救援基地、全国中医药文化宣传教育基地，是全国首批三级甲等医院、全国百佳医院、全国百姓放心示范医院。

医院现有南开院区、西青院区、静海院区三个院区，总占地面积537.37亩，设45个临床和技术科室。医院编制床位2600张，年门急诊量303万余人次，年出院患者7万余人次。

医院在职员工3200余人，拥有中国工程院院士2名，国医大师3名，全国名中医5名，岐黄学者5名，青年岐黄学者4名，国务院政府特殊津贴专家20名，国家级突出贡献中青年专家8名，全国老中医药专家学术经验继承工作指导老师37名，全国中医临床优秀人才23名，天津市政府授衔专家5名，天津市名中医33名。教育部创新团队2个，国家中医药传承创新团队1个。博士研究生导师48名，硕士研究生导师234名。

医院坚持以人民健康为中心，关注全生命周期健康管理，坚持以预防、医疗、康复为一体，坚持中西医并重，坚持五专道路，突出中医药特色，广泛开展中医特色诊疗技术，全面提升中西医结合诊疗能力，形成了一批针对脑卒中及其并发症、冠心病等疑难疾病的独具特色的中西医结合诊疗方案，充分发挥了中医药在常见病、多发病和慢性病防治中的独特作用。

医院着力打造学（专）科高峰，形成了以针灸学科为龙头的学科集群，拥有国家重点学科2个，国家临床重点专科4个，国家中医药管理局高水平中医药重点学科3个，国家中医药管理局区域中医（专科）诊疗中心6个，国家中医药管理局重点学科10个，国家中医药管理局中医优势专科13个，国家中医药管理局重点专科13个。

医院设立中医学博士后科研工作站，是国务院批准的中医学一级学科博士学位授

编委会

顾　　问　Gordon H. Guyatt

主　　编　刘保延

副 主 编　张艳军　王金贵　杨金生　杨龙会　许能贵　杨宇洋
　　　　　石江伟　陆丽明　沈　燕

编　　委（按姓氏笔画排序）

王　伟（中国·武汉）　王　华　王　舒　王金贵
王胜锋　王富春　方剑乔　石广霞　石江伟　刘存志
刘志顺　刘炜宏　刘建平　刘保延　闫世艳　许能贵
孙　凤　孙　鑫　孙元杰　孙建华　芦文丽　苏同生
杜元灏　杜志成　李　瑛　杨　骏　杨　硕　杨龙会
杨宇洋　杨金生　吴佳霓　吴焕淦　岗卫娟　何丽云
余勇夫　余曙光　沈　燕　张王剑　张永刚　张汝阳
张艳军　陆丽明　陈　征　陈　波　陈　雯　周　旭
房繄恭　孟智宏　赵　宏　赵　星　赵　凌　赵吉平
郝　洋　荣培晶　胡思源　费宇彤　姚　晨　秦国友
倪光夏　殷海波　郭　义　郭盛楠　陶立元　崔　壮
章　薇　阎小妍　梁繁荣　葛　龙　曾　芳　雷　黎
翟静波

学术支持　《中华针灸电子杂志》《世界针灸杂志》

参编人员（按姓氏笔画排序）

马庆韬　王　伟（中国·天津）　王　松　邓士哲
邢晶晶　刘　健　刘　巍　刘超达　孙　淳　杜世豪
李波漩　杨红玲　张亚男　陈雅琼　范宝超　聂德慧
徐　帆　徐志杰　黄泓文　董　昱

世界针灸学会联合会

世界针灸学会联合会（简称"世界针联"），自1984年开始筹备，由中国原卫生部、中国科学技术协会、中国外交部和中国原国家科学技术委员会四大部委联名报请中华人民共和国国务院，经国务院批准后，由中国方面牵头，在世界卫生组织的指导下，于1987年11月成立，总部设在中国北京。

世界针联是非政府性针灸团体的国际联合组织，1998年与世界卫生组织建立非政府组织正式工作关系，是国际标准化组织中医药技术委员会（ISO/TC249）A级联络组织，享有联合国经济与社会理事会特别咨商地位。其现有272个团体会员，分布在全球70个国家和地区。

世界针联的宗旨：促进世界针灸界之间的了解和合作，加强国际学术交流，进一步发展针灸医学，不断提高针灸医学在世界医疗卫生保健工作中的地位和作用，为人类的健康作出贡献。

世界针联的任务：组织世界针灸学术大会、中型学术研讨会和专题学术讨论会；促进国际针灸界之间的友好往来，鼓励各种针灸学术交流；完成与世界卫生组织建立正式关系所承担的工作，实施世界卫生组织传统医学战略；宣传和推广针灸医学，争取各国针灸合法地位；发展针灸教育，提高从业人员水平；开展针灸医疗服务；出版针灸学术刊物，提供针灸信息服务；制定和推广有关针灸的国际标准；为实现本会宗旨所必须承担的其他任务。

世界针灸学会联合会科技工作委员会（简称"科技工作委员会"）是世界针联下属工作委员会之一，由中国许能贵教授、加拿大 Gordon H. Guyatt 教授担任主任委员，澳大利亚韦国庆教授、美国张誉清教授、美国王少白教授、中国唐纯志教授、中国陆丽明教授、中国石江伟教授担任副主任委员。

在过去的几年里，科技工作委员会紧紧围绕国家科技发展战略，积极开展各项工作，多项研究发表于 *The BMJ*、*Annals of Internal Medicine*、*Autophagy*、*Nature Communications* 等国际著名医学期刊，展示了团队在针灸领域的突出成绩。科技工作委员会在国内开展了30余次学术培训及义诊活动，在增进学术交流的同时，推动了岭南中医特色针灸传承传播。此外，与云南省昭通市中医医院、广东省广州市中医医院、广东省中山市第三人民医院、深圳市宝安纯中医治疗医院等多家医院联合开展科研工作与新技术推广应用；与深圳市宝安纯中医治疗医院开展"三名工程"推广新技术及联合科研；与西安电子科技大学广州研究院、哈尔滨工业大学（深圳）等单位联合开展多学科交叉科研，打造了一支针灸治疗、临床研究方法学、计算机、人工智能、生物医学、临床医学等跨学科、多层次、国内领先的研究团队，促进针灸影像交叉学科发展；联合国内外多所高校建立了广东省教育厅重点实验室、粤港澳大湾区针药干细胞结合治疗中枢神经退行性疾病重点实验室，取得丰硕成果。

未来，在世界针联的指导下，科技工作委员会将继续推进针灸的科研工作创新和交流合作，搭建国内外针灸科技研究工作者的沟通和合作桥梁。通过科研创新工作促进针灸的临床应用和推广，促进针灸的国际化，提升针灸研究的国内外影响力。重视青年科技工作者的培养，给予必要的支持和激励举措，为青年针灸科技工作者搭建施展才华的舞台。

图书在版编目（CIP）数据

针灸临床研究证据蓝皮书：2015—2024 / 刘保延主编. -- 北京：中华医学电子音像出版社, 2024.12.

ISBN 978-7-83005-483-0

Ⅰ.R245

中国国家版本馆CIP数据核字第2024QN7789号

针灸临床研究证据蓝皮书（2015—2024）

ZHENJIU LINCHUANG YANJIU ZHENGJU LANPISHU（2015—2024）

主　　编：刘保延
策划编辑：裴　燕
责任编辑：李雪丽　崔晓鸥　封艳辉
校　　对：刘　欢
责任印刷：李振坤
出版发行：中华医学电子音像出版社
通信地址：北京市西城区东河沿街69号中华医学会610室
邮　　编：100052
E - mail：cma-cmc@cma.org.cn
购书热线：010-51322635
经　　销：新华书店
印　　刷：北京虎彩文化传播有限公司
开　　本：889 mm×1194 mm，1/16
印　　张：18.5
字　　数：607千字
版　　次：2024年12月第1版　　2024年12月第1次印刷
定　　价：198.00元

版权所有　侵权必究

购买本社图书，凡有缺、倒、脱页者，本社负责调换

针灸临床研究证据蓝皮书

(2015—2024)

世界针灸学会联合会
国家中医针灸临床医学研究中心

主编 刘保延